MEDICAL ETHICS

MEDICAL

ETHICS

by EDWIN F. HEALY, S.J.

LOYOLA UNIVERSITY PRESS

Chicago 1956

IMPRIMI POTEST:
William J. Schmidt, S.J.
Provincial of the Chicago Province
May 31, 1956

NIHIL OBSTAT:
Austin G. Schmidt, S.J.
Censor Deputatus
June 4, 1956

IMPRIMATUR:
✠ Samuel Cardinal Stritch
Archbishop of Chicago
June 7, 1956

416

To the numberless justly revered physicians

of the United States of America

who have accomplished so much for this nation

in consecrating themselves to the preservation of life

and to the alleviation of suffering,

in devoting so generously and conscientiously

to the care of others

their skill, their learning, and their convenience

in a measure always adequate and not rarely heroic,

this book, on behalf of those thus aided,

is gratefully dedicated

WHILE this work on medical ethics has been written primarily as a textbook for use in Catholic medical schools and as a reference book for use in Catholic hospitals, the author from the beginning had in mind the many thousands of non-Catholic physicians to whom the book might be helpful. The non-Catholic physician will in practically all cases have a number, perhaps a large number, of Catholic patients. He will gain their confidence and treat them more successfully if in matters involving ethical and moral issues he understands what they accept and why they accept it. As a scholar and as a believer in freedom of conscience, he will wish to respect the ethical convictions of his patients and to refrain from using or suggesting procedures which they cannot in conscience approve. To all such non-Catholic physicians this book should be helpful, not as something to be studied from cover to cover, but as a reference to be used as occasion arises.

To both non-Catholic and Catholic physicians this book should prove helpful in still another way. There may be patients who, because of misinformation or prejudice, refuse to accept the recommendations of their physician on the ground that the action proposed is not permissible. Delays occasioned by the desire of patients to make inquiries or to seek advice elsewhere could at times be costly or even fatal. If the physician can satisfy them that he has good authority for using the procedure he considers best, he can set their minds at rest and begin at once to treat the case.

The purpose of the author, then, has been to state what may be done as well as what should not be done. He has aimed at granting the greatest possible amount of freedom. Even those who believe in greater freedom than he can grant should find the material helpful when dealing with patients whose philosophy is the same as that of the author.

The ethician seeks to discover the same truth which is sought by the conscientious physician. Truth in the science of ethics cannot contradict truth in the science of medicine, for the source of all truth is the same all-knowing, all-wise God. God is the source of all truth, whether the truth in question refer to matters of religion, ethics, mathematics, physics, chemistry, or medicine. It is the study of this truth which is the objective common to every sincere scholar, be he moralist or physician.

The physician who uses this book may discover here and there references to types of therapy that he considers obsolete. In some cases this will be due to the fact that the physician himself belongs to a school of thought which looks with disfavor upon certain procedures still in good repute. In other cases the procedure may be indeed obsolete or almost obsolete. While the author has made every possible effort to acquaint himself with what is most recent in medical science, he has in a few places referred to procedures which he knows are not frequently used today. It must be remembered, for one thing, that there are old practitioners who have not kept abreast of the times and who continue to use procedures which they found satisfactory when they were younger. If such men are uncertain concerning the morality of a procedure, it is the duty of the ethician to solve the difficulty. In addition to these older practitioners we find younger men who are following their profession in small and isolated communities, where they do not have the opportunity to become acquainted with what is most recent that is enjoyed by physicians in larger centers. Again, it could easily happen that a procedure looked upon at one time as obsolete began after some years to be used again. Finally, the ethical principles applicable to one procedure, whether or not it is in common use, point the way to the solution of problems connected with other procedures of a similar nature. For these reasons the author did not consider it wise rigorously to exclude mention of every procedure that is not recommended today by specialists of the highest rank.

Because of newly discovered drugs, new methods of treatment, and new procedures in surgery the medication and surgical operations indicated may, within a few years, be quite different from those specified in the cases discussed in MEDICAL ETHICS. Nevertheless, the principles on which the solutions to the cases are based remain ever the same. These same principles will then be applied by the ethician to the changed conditions of the case.

CONTENTS

LIST OF CASES

FUNDAMENTAL ETHICAL PRINCIPLES

THERE is a conviction among all civilized and educated men, and even among primitives who are neither civilized nor well educated, that there is a fixed difference between good and evil. There is, moreover, a general contempt for evil and a general admiration for what is good. The habitual liar is despised. The man who breaks his word is held in low respect. Murder is condemned as a wicked thing. On the other hand, the soldier who renders heroic service in time of war is honored with some decoration, such as a medal. The physician who serves at the risk of his own life during a pestilence is admired and praised. In general, the good citizen is held in esteem; the criminal and the traitor are looked upon as being objectively out of order, even though their actions may to some extent be excused on the ground that they are the unwilling victims of a poor environment.

If there is a difference between what is ethically good and what is ethically evil, there must be a reason for the difference, and the reason ought to be discoverable. The writers of our Declaration of Independence believed that certain facts concerning man, his rights, his duties, and his destiny could be known with certainty. They said: "We hold these truths to be self-evident: That all men are created equal; that they are endowed by their Creator with certain unalienable rights; that among these are life, liberty, and the pursuit of happiness." If such facts were discoverable by reason in 1776, they are discoverable today, and man by the exercise of his reason can know what is right and why it is right.

The responsibility of the physician in ethical matters is an exceptionally heavy one. He is present at the time of birth, and he is present when life ends. His entire task revolves around life: that life may begin to be, that life may be preserved, that life may be richer and fuller. Because he has freely assumed this task and because he accepts a compensation for doing what he does, he has a far graver responsibility in the matter than does the ordinary layman. He is responsible for what he himself does, and he is responsible for what he advises others to do. This responsibility is heavier today than it was in the past because the physician of today does not always treat bodies only. He often feels the need to treat minds as well as bodies.

Every physician has a code of ethics of his own that governs him in his relations with his patients and the public. These codes are often admirable from every point of view. Our purpose, then, in speaking of the fundamental principles on which a code of ethics should be based is merely to make our treatment of the subject logical and complete. We begin with three postulates accepted by ethicians as truths already established by other sciences. These postulates are: (1) There exists an infinitely wise and good Creator. (2) God rewards men for their good acts and punishes them for their evil acts. (3) Man possesses an immortal soul and enjoys the use of what is known as free will.

THE FIRST POSTULATE

THE ethician accepts the existence of a Creator as a truth proved in philosophy. The truth may be said in general to represent a universal conviction on the part of mankind. The conviction is based for one thing on the design and purposefulness seen everywhere in nature. The physician sees this

2

design and purposefulness in the single small cell which in time develops into the wonderfully complicated human organism. Purpose rather than accident or chance is the only logical explanation of the order found in the universe and of the powers and properties of living and nonliving things. The conviction is based, again, on the truth that a universe of limited and perishable things could not be the cause of its own existence and on the necessity of a cause outside the universe that exists in virtue of its own power.

The Creator is the First Cause, a being uncreated, the cause of all other causes, eternal, infinite, living, intelligent, and existing separately from the world. We call this being God. Since God must possess in an eminent degree all the perfections that He creates, He must be wise and good.

THE SECOND POSTULATE

THE second postulate, that God rewards men for their good acts and punishes them for their evil acts, is likewise accepted as having been demonstrated in philosophy. If God is indeed wise and good, He must have had a purpose in creating. He must wish right order to be observed by mankind. He must do something effective to make the observance of right order worth while to the individual. Since man has an inborn desire of immortality and since in this life those who are good often receive little or no reward (the man who dies for a good cause receives nothing in this life for making the supreme sacrifice), we conclude that adequate rewards and punishments will follow in the life after death.

THE THIRD POSTULATE

THE third postulate, that man possesses an immortal soul and enjoys the use of what is known as free will, is accepted as having been demonstrated in psychology. Unless this postulate is accepted, it is useless to speak of a code of ethics as something to be chosen as one's own. Man, if not endowed with a soul and with free will, is merely a superior animal. He is not free to choose but acts as a result of some inner compulsion. It is vain to tell him what he ought to do and it is unreasonable to reproach him if he fails to do it.

In general, there can be no science of ethics if any one of these three postulates is denied. We cannot tell men what they ought to do if they are not free and if there is no lawgiver to whom they are responsible. Mere human law, if we do not believe that God requires us to obey legitimate authority, can prescribe rewards and punishments, but it cannot impose a true obligation. If God does not exist, those who wish to violate human laws are free in conscience to do so. If there is no God, the outlaw who acts without respect for what society desires has done no moral wrong. If he can outwit society and elude society's police force, all is well with him.

THE NATURAL LAW

W HEREVER there is to be order in things that manifest activity, there must exist uniform modes of acting. Unless things act in a manner that is constant and dependable, chaos, not harmony, will result. If, for example, a stone tossed into the air might on one occasion fall to the ground, and at another time rise higher and higher until it disappeared into the stratosphere, and on a third occasion travel perpetually in an easterly or westerly direction, the unpredictable irregularity in its activity would lead to confusion and would create untold problems.

God has established order in the physical universe by means of laws which we call the physical laws of nature. All nonliving things have certain qualities or properties because of which they consistently act in a given manner under a given set of conditions. A stone dropped into a lake will sink to the bottom; gunpowder to which a flame is applied will explode; water raised to a certain temperature is converted into steam. Night follows day and spring succeeds winter because of the

4

physical laws of nature. As to living things without the power to feel, the plants, they too are governed by certain laws. The brute animals act without freedom in response to stimuli. Thus all nonrational beings are guided to their destiny by a necessary conformity to the physical laws of nature.

There is another class of beings, however, which are not directed to their end by means of physical necessity. The creatures in this class are rational; that is, they are gifted with understanding and free will. This second category as found upon earth is made up exclusively of human beings, who have the power to act freely, who are able deliberately to choose to do this action and to avoid that one. In keeping with their rational nature human beings are directed to their eternal destiny by moral precepts. God imposes on them the obligation to conduct themselves in a reasonable way, in a manner which befits their nature. He has given them certain commands and prohibitions, the observance of which will enable them to accomplish the purpose for which He brought them into being. These fundamental commands and prohibitions form what is called the moral law of nature and are commonly referred to as the natural law.

The principles of the natural law fall into two categories: (1) the primary principles and (2) the secondary principles. The *primary principles* are general rules of conduct which are so fundamental that there can be little disagreement about their existence. "Evil is to be avoided" and "Parents should be respected by their children" are examples of primary principles. The *secondary principles* are particular conclusions drawn from the primary principles. "Adultery is forbidden" and "Stealing is wrong" are examples of secondary principles. The science of ethics investigates the nature of these precepts, explains their origin, and enumerates the more important primary and secondary principles.

Many today defend the theory that the principles of moral conduct change from time to time, and that they are not the same throughout the world but vary according to local conditions and under the influence of changes in society. "It is a mistake to suppose that moral principles alone remain fixed and unchangeable while everything else around us grows and develops," contends Professor Hollingworth of Columbia University. "Traditional systems of ethical doctrine do not relate very closely to contemporary activities and ideals, and they are often based on antiquated descriptions of our minds and misguided accounts of human motives."[1]

In his criticism of "traditional systems of ethical doctrine" Professor Hollingworth presupposes that "everything else around us" changes. This supposition all but the intellectually blind will deny. Do the physical laws of nature—the law, for example, of gravitation or the law of combustion—vary from century to century? In order to solve his problems must the mathematician follow one set of principles today and completely different principles ten years from now? The moral law, like the laws of mathematics, is intrinsically unchangeable. If it is unthinkable that two and two should equal four today and five tomorrow, it is likewise inconceivable that the law which forbids lying should be true today and false tomorrow. Actually, the fundamental principles are recognized as such by savage and civilized alike. Barbarians, it is true, have had moral codes which differed somewhat from the code of civilized nations, but the few differences in the savages' codes stemmed from their having falsely applied the teaching of the universally accepted general principles.[2]

It is true that the moral code of all civilized peoples is not identical in every detail. Within our own century there have been places in North America where fishing on Sunday was

[1] Harry L. Hollingworth, *Psychology and Ethics*, p. v (New York: The Ronald Press Company, 1949). Professor Hollingworth seems to classify under "principles" the Ten Commandments. See p. 130.

[2] For a detailed study of this question see Michael Cronin, *The Science of Ethics*, vol. I, chap. 5, "The Moral Criteria," pp. 124-74 (New York: Benziger Brothers, 1949).

forbidden by law, and there are groups today which consider such things as dancing, card playing, and gambling evil in themselves. Others do not consider any of these things necessarily evil. But the fact that there are differences of opinion in regard to details of the code does not prove that there is nothing in the code that is fixed and unchangeable. Behind all these prohibitions are such absolute and constant principles as these: that nothing should be permitted to interfere with the worship and service of God; that our time should be used for some good purpose; that recreational activities should be decent; that things leading us into moral wrongdoing must be avoided. The rigorist can be too strict in his application of these principles, and the laxist can grant too much freedom; but both rigorist and laxist accept the same fundamental principles, and both make the same applications of the principles in very many matters. It is a common thing today for men to build up from instances of these opposed applications of fundamental principles an argument to the effect that nothing in the moral code is absolute, that the natural law is a mere fiction. The very fact that codes continue to exist and that applications continue to be made is an argument to the contrary, for every application presupposes the existence of the principle from which it is thought to follow. It is to be expected that some differences of opinion in regard to details should be found, especially among those who do not accept the existence of any authority competent to pass upon the soundness of their personal conclusions.

All men, then, are called upon to obey the natural law. Hence it matters not whether one be a Roman Catholic, a Protestant, a Jew, a pagan, or a person who has no religious affiliations whatsoever; he is nevertheless obliged to become acquainted with and to observe the teachings of the law of nature. In the present volume all the obligations which are mentioned flow from the natural law, unless the contrary is evident from the context.

If an action is evil in itself and so prohibited by the law of nature (for example, lying, stealing, or murder), no authority on earth, be it civil or ecclesiastical, can under any conceivable circumstances legitimately grant permission to perform that action. Nor can any authority on earth legitimately forbid an individual to perform an action that is clearly and under the circumstances required by the natural law. It follows that a work on medical ethics written by a Catholic is not merely a collection of rulings of an arbitrary nature made by his Church. It is rather an application to the practice of medicine of the principles of the natural law. The Catholic looks to his Church for guidance in his interpretation of the natural law, for in her role of teacher she has the right to explain and interpret difficult principles of the natural law and to pass judgment on applications of these principles. Because of confused notions which have at times arisen with regard to certain prescriptions of the natural law, the Church has issued clarifying and authoritative pronouncements which serve to protect her subjects from error.

An example of such an official interpretation of one point of the law of nature is the decision of the Sacred Congregation of the Holy Office which condemned the direct killing of persons who had committed no crime worthy of death, though because of mental and physical defects some judged them to be useless to the nation.[3] This pronouncement contained nothing not already found in the natural law, nor was the principle on which it was based unknown to men in general. The Church, however, knowing that dictators were unjustly condemning to death allegedly useless members of society and that some scholars of standing were defending the action on philosophical grounds, felt obliged to speak out in defense of the rights of humanity. To have remained silent might have created the impression that she tolerated or even approved the action. The Church, as a matter of fact, has issued only a lim-

[3] See *Acta Apostolicae Sedis* 32:553-54, January 22, 1940.

8

ited number of pronouncements on the subject of medical ethics, and these in general were either inspired by conditions such as that described or were issued in response to requests for a decision on difficult and doubtful points.

THE CRITERION OF ETHICAL GOODNESS

How are we to proceed in determining what is ethically good or ethically evil? What criterion are we to use? Must we be guided by custom, by popular opinion, by utility, by mere sentiment, or do we have some better standard? Mere sentiment and the selfish advantage of the individual can be rejected at once as determinants of moral goodness. If custom and popular opinion are ever safe guides, the reason must be that they are seen to conform to some acceptable standard. How is any custom, opinion, or standard to be appraised?

The proximate objective criterion of ethical goodness is man's rational nature as such, considered completely in itself and in its relationships. Inner consciousness tells man that he is capable of arriving at truth and that he is free. Reason makes known to him that he is a created being, made for a purpose, and that all other men were created with the same rights that he enjoys. Toward his Creator he has an obligation of worship, of obedience, and of service. Toward his fellow man he has an obligation of justice and, at times, of charity. An act is ethically good if it befits man's rational nature thus considered in itself and in its relationships.

For example, to curse God is an act opposed to man's rational nature. It is an act prompted only by ignorance, passion, pride, or rebellion, and is therefore unworthy of man and ethically wrong. To refuse to pay a worker the sum agreed upon after he has faithfully done his work is an act opposed to man's rational nature and hence ethically wrong, for man's rational nature requires that he should keep promises made and that he should not deprive a fellow man of the fruits of his labor. All ethical problems are solved on the same basis.

9

What is in harmony with man's rational nature is good. What is opposed to man's rational nature is evil.

SIX FUNDAMENTAL PRINCIPLES

O N THE basis of this criterion we can lay down six general principles that will serve as guides in solving the various special problems of medical ethics. The six principles are as follows.

1. Every human being has a right to life. Deliberate murder is therefore wrong. It violates four important rights: God's right over human life, the right of the murdered man to his own life, the right of society to public peace and order, and the right of the relatives and friends of the murdered man to his love and service.

This right of a human being to his own life, however, is not absolute and unlimited. In the first place, he is not free to end his life by suicide. In the second place, he may be deprived of his life by public authority if by serious crime he becomes a menace to society, or even by a private individual if he unjustly assails a fellow man and can be restrained only by violent means resulting in death.

The right to life applies to life in its full sense. Not only is murder wrong, but mutilation and physical injury to another are likewise wrong. Injury to one's character, to his spiritual or religious life, is likewise wrong. Hence to encourage another to do evil or to subject him needlessly to temptation is wrong. Finally, every man has a right to his reputation or good name, essential to him as a means of living successfully and happily.

2. Every human being has a right to the truth. The evident purpose of the power of communication is that truth should be conveyed from man to man. A lie is therefore of its nature wrong because it is opposed to the rational nature of man. The right to truth, however, does not necessarily include the right to know the full and entire truth. We are not always obliged to tell everything that we know, nor are we always free to do

so should we wish. The right to truth means that every man has a right to know those things which in justice or charity he should be told, and that in no case should he be deceived by a lie.

3. Justice is due to every human being. He possesses a right to those things that properly belong to him by nature, by birth, by gift, by contract, or in virtue of any other circumstance by which rights are established. Hence a newborn child has a right to the care and protection of his parents, who are responsible for his welfare because they freely brought him into the world. Hence, too, a patient has a right to the competent and conscientious care of the physician who has accepted him as a patient.

4. The faculties and powers of man must be used according to the purpose for which they were evidently intended by nature and in the manner evidently intended by nature. Hence the faculty of speech is perverted if used to communicate to another as one's judgment what is directly contradictory to one's true thought in the matter. Hence the sex powers of man are perverted if used outside the licit marriage act.

5. If an act is ethically wrong, one is not only obliged to refrain from it himself, but he is also obliged to refrain from formal cooperation with another in the performance of the act. Both of two bandits who rob an autoist are guilty of robbery. There are types of cooperation, however, which may be permitted. These will be discussed in their proper place.

6. Evil may never be done that good may result from it. The end does not justify the means. Unless this principle is accepted, there is no limit to the disorder that would result. Wives would be free to murder alcoholic husbands as a means of preventing discord and physical violence in the home and of removing a bad example for the sake of the children. A man with an invalid wife urgently in need of a trip to Florida would, in order to finance her trip, be free to steal money wherever he could find it. In general, some real or imagined good results from every evil deed. The robber becomes richer, the murderer is rid of someone who interferes with him. The principle that the end does not justify the means must be accepted as essential to any sound system of ethics.

If anyone feels inclined to doubt the validity of these six basic principles, let him ask himself what his own life would become if the society in which he lives did not accept them. He would find himself deprived, as men are actually being deprived in some nations of the world today, of his most precious rights. His right to the property acquired through his industry, his right to justice in the courts of law, his right to follow the dictates of his conscience, his right to fair dealing on the part of his neighbors, his right even to life itself, would be lost. It is therefore the duty of all individuals to do what they can for the general acceptance and observance of these six principles. The discussion of certain problems connected with their practical application is begun in the next chapter.

REFERENCES

Bruehl, Charles P. *This Way Happiness.* Milwaukee: Bruce Publishing Company, 1941.

Coppens, Charles, S.J. *Brief Text-Book of Moral Philosophy,* revised by Henry S. Spalding, S.J. New York: Schwartz, Kirwin and Fauss, 1924.

Cronin, Michael. *The Science of Ethics.* 2 vols. New York: Benziger Brothers, 1949.

Frenay, Adolph Dominic, O.P. "The Natural Law." *Ecclesiastical Review* 97:1-17, July 1937.

Hull, Ernest R., S.J. *Practical Philosophy of Life,* third edition. St. Louis: B. Herder Book Company, 1937.

———— *Why Should I Be Moral?* second edition. St. Louis: B. Herder Book Company, 1923.

MacGillivray, G. J., editor. *Moral Principles and Practices,* chaps. 1-6 and 9. London: Sheed and Ward, 1933.

Rickaby, Joseph, S.J. *Aquinas Ethicus.* London: Burns and Oates, 1892.

THE OBLIGATIONS OF PHYSICIANS

IN GENERAL

ETHICS in its strict sense is the science of moral duty. In a broader sense it is the science of the ideal human character. The man who aims at becoming an ideal character always does much that is not required of him as a duty. This book, except for the chapter on the physician as counselor, in which some of the things that are suggested are excellent but not obligatory, discusses medical ethics in the strict sense and not in the broader sense. When physicians, surgeons, and hospital personnel refer to the ethician questions concerning practices and procedures, what they wish to know is whether the practice or procedure is morally permissible. The ethician is therefore concerned with obligation rather than with ideals that transcend what is of obligation.

This will explain why the present chapter says nothing concerning certain practices that are either approved or condemned in codes to which members of the profession are asked to subscribe, such as the code of ethics of the American Medical Association. These practices may set an ideal which is in every way to be commended; but if they do not involve a strictly moral issue, they do not fall within the scope of the present work. Nor are we concerned with those attitudes toward their work that physicians are sometimes urged to make their own, unless these attitudes are a matter of duty. As the title of the chapter indicates, we are concerned with the obligations of physicians; and the first and most obvious obligation of every physician is this, that he should be competent to render those services which he offers to the public.

PROFESSIONAL COMPETENCE

BEFORE a physician practices his professional duties, he is obliged to be reasonably competent. He must have at least enough knowledge of his science to care for the ordinary cases with which he is to deal, and he must be able to recognize in a patient the need of a specialist's skill. Although it would be asking too much to require that he be highly qualified in every branch of medicine, still the physician must endeavor to keep himself informed about the most recent types of successful therapy.[1] He can fulfill his duty in this regard by reading well-selected medical journals. The general practitioner must not remain satisfied with his medical-school training, but should maintain the competence which he professes to possess. If he continually neglects his medical education after he receives his professional degree, he will soon be ignorant of advances that have been made in methods of diagnosis and treatment. If he has the opportunity of taking postgraduate courses, he will find these more beneficial than merely reading contemporaneous literature.[2]

Unless a physician is qualified to do surgery, he should not engage in this practice. Not a few young physicians who have no special competence in this field undertake to perform deli-

---

[1] In making application for fellowship in the American College of Surgeons the candidate pledges himself "to advance constantly in knowledge by the study of surgical literature, instruction by competent teachers, interchange of opinion among associates, and attendance on sessions of the important societies and at clinics" (*Requirements for Fellowship, American College of Surgeons.* Chicago: American College of Surgeons, July 1, 1954).

[2] See *American Medicine: Expert Testimony out of Court,* vol. I, pp. 392-427 (New York: American Foundation, 1937); Paul de Kruif, "Family Doctor: Model 1955," *GP* 11:127-31, January 1955.

cate and intricate operations. Some of these imprudent men are motivated by a desire to obtain experience in surgery. The foolhardiness of others stems from their greed for money. Such physicians can be guilty of grave fault in unnecessarily exposing the patient to very serious danger.

The physician's competency includes knowledge of ethics as well as skill in his profession. His patients depend upon him for their physical well-being and even for their very lives. He can be guilty of wrongdoing by neglect and by using procedures that are not permissible. He therefore needs to have a code of ethics that will guide him in the performance of his everyday duties.

When analyzing the morality of a medical case, the physician must be guided by reason and not by sentiment, expediency, or the actions of others. Under no conditions should one's solution be based on mere sentiment. The obstetrician, for example, probably feels greater sympathy for the mother, whom he has known and treated perhaps for years, than for her unborn baby, who is wholly unknown to him. He must nevertheless refrain from letting this sympathy for the mother interfere with his according equal justice to the child. When the danger of death hovers over a patient who is very dear to the physician, his deep emotional reaction may exert a very undesirable influence on his moral judgment. Strong emotion may becloud his reason and tempt him to follow what his heart rather than what his intellect dictates. Not long ago a physician who opposed therapeutic abortion on principle was heard to remark: "If my wife needed an abortion to save her life, I would not hesitate to empty her uterus." This physician lived up to the moral code in dealing with strangers; but if the natural law were to prohibit what he considered to be necessary for safeguarding the physical health of his own wife, he was willing to act against the law. Physicians, then, should beware of permitting sentiment to have any part in determining the morality of an action.

The physician, moreover, should not be guided by expediency in performing the duties of his office. Conscientious observance of the natural law may cost the physician large sums of money. Immoral operations often bring fat fees. Older physicians have mentioned how difficult it is for a struggling young physician to refuse to handle a lucrative but illicit case. In the case of a rich unmarried girl who is with child, a physician may be offered a large fee to effect an abortion to save the girl's good name. The natural law, however, and not expediency must determine his reply to such a request.

We are well aware of the fact that there are physicians and surgeons who are in perfect good faith when they use treatments or perform operations which we shall feel forced to describe as opposed to the natural law and hence as illicit. Nothing that we may say should be interpreted as indicating that we consider these members of the profession necessarily guilty of deliberate and culpable wrongdoing. One may do what is objectively wrong and still be subjectively guiltless. Any act, considered objectively in itself, is either good or bad quite independently of what one may think of it. We cannot make a wicked act good by thinking that it is good or by calling it good. It is quite possible, however, that we may be sincerely convinced that it is good; and if we then perform the act in question, we are subjectively guiltless while doing what is objectively wrong.

A striking example of an action objectively blameworthy but subjectively blameless was encountered on an island of the New Hebrides during World War II by a Red Cross nurse. She thus describes what she learned: "When a person [on this island] gets old—when he passes the age of usefulness to himself or to the community—his relatives dig a hole, stand him up in it, fill the hole in with dirt right up to his chin, and then go away and leave him to starve to death."[3] These barbarians

<hr>

[3] Wanda Burnett, "Yank Meets Native." *National Geographic Magazine* 88:107, July 1945.

believed that it was the filial duty of the relatives to kill off their kin when old age had supposedly deprived them of all usefulness. In this killing of the old person the natives were objectively committing murder; subjectively, however, their action was blameless.

In determining the morality of an action, then, one must not be guided by mere sentiment nor by expediency nor by the actions of others, but should follow the direction of reason. The principles expounded in the science of ethics often enable a person to judge quickly whether a proposed action is good or bad or indifferent. If because of its involved nature it is difficult to ascertain an action's morality, one wisely has recourse to the pronouncements of the Church and to the teachings of ethicians.

The physician, because of his desire to help his patients, may become so absorbed in the medical problems of a case that he loses sight of its moral aspect. Even conscientious physicians sometimes use or advocate measures clearly prohibited by the law of nature. Physicians must avoid thinking that a good end or purpose can dispense from the obligation of considering the morality of the means to be used.

THE OBLIGATION TO ATTEND PATIENTS

THE physician's obligations toward patients vary according to circumstances. They may bind him to care for the patient either in justice, in charity only, or in both.

Obligations of the Physician in Justice

Under certain circumstances the obligation of a physician to care for a patient is one that binds in justice.

1. If the physician is under contract to the patient (hired by an annual fee, and so forth), he must in justice:

    a. Go to his patient's aid at any hour of the day or night, even at the cost of grave inconvenience, unless he knows that his delay will cause no harm to the patient.

b. Care for the patient even though the latter is afflicted with a highly contagious disease or proves almost unbearable because of his character and his temperamental behavior.

2. If a physician has already begun the care of a patient, a contract, at least a tacit contract, is thus entered into and so he must in justice:

a. Cure the patient as best he can.

b. Not desert the patient, even though the disease turns out to be contagious, unless he makes satisfactory provision for the care of the patient elsewhere (for example, in the isolation ward of a hospital).

Obligations of the Physician in Charity

The physician is bound only in charity in cases that do not come under the above-mentioned circumstances.[4] He is under no obligation to seek out the sick among the poor, but he may have an obligation in charity of attending those who ask his help, even though they are unable to reimburse him at all, and of attending victims of accident or disease whom he knows to be in grave need of help but who are unable to ask for it. These obligations may be summarized as follows.

1. If the patient is *in extreme need* of medical attention, the physician has the grave obligation to aid him even though he finds it seriously inconvenient to do so.

When we say that the patient is *in extreme need* we mean that he is in a dying condition and that, unless the physician undertakes his care, death will probably ensue or that some very grave physical harm will follow, such as the complete loss of sight or an injury of equivalent severity. An example of such a patient is one who is running a very high fever which may cause death, or who is hemorrhaging severely, or who

[4] See Theodore Wiprud, M.D., *The Business Side of Medical Practice,* second edition, chap. 8, "The Charity Patient," pp. 95-102 (Philadelphia: W. B. Saunders Company, 1949); Timothy O'Connell, "The Physician's Obligation To Give Spiritual Advice," *Linacre Quarterly* 17:11-22, February 1950.

would become a permanent invalid if he is deprived of the help of a physician.

2. If the patient is *in serious need* of medical attention, the physician is not obliged to help him if he would find it gravely inconvenient to do so.

When we say that the patient is *in serious need* we mean that he is gravely afflicted with some bodily disease or injury which requires the services of a physician. Danger of death is not present at the moment, but the patient's condition is such that, without professional care, danger of death may result as could happen in the case of one who has incipient pneumonia.

3. If the patient is *in ordinary need* of medical attention, the physician is obliged to give him only that time which he has free after his regular work is done. Moreover, his obligation to do this is slight.

When we say that the patient is *in ordinary need* we mean that his condition is such that depriving him of professional medical care will cause him inconvenience only, not danger of death. An example of this is the case of a person who is suffering from bursitis.

Because physicians are, as a rule, always ready to attend a patient even at the cost of their own comfort and health, it is unnecessary to point out that every patient must be accorded at least ordinary care. The fact that the one whom the physician is treating is a mental defective or is being administered to out of charity does not justify the physician in being hasty or slipshod in his treatment. The competent physician will have due regard for the patient's feelings and will not offend by too brusque a manner, by unnecessary roughness, or by needlessly causing mental torment to the patient. It happens at times, for example, that a mother finds her young baby dead in his crib, to all appearances smothered by the bedclothes. Physicians have been known bluntly to inform the sorrowing mother that the child's death was due to her negligence. Apart from the fact that the infant's death in such cases is rarely due to his being suffocated by pillow or bedclothing,[5] physicians act with great imprudence if they openly condemn the mother for gross negligence.

Emergency Cases

A physician who makes it a practice not to attend patients in their homes may be appealed to in an emergency when the stricken person can find no other physician. There are not a few cases on record in which physicians who specialized in office cases refused to go to the patient's home despite the fact that the latter was in acute need of medical attention. A physician, appealed to in such cases, is obliged to take the home call if (1) he judges the patient's need to be extreme and (2) no other physician is available. The obligation would be present even though going to the other's assistance would be gravely inconvenient, for the patient's danger of death is rightly considered to outweigh in importance the physician's serious inconvenience. If, however, the patient's need were merely grave, the physician would not be obliged to visit him at the cost of grave inconvenience to himself.

THE SELECTION OF REMEDIES

IN CARING for his patient the physician must always use the best remedy at hand. The best remedy means that which most benefits the patient; that is, the one which is the most effective, the safest, the quickest, and the least costly. If a particular kind of treatment is very expensive, it is looked upon as extraordinary means of preserving one's health, and therefore the patient, if he so wishes, may rightfully refuse to use it.[6] In

[5] See Keith Bowden, "Sudden Death or Alleged Accidental Suffocation," *Medical Journal of Australia* 1:65-72, January 21, 1950. "The fear of accidental suffocation causes unnecessary maternal anxiety. . . . There will continue to be instances in which babies are found dead face downwards in their cots; but few, if any, will be accidental suffocation in my opinion, but instances of the appalling swiftness with which death in the form of natural disease snatches young life" (p. 72).

[6] See "Extraordinary Means of Preserving Life," pp. 67-72.

20

such a case the physician may of course administer, with the patient's consent, a remedy that is less costly and less effective.

If there is at hand a remedy which is not too expensive and certainly effective, the physician may not try uncertain ones on his patient with the danger of causing his death or serious injury to his health, even though the patient has given him permission to do this. The patient actually cannot accord him permission for such experiments, since he is not master of his own life. The physician, moreover, may not rightly argue that such a remedy, if once proved effective, would undoubtedly save many others and that, though one or two individuals would perhaps be sacrificed during the experiments, a large number would be benefited afterward. To use such an argument would be equivalent to defending the commission of evil in order to accomplish some good—a principle that must always be condemned as immoral. If, however, there is no safer remedy available, the physician may, in cases where death would otherwise result, employ such uncertain remedies, for then he is doing all that he possibly can to save the patient. He is using this means only as a last resort. In these circumstances the physician must have the patient's consent, either explicit or implicit,[7] and there must be due proportion between the risk that is run and the good which is hoped for. If possible, the remedy should be first sufficiently tested on animals. A discussion of special aspects of this question will be found under "The Experimental Use of Drugs and Germs," pages 259-63.

Case 1
Remedies for Patients in Public Institutions
The patient has been received in a county hospital. Is the physician permitted to use any treatment, no matter how expensive, or must his remedies be those which a person of average means would request?

---

[7] For an excellent explanation of cases in which the consent of the patient may be licitly presumed see Gerald Kelly, S.J., *Medico-Moral Problems*, pt. 4, "Consent of the Patient," pp. 9-12 (St. Louis: Catholic Hospital Association of the United States and Canada, 1952).

Solution. The physician is obliged to give his patient the care which the ordinary patient would receive. If the patient demands that he use very expensive medication, the physician is obliged to accede to the request to the extent permitted by the civil law. The solution here given for patients in public institutions applies also to patients receiving free medical care in countries such as Great Britain.

Explanation. The extent of the rights of the patient in this case should be clear from the civil law. If the law grants such patients the right to medical care without limitation, the physician may not justly deny them even very expensive medication. If, however, less costly medication will prove equally effective and if it can be employed without causing grave inconvenience to the patient, it seems only reasonable that the physician should begin his treatment by using such medication.

THE USE OF TOXIC AND HABIT-FORMING DRUGS

THERE are two types of remedy which can involve danger for the patient: those which are toxic and those which are narcotic. If toxic medication is given in too large dosage, it can prove fatal. If narcotic medication is used too freely, it can develop in the patient a habit which is extremely difficult to overcome. Hence the physician must prescribe sparingly in such cases and use all diligence to avoid erring in so important a matter. Some persons are what are known as addictive personalities. They are liable to become addicts much more readily than the normal individual. Although the physician will find it very difficult to identify this type of patient beforehand, he should not forget that some persons are especially susceptible to drugs.

It is of course permitted to use morphine, cocaine, codeine, and other similar drugs in order to prevent, alleviate, or end pain. If the sickness or pain is severe, drugs may in general be administered even though loss of consciousness results. To prescribe without sufficient cause drugs that would deprive the patient of the use of reason for some time (according to some theologians, for an hour or more) would be gravely illicit. In the altogether unlikely case where a physician gave the patient, for example, a strong dose of opium for a slight headache, he would not only be going against proper medical procedure; he would also be violating the moral law.

Case 2

Illicit Use of a Habit-Forming Drug

The patient, a woman who is passing through her menopause, is suffering from involutional melancholia. Her husband complains to the physician because no improvement occurs after months of costly treatment. The physician thereupon gives her morphine to be taken as often as she feels the need of it but without letting her know what drug she is taking. The patient recovers but is now a drug addict. Was the physician justified in prescribing morphine?

Solution. The use of morphine and other narcotics is what is called symptomatic therapy. Narcotics do not cure the basic disease but may alleviate pain and produce a feeling of euphoria. It is the duty of the physician to evaluate the psychological status of patients for whom he is thinking of prescribing narcotics. While he can seldom if ever be certain that an individual will never become an addict, he will meet cases in which it is evident to him that addiction will very probably result, and in such cases he must use narcotics sparingly if at all. Greater freedom is permitted in postoperative and other cases of short duration and in terminal cases. In the case described the physician did wrong in acting as he did.

Explanation. The drug habit involves moral evil; once contracted, it causes the addict to neglect his ordinary duties, to lie, to steal, and perhaps to commit still more serious faults. The drug addict is a source of scandal to others. These are moral evils. There is also the physical evil resulting from the undermining of the addict's health.

The giving of opiates to a dying patient who is suffering intensely presents special problems. To administer drugs to a dying man so that he will die in the state of unconsciousness and thus escape the agony that usually accompanies death is illicit if any one of the following five conditions is verified.

1. If the drug would notably accelerate the patient's death. In that event the action would violate the Fifth Commandment and would partake of the nature of mercy killing.

2. If there is reason for believing that the patient is not in the state of grace, for then this action would deprive him of the opportunity of making his peace with God and of receiving the last sacraments.

3. If the temporal affairs of the patient are not in order and if he could and would attend to them were he not unconscious. By temporal affairs is here meant the patient's last will and testament, business matters which he alone can properly take care of, and so forth.

4. Even when the patient is in the state of grace and his temporal affairs have been duly cared for, if the pain is not severe, for this would be taking from him a valuable occasion for meriting.

5. If the patient does not consent, at least implicitly, to this act.

Instead of giving the patient a dosage of the drug which will bring on prolonged coma, it is preferable, from a spiritual viewpoint, that he be kept conscious so that he may have the opportunity of gaining merit during the hours immediately preceding his death.[8]

THE OBLIGATION OF CORRECTING ERRORS

IT CAN happen, and indeed has happened, that a physician in good faith prescribes for his patient something which will prove gravely harmful to him. When this occurs the physician must recall the prescription as soon as he possibly can. If, however, this cannot be done without grave injury to himself or without causing himself very serious difficulty, his obligation to correct his mistake is at an end.

It is very difficult to imagine a situation in which the physician could not correct such a mistake without even slight embarrassment to himself. The physician, whether he is giving his instructions to the patient himself or to the hospital where

[8] See John McCarthy, "The Giving of Drugs to the Dying." *Irish Ecclesiastical Record* 61:345-46, May 1943.

the patient is confined, need say no more than that he wishes to change his instructions or that he has thought of something that will be better for the patient. It is equally difficult to imagine a situation in which the correcting of the mistake would cause such grave injury or difficulty to the physician as to justify him in permitting the patient to suffer injury. The ethician, however, is obliged to answer frankly when asked what must be done should such situations occur. If under any circumstances he releases the physician from the obligation of correcting a mistake which was accidental rather than malicious or inexcusable, he does not by any means wish to discourage him from accepting the greatest conceivable injury or loss rather than permit his patient to suffer. As has been said before (see pages 9-10), ethics in its strict sense tells men what they must do to avoid guilt or moral wrongdoing. The ideals proposed by medical ethics in its broader sense go far beyond what is a matter of strict obligation.

GHOST SURGERY

G HOST surgery is the practice in which Dr. B performs a surgical operation as the agent of Dr. A, who the patient believes is actually doing the surgery. Dr. A is as a rule a general practitioner and, as a general practitioner, he collects fees which are comparatively small. When one of his patients is in need of an operation, Dr. A agrees to do the surgery, but because of his lack of special skill in this field, he wisely hesitates to perform the operation. In order, however, that he may share in the richer revenue of the surgeon, Dr. A then has Dr. B, a specialist with whom he has a standing agreement, perform the operation. The patient, ignorant of the substitution, never sees Dr. B, for the latter deals with the patient only during the time when he is under anesthesia.

What is to be said of the morality of ghost surgery? Besides the fact that the patient is deceived as to the physician who performs the operation, there are many abuses which are closely connected with ghost surgery.[9] In this practice it generally happens that Dr. B sees the patient for the first time in the operating room. Hence, unable to make a personal diagnosis of the case, he accepts without question the diagnosis which has been charted by Dr. A. Dr. A may be incompetent and may prescribe what is certainly or at least probably injurious to the patient. In order to avoid incurring the disfavor of Dr. A or losing his lucrative referrals, it often happens that Dr. B performs the recommended surgery in spite of the fact that all the evidence before him proves clearly that Dr. A is either grossly incompetent or is motivated solely by pecuniary considerations. After the surgery, moreover, the patient will be deprived of the specialist's postoperative care, for the identity of Dr. B must not be revealed. It seems clear, therefore, that the physician should keep himself free from a practice of this kind. Referrals are of course necessary, but the identity of the surgeon should not be kept secret.

SAFEGUARDING THE HEALTH OF ASSISTANTS

THE physician is under an obligation of safeguarding the health of those whom he uses as professional assistants. If, for example, a patient who is being treated at home has sometimes become violent and attacked those attending him, the physician should not employ a trained nurse without taking whatever steps are necessary to have her warned.

Case 3
Failing To Protect a Nurse against the Danger of Infection

Dr. N obtains the services of a graduate nurse for a patient who is ill at home. He does not make known to the nurse the fact that the maculopapular lesions over the entire body of the patient are secondary syphilitic lesions.

Solution. Dr. N was at fault in failing to warn the nurse.

---

[9] See the suggestions made by Dr. I. S. Ravdin of Philadelphia at a meeting of the American Medical Association, reported in *Journal of the American Medical Association* 147:535-37, October 6, 1951.

Explanation. The nurse will probably become infected if she fails to take the proper precautions. While it is true that she should be able to recognize secondary luetic lesions, Dr. N cannot be certain that she will not mistake them for another dermatitis. In addition, his failure to warn the nurse may create in her mind the impression that no danger is present.

THE FEES OF PHYSICIANS

A physician may of course accept for his professional services any amount of money which is freely and spontaneously offered him by the patient. If a patient not only intends to pay what is strictly due but desires generously to show his gratitude for the care which he received, the physician may without scruple profit by this act of generosity, no matter how large the sum may be.

A more difficult question is this: How much may a physician licitly *exact* for services rendered? In answering this query it would be best to distinguish between the following two cases: (1) when the amount of the fee is definitely determined beforehand and (2) when the amount of the fee is not fixed in advance.

1. *Fee Determined Beforehand.* If a patient approaches a physician before the professional services are rendered and wishes to come to an agreement about the size of the honorarium to be paid, is there any limit to the sum which the physician may demand?

We here assume that there are other competent physicians available in the vicinity to whom the patient could go without too much inconvenience. In this case the physician may fix as the price of his services any fee within reason. Even though the sum he asks be far in excess of that which other physicians demand for the same work, he is guilty of no injustice, for the patient is perfectly free to pay that price or not. The patient is not compelled by circumstances to request the services of this physician and can, if he so desires, have the same work done by another skilled physician at less cost to himself.

27

2. *Fee Not Determined Beforehand.* If the professional services have already been rendered, what should be the sum which a physician fixes upon as his fee? In general we may say that he should charge no more than is customary among those of his professional standing in his own community. It does not seem possible to define the exact limits of a just fee. When one tries to place a value on the services rendered in a particular case by a physician, one must take into consideration the years of arduous study, costly schooling, carefully acquired skill, and long training demanded of every physician; the cost of office and attendants, of many expensive instruments which physicians must have at hand, of books and periodicals with which they keep abreast of the most recent medical progress; the complexity of the treatment required; the gravity of the patient's condition and the corresponding degree of responsibility which the physician must assume; and the nature of the rightful reputation of the particular physician.[10] The fee may obviously include the expenses of travel to which the physician is put in visiting a patient and any extraordinary care which the case requires. A physician may justly proportion his fee to the wealth of the patient. Many physicians praiseworthily ask for but a minimum fee from those who are in moderate circumstances, though they very properly demand the full just price of their professional services from the wealthy. The best norm for determining a fair honorarium is the practice of conscientious doctors in that part of the country where the physician is practicing.

THE AVOIDANCE OF NEEDLESS EXPENSE

THE physician may not make useless visits to his patients, for this would be demanding payment for what is valueless. Visits, however, though of no value physically, may be quite helpful to the patient psychologically, as happens in the

---

[10] See Theodore Wiprud, M.D., *The Business Side of Medical Practice,* second edition, p. 86. Philadelphia: W. B. Saunders Company, 1949.

case of some slowly dying patients who are beyond the aid of physicians but who would be greatly worried if the physician did not visit them and prescribe medicine for them. The physician may call on such patients, prescribe harmless pills, and charge for his service. As long as he does not foster this kind of dependence through selfish and unworthy motives, the practice will be justified.

A physician may not call in other medical men for consultation at the expense of the patient unless there is real need for doing so. On the other hand, a physician commits a moral wrong if in difficult cases he refuses to allow other physicians to be called in for advice or if in selecting consultants he considers friendship in preference to competency.

FEE SPLITTING

Fee splitting is the practice in which surgeons and physicians who are specialists give a share of the fee accepted from a client to the physician who has referred the patient to them. The share which is given to the referring physician may vary from perhaps 10 per cent to 50 per cent or more. The American Medical Association says: "Included among unethical inducements are split fees, rebates, 'kickbacks,' discounts, loans, favors, gifts, and emoluments with or without the knowledge of the patient. Fee splitting violates the patient's trust that his physician will not exploit his dependence upon him and invites physicians to place the desire for profit above the opportunity to render appropriate medical service."[11] The same norm is accepted by the American College of Surgeons.[12] In England, it is said, the General Medical Council makes fee splitting or dichotomy punishable with erasure from the medical register.[13] Most physicians will agree that today there

[11] "Principles of Medical Ethics." In *Guide to Services,* chap. 1, sec. 6, p. 103. Chicago: The American Medical Association, 1955.

[12] See "Principles of Financial Relations in the Professional Care of the Patient." *Bulletin of the American College of Surgeons* 35:8, January 1950.

[13] "Fee-Splitting Is a Sin." *America* 82:684, March 18, 1950.

are in the United States many cases of fee splitting. With regard to this practice Dr. Bernheim says that "the general impression is that the custom is widespread throughout the country and is growing."[14]

Is it ethically wrong for a physician thus to share the fee which he receives with another physician? Fee splitting, it is true, tends to reflect discredit on the medical profession and to throw unwholesome suspicion on physicians in general.[15] It is tantamount to making the general practitioner a sort of sales agent for the specialist. Considered apart from the ethical code of any medical association, what is to be thought of the morality of this manner of acting?

The morality of fee splitting is as follows.

1. The referring physician, Dr. A, is not permitted to *exact* from the patient more than his patient owes him for the visit itself. The reason is that, when Dr. A imparts to the patient the knowledge about the proficiency of Dr. B as a specialist, he is administering merely the ordinary care to which the patient has a right. A physician is expected to recognize the need which his patient has of a specialist's skill and to inform the patient of this need. It is also part of a physician's ordinary duty to recommend to the patient specialists who are trustworthy. Hence it would be unjust if the physician, Dr. A, were to exact from the patient a fee for this information over and above the one given for the professional visit to him.

2. The specialist, Dr. B, cannot exact from the patient thus referred more than he would have demanded if the patient had come to him directly without the recommendation of Dr. A.

3. If Dr. A refers the patient to Dr. B without necessity or without proportionate utility, he offends against justice, for he

[14] Bertram M. Bernheim, M.D., *A Surgeon's Domain*, p. 219. New York: W. W. Norton and Company, 1947.

[15] See Theodore Wiprud, M.D., *The Business Side of Medical Practice*, second edition, pp. 199-202 (Philadelphia: W. B. Saunders Company, 1949); Norman Barnesby, *Medical Chaos and Crime*, Appendix F, "Conservative Surgery and Fee-Splitting," pp. 338-45 (New York: Mitchell Kennerly, 1910).

unjustly causes financial loss to the patient. Dr. A is likewise guilty of injustice if he sends the patient to an unskilled physician or to one who is notably excessive in his fees.

4. If Dr. A could refer the patient to other specialists who are equally as skilled and whose services are no more expensive, he could without injustice demand from Dr. B beforehand some share of the fee which the latter collects from the patients whom he refers to him. Dr. A by his referrals is conferring on Dr. B a genuine benefit which has money value, and by exacting compensation for this he does not act unjustly.

5. If Dr. B, the specialist, voluntarily offers to give Dr. A, the referring physician, a percentage of the just fees collected from the patients whom he refers to him, this practice is not unjust and in some circumstances might be licit.

6. Although this latter manner of acting (nos. 4 and 5) is in itself morally unobjectionable, there can be, and very often are, grave abuses which attend it. The danger is that the specialist who receives the patient will increase his fee in order to pay the referring physician a sizable sum for the referral, or that the referring physician may send him cases which do not require a specialist's care. The general practitioner may send patients to the specialist for useless X-ray work, cardiograms, blood tests, and so forth. In such cases as these the referring physician does the patient an injustice, and he is obliged to make reparation for any foreseen and intentional injury which he has caused by such referrals.

7. If a physician is convinced that, unless he engages in the practice described under no. 5, he will suffer grave harm, he may, scandal apart, act in this manner. It may happen in some communities that, if a physician refuses to have anything to do with fee-splitting arrangements with other physicians, he will suffer a great decrease of income, for the others will carefully avoid ever sending him patients whom he is qualified to treat. In order to protect himself against these gravely injurious effects, a physician is justified in acting as outlined in no. 5.

31

Obviously he must take every precaution against doing the patient any injustice.

The doctrine in regard to fee splitting which we have explained above takes into consideration only the obligation imposed by the natural law in all cases and independently of special circumstances. There is another thing which the physician must keep in mind, and that is the promise which is usually made at the time of graduation from medical school. On that occasion the young physician, as a rule, gives his word that he will not engage in the practice of fee splitting. The binding force of the promise depends upon the intention of the one who makes it. It may perhaps be assumed that the physician here intends no obligation beyond that which arises from the natural law itself.

Case 4
Unnecessary Referral

Dr. A, the family physician, says to his patient, Miss X: "I don't like the looks of that skin infection at all. You had better go over to see Dr. B. He'll fix you up. He specializes in skin ailments." Actually, Dr. A himself has diagnosed the case without any difficulty and is certain about the remedy that should be employed, for the infection is of a common type.

Solution. Dr. A is guilty of a violation of justice.

Explanation. Dr. A is effectively persuading Miss X to pay for the unneeded services of his friend, Dr. B, and he is neglecting to give the professional service for which his patient is paying him.

Case 5
Fee Splitting

Dr. A is the family physician of Mrs. X. After notifying her that she must undergo a caesarean section, he makes arrangements to have Dr. B perform the operation. Dr. B afterward collects $250 from Mr. X for his services and, as usual, gives Dr. A 20 per cent of the fee.

Solution. If Dr. B does not add to his fee the 20 per cent which he gives to Dr. A, his action is not dishonest.

Explanation. Dr. A might have had any one of several competent surgeons do the operating, but he actually chose Dr. B. This favor has

32

money value, and Dr. B may reward Dr. A by sharing with him the fee which he collects. For the reasons mentioned above, however, this procedure is to be frowned upon. Dr. A must of course beware of the evil practice of referring his patients to a surgeon who, though less competent than others who are readily available, offers him a more generous sum. The solution here given considers only whether the act of the physician is good or bad; it does not state what is the better thing to do. It assumes that the physician has not signed a pledge or taken an oath by which he intended to bind himself to avoid all fee splitting.

Case 6
Commissions Accepted from Pharmacies

Dr. A writes out a prescription for his patient and gives it to her with the words: "Take this over to the Newcomb Pharmacy at the corner. They'll have it ready for you in a short time." Dr. A is careful to encourage his patients to go to this pharmacy, for he receives 10 per cent of what it collects from those whom he sends there.

Solution. Insofar as the natural law is concerned, this practice is licit provided the druggist sells the medicine at the usual current price and does not add to his price the 10 per cent which he must pay the physician. The practice could be morally wrong in the case of physicians who have signed a pledge to avoid the practice.

Explanation. Dr. A has not committed an injustice against his patient, for she pays only the regular price for what she receives. He does not commit an injustice against the druggist, who willingly enters into what he considers a good business arrangement.

THE OBLIGATION OF TRUTHFULNESS

TRUTHFULNESS or veracity is a moral virtue that inclines one fittingly to speak the truth. We say "fittingly" because the virtue of truthfulness does not require one to tell the entire truth on all occasions. Were this the case, the physician would offend against the virtue of truthfulness by refusing to tell others what he knows about the limitations of his colleagues or by considering sacred secrets committed to him in his professional capacity. Belonging to the virtue of truthfulness are the virtue of simplicity, which excludes all hypocrisy and double-dealing, and the virtue of fidelity, which inclines one

[handwritten marginal note: wrong! from the standpoint of medical ethics]

faithfully to execute his promises. The physician, perhaps more than many others, has need to cultivate the virtue of veracity. He must endeavor always to be truthful with others and, above all, with himself. In the discharge of his professional duties honest judgment without exaggeration should be his invariable rule of conduct.[16]

We have said that the physician must be truthful, above all, with himself. There will be occasions when not a little courage on his part is required in order to live up to this rule of conduct, but he must be ready frankly to face the truth. If he occasionally discovers that his diagnosis was erroneous, he must honestly acknowledge his mistake unless excused from so doing by the principles explained on pages 24-25. To err at times in diagnosing a patient's ailment is not an unpardonable fault, for the symptoms observed in a patient are often misleading. How many physicians are there who have never been mistaken? It may happen, for example, that the surgeon who has charted the patient for a hysterectomy discovers after opening the abdomen that the uterus is entirely healthy. In such a case there is nothing to do but admit the error in diagnosis and close the incision.

In order to safeguard their reputation in the eyes of others in the operating room, some surgeons have in these circumstances removed the healthy organ. It might be well for such surgeons to remember, however, that the unprejudiced eye of the pathologist will observe the objective condition of the excised part. If the records show that a certain surgeon has on one or two occasions removed a healthy organ, the blameworthy mutilation, though recognized as objectively illicit, will very probably be ascribed to a mistake which anyone might make. If, however, that same surgeon does this sort of surgery frequently, the hospital authorities will know that it

---

[16] "The physician should neither exaggerate nor minimize the gravity of a patient's condition" ("Principles of Medical Ethics." In *Guide to Services*, chap. 2, sec. 3, p. 105. Chicago: The American Medical Association, 1955).

is not due merely to an excusable error, but to unpardonable incompetence or to an immoral attitude.

Definition of Lying

Lying is speaking deliberately against one's mind. In order to understand well this important definition, we shall analyze it accurately.

1. By *speaking* is meant communicating ideas to another person. If one who is entirely alone talks to himself, or if one talks to his dog, to his horse, or to an infant, there is no sharing of his ideas with another, and so there can be no lying involved, even though the speaker is saying what he knows to be false. Speaking, which we use here in the broad sense of communicating ideas, is effected not only by means of words, spoken or written, but also by gestures. A wave of the hand or a nod of the head could involve sufficient imparting of ideas to constitute a lie.

2. By speaking *deliberately* is meant that the speaker must realize what he is saying. Hence if one in a fit of distraction speaks what he habitually knows to be false, though here and now he does not advert to the significance of his words, he is not telling a lie. He is merely guilty of a misstatement. One who utters falsehoods in his sleep does not tell a lie.

3. When we say that lying consists in speaking deliberately *against one's mind* we mean that there must be real opposition between what one says and what one thinks. The speaking must be contrary to one's judgment in the matter. Therefore one lies if he speaks the truth, thinking that the statement is false. On the other hand, one does not lie if he says what is actually false, believing it to be true.

Circumstances That Modify the Meaning

The meaning of the speaker's words is colored by the particular circumstances in which the words are pronounced. These various circumstances modify the meaning of what is said and are rightly considered as part of the speaking. Such circumstances are the time, the place, the manner of speaking, the persons involved, and so forth. The following examples illustrate the manner in which circumstances form part of the speaking and help to determine the meaning of what is said.

Example 1. Dr. A, leaving the room of a patient, meets a nurse and asks, "Have you seen Dr. B?" The nurse answers, "No, I haven't." She has of course seen Dr. B many times, but she knows that Dr. A does not wish to ask whether she has ever seen Dr. B but whether she has seen him recently.

Example 2. The hospital reserves a certain number of rooms for emergency cases and for the use of older and privileged members of the staff. The clerk in the admissions office says to a physician who wishes to hospitalize a patient, "I am sorry, but we do not have a room." Under the circumstances the physician's question means, "Do you have a room that you can let me have?" and so the clerk's reply is truthful.

We may here say a word about the persuasive remarks used by physicians when dealing with young patients who are reluctant to take the medicine prescribed.

Example. Dr. A, a pediatrician, persuades his young patients to take the medicine he prescribes by telling them: "This will make you as strong as Popeye"; "This will make you grow"; "If you want to be a real cowboy, take this." Dr. A's remarks do not offend against the virtue of veracity, for the medicine will, it is hoped, make the young patient strong and help his growth. The references to Popeye and cowboys are merely emphatic ways of expressing the truth. Moreover, the remarks are intended as distractions rather than as expressions of the truth, and the youngster himself probably recognizes them for what they are.

Hyperboles, Irony, Fiction, and Jokes

Hyperboles are not necessarily lies. One man asks, "What kind of a fellow is Jones?" and the other answers, "Jones is the best man in the state." This is an exaggeration, and since it is easily understood as such, it is not a lie. It is merely another way of saying that Jones is a very fine fellow. Ironical expressions are not necessarily lies. James, noticing Mary Brown stumbling awkwardly during her dancing, whispers to her as she whirls by: "You surely are graceful." His meaning that she is anything but graceful is clear from the circumstances and from his tone of voice. Fictitious narratives presented as such are not lies. Jokes are not lies if their jocose nature is clear. The evident attempt at humor, the twinkle of the eye, the smile, the manner of saying a thing—these are circumstances which show clearly that remarks are meant to be fiction and not fact.

The Malice of Lying

A lie is intrinsically evil because it involves using a natural faculty in a way that is directly contrary to its natural end or purpose. The primary purpose of the faculty of speech is to manifest to others one's thoughts and judgments. Since we are by nature obviously destined to live, not each in utter seclusion, but with other human beings, God evidently intended us to exchange ideas with them, and the means given us for this is the faculty of speech. The right use of this faculty is to reveal to others the thoughts of one's mind. To employ this faculty in order to manifest as the thought of one's mind what is not the thought of one's mind is contrary to the primary end of speech. The intention to deceive does not pertain to the essence of lying, and a lie is properly defined as "speaking deliberately against one's mind."

The Seriousness of the Malice of Lying

A lie in itself is not a seriously grave moral fault. The gravity of the malice of lying is measured by the seriousness of the disturbance of the order of nature, and this disturbance is ordinarily not great. Jocose lies, which are uttered merely to amuse, and lies of excuse, sometimes called white lies, are likewise not considered serious offenses. A jocose lie differs from a joke in this, that the jocose nature of the speaker's words is not evident and that as a consequence what he is saying contradicts what he is thinking.

At times, because of other circumstances, a lie may involve grave guilt. These other circumstances would introduce an additional fault joined to the violation of veracity.

Example 1. Dr. A, under oath in court to tell nothing but the truth, tells a deliberate lie. Here we have the grave fault of perjury.

Example 2. Dr. B, who is intensely jealous of Dr. C, invents stories to prove that Dr. C is incompetent when the latter's application for staff membership is under discussion. Here we find a grave moral wrong of injustice.

Example 3. Nurse D forgets to give his medication to a patient who is critically ill. She later makes a false entry on the patient's chart to conceal her mistake. The physician, finding that the patient's reaction to the medication was not what he expected, abandons it for something else to the serious injury of the patient. Nurse D was guilty of grave misconduct because her false entry exposed the patient to serious harm.

THE USE OF MENTAL RESERVATIONS

ONE is never justified in telling a lie. Still, one is at times obliged in conscience to veil the truth, for there are secrets to be guarded and detractions to be avoided. Sometimes silence will not suffice to conceal the secret which one is trying to guard. In fact, it may happen that silence would betray the secret. Hence there must be some licit means of concealing the truth when necessary. This licit means is the broad mental reservation or restriction.

Mental reservation consists in limiting the common and obvious sense of one's words to a particular meaning. Mental reservations are of two kinds: (1) strict mental reservations and (2) broad mental reservations.

1. A *strict* mental reservation is one that limits the meaning and gives no clue to the particular sense intended. This type of mental reservation is a lie, and so is never allowed. For example, A asks B: "Are you going to New York this summer?" B answers: "Yes," meaning that he is going there merely in imagination. This is a lie, for no clue is given to the sense that is intended.

2. A *broad* mental reservation is one that limits the meaning and contains some clue to the sense intended. Here the speaker is not guilty of a lie, for what is said has two meanings. These two meanings are present either by reason of the words themselves or by reason of the circumstances attending their utterance. One who employs a broad mental reservation actually expresses what he thinks and uses words according to the meaning that they really have. The words, however, have another meaning also, and the speaker foresees that it is in this other meaning that the one spoken to will probably understand them. For a sufficient reason we may permit others to deceive themselves by taking the wrong meaning out of what is said, even though the listener does not know that there is another meaning to the word that is employed.

Example 1. Mr. and Mrs. Smith, gravely injured in an automobile accident, are hurried to a hospital. Mrs. Smith died shortly after being admitted, but this fact is unknown to her husband. The following day Mr. Smith asks his brother how his wife, Martha, is getting along. His brother, afraid that the knowledge of her death will retard Mr. Smith's recovery, replies: "She is all right. Don't you worry about Martha." This reply is justifiable as a mental reservation. "She is all right" will no doubt be understood by Mr. Smith to mean that his wife is recovering from the accident, but the phrase can also be used in the sense that, now in eternity, she is released by death from the misery and trials of life.

Example 2. "Mrs. Smith is not at home now." Custom has given this phrase two meanings: (1) She is not now in the house. (2) She is not receiving visitors at this time. If a visitor, being told that Mrs. Smith is not at home, concludes that she is not in the house, he may be deceived. The butler has not lied, even though Mrs. Smith is in the next room listening to the visitor's inquiries.

Example 3. A murderer in court pleads not guilty. To the ordinary meaning of the phrase the qualification "not juridically guilty" is added by the circumstances.

Example 4. A priest, asked if a certain individual committed a murder, may (and must) answer, "I don't know," even though the individual confessed the murder to him. The circumstance of his priesthood colors his answer so that it means, "I have no communicable knowledge on that subject." The same holds true for lawyers, physicians, nurses, and others who are asked questions concerning knowledge acquired in the fulfillment of their duties. Even if the questioner does not know that he is addressing a priest, a physician, or a lawyer, the answer may still be, "I don't know," for the other's ignorance does not make this additional circumstance (namely, that of the professional standing of the speaker) less real. It is actually present in spite of the fact that the other does not realize it, and it could be known.

Example 5. If somebody we cannot trust asks us for the loan of $100, we would be justified in saying, "I haven't any money," meaning "any money that I wish to lend you."

Example 6. If in answer to an invitation to some social gathering one writes, "I accept with pleasure," "I am happy to be invited," and so forth, there is no question of a lie, even though one really feels just the opposite about the invitation. These formulas are merely conventional replies and are not intended to indicate the writer's genuine sentiments. The same is true of phrases addressed to an elderly woman that praise her youth and beauty. This is mere urbanity.

Example 7. If a suspicious husband asks his wife whether or not she has committed adultery, she may licitly answer no, even though she has actually done so many times. Her answer really means: "No, I have committed no crime of adultery that I must reveal." The question ought to be aimed only at knowledge that is not secret, and so the wife may reply accordingly.

The Licitness of Broad Mental Reservation

Unless one has a good reason for concealing some fact, he may not licitly use a broad mental reservation. If broad mental reservations could be employed without some justifying reason, there would result general loss of security and confidence in our social relations. Thus there would be engendered widespread mistrust and suspicion. We would not accept the word of others at its face value, but would constantly be obliged to try to uncover some hidden meaning.

A sufficient reason for using a broad mental reservation is genuine utility for oneself or others, and this is graded according to the degree of importance of concealing the truth of which there is question.

While under oath in a court of law, one may use broad mental reservations, though he must have a very good reason for doing so. One who uses broad mental reservations when on trial does not violate his obligation as a witness "to tell the truth, the whole truth, and nothing but the truth," for to the words of the oath is attached the tacit limitation "insofar as the law obliges me to reveal it." Hence the defendant may use broad mental reservations to avoid incriminating himself, since he need not give proof of his own guilt.

It is very important for the physician to have clear and correct ideas on the subject of truthfulness and the use of mental reservations. A physician may seldom if ever have to ask himself whether a certain therapy or a certain surgical operation is licit or illicit, but the question of what to tell patients about their condition is one that arises constantly. Truthfulness is a virtue that is extremely necessary for the good order of society, and physicians are not exempt from the obligations that bind men in general. Hence we will conclude this section by laying down certain principles and illustrating them by means of practical cases.

1. Not only physicians, but all individuals, may licitly answer "No" or "I do not know" to a question asked by one who has no right to ask it. Such an answer must be given whenever the revelation of the facts in the case might do injury to another or cause him embarrassment. An answer of this kind is not a lie, for all men understand that, when one says he does not know, he may mean that he does not choose to answer. There may be individuals who are so ignorant of the conventions of society that they do not understand this point; but in the first place one may assume in any particular case that such gross ignorance does not exist, and in the second place its existence does not impose upon the one who is asked a question an obligation of telling the ignorant person more than he would tell anyone else. We may use words in their ordinary meanings whether or not they are properly understood.

2. Patients have in general a right to know the nature of their ailment. They consult their physician in order to learn what their ailment is and to obtain treatment for it, and the physician accepts a fee for rendering this service. Knowledge of their condition is often necessary if they are to take the proper precautions during their illness, and it may help them avoid recurrences. If they are ever hospitalized, it will be assumed, when their case histories are taken, that they know from what illnesses they have suffered, and the information that they are able to give will have an influence on the therapy that they receive. If the illness is a serious one, the patient and his family will as a rule need to make plans and arrangements for the future. If, then, a patient with cancer suspects the nature of his disease and asks, "Do I have cancer?" the physician is not justified in answering no.[17]

---

[17] The obligation of warning patients of approaching death is discussed in the chapter on the spiritual care of patients, pp. 378-79.

3. If neither the patient himself nor any member of his family inquires about the nature of the illness, the physician is not obliged to volunteer information unless by withholding it he would do injury, spiritual or otherwise, to the patient, to his family, or to others. Injury to others might result if, for example, the patient had business obligations to which he would attend if he knew that his illness was to be of long duration or fatal.

4. If a patient inquires about the nature of his illness, the physician is obliged to state the facts unless he has good reason for believing that their revelation would either retard the recovery of the patient or cause him acute and needless mental suffering. If the physician is sincerely convinced that the facts should not under the circumstances be revealed, he should endeavor if possible to satisfy the patient by means of some vague and general statement such as, "Let's not worry about what we have; let's try as hard as we can to get well"; "I'd rather not answer that question until we have made a few more tests," and so forth. When the patient refuses to be put off by such statements and persists in asking questions, the physician may use a mental reservation.

Physicians sometimes accuse ethicians of quibbling when ethicians sanction the use of mental reservations in such circumstances. It is better, physicians sometimes contend, to answer an inquiry with what moralists term an outright lie than to resort to clever mental reservations, the real purpose of which is to deceive the patient. To this the ethician answers that the purpose is not to deceive the patient but primarily to conceal from him certain information which it is better for him not to have. The ethician cannot defend or excuse the practice of lying, which is an evil thing in itself and the source of great disorders in society. He can permit mental reservations because they are not lies, but he permits them only when there is a very solid reason for their use, since they too, if used without some good reason, would undermine the confidence that

men need to have in the trustworthiness of what their fellow
men say.

Case 7

Concealing a Patient's Disease from a Third Party

Dr. A is asked by a friend of his patient, B, whether the latter has a
cancer. Actually the patient has carcinoma of the stomach, but Dr. A
replies, "No, he hasn't."

Solution. This is a justifiable mental reservation.

Explanation. Every well-informed person should know that a physician
is not free to reveal the nature of a patient's disease to every casual
inquirer, and that any negative answer which is given is equivalent
to saying that the physician is not free to reveal what he knows.

Case 8

Concealing a Patient's Condition from a Third Party

"How is he doing, Doctor?" a visitor asks Dr. A about his gravely ill
patient. "He is doing all right," replies Dr. A, though the patient has
shown no improvement at all during the last three days.

Solution. The reply of Dr. A is not morally objectionable.

Explanation. Dr. A's reply is to be interpreted by the visitor in the light
of the present circumstances. He should realize that the physician is
bound by professional secrecy and that the answers which he gives
to questions about his patients are to be qualified and interpreted in
the light of that obligation.

Case 9

Concealing the Result of a Test from the Patient

Mrs. A has hypertension and visits her physician every two weeks for
an examination. The physician finds that her systolic blood pressure
is 218. "What is it today, Doctor?" asks Mrs. A. The physician,
knowing that Mrs. A is extremely nervous and excitable and that
knowledge of what her blood pressure really is will make her condition worse and possibly result in a stroke, cheerfully replies, "Over
one seventy-eight."

Solution. The physician's answer is not morally wrong.

Explanation. In saying that the patient's blood pressure reached a point
over 178 the physician did not affirm that it was not a great deal
higher than 178. What he said was true, although the patient will no
doubt conclude that her blood pressure is about 178 only.

Case **10**

Concealing the Nature of His Disease from a Patient

Miss A has chondrosarcoma. "Tell me," she pleads with Dr. B, "do I
really have a cancer?" Dr. B, knowing that Miss A has ample time in
which to prepare for death and wishing to spare her needless mental
suffering, answers, "Your pains are due to arthritis."

Solution. If Miss A actually has arthritis, or if Dr. B is convinced that
everyone at her age does have at least a mild case of arthritis, his
answer is not morally wrong.

Explanation. Dr. B does not affirm that Miss A's pains are due *solely* to
arthritis. If she does have arthritis even in a mild form, Dr. B is
justified in thinking that her pain is due in part to the arthritis, and
hence his answer is not a lie. If Miss A really wanted the entire
truth, she would ask, "Are *all* my pains due to arthritis?" In such
cases patients often do not wish to pursue the matter, preferring to
accept an answer which leaves them with some ray of hope, even
though in their hearts they know what the facts are.

THE OBLIGATION OF RESPECTING SECRETS

To the physician will be given much information which is
of a strictly confidential nature. It should prove profitable,
therefore, to outline briefly the physician's duties with regard
to secret communications.

A secret is hidden knowledge which may not be revealed.
It may concern an invention (television) or some incident
(a murder or a clandestine marriage). There are three types
of secret.

1. A *natural* secret is one which the natural law itself binds
its possessor to keep hidden.

Example. A knows that B, the reputedly legitimate son of
C, is illegitimate.

2. A *promised* secret is one which a gratuitous promise,
made after one already knows the secret, obliges one to refrain
from revealing.

Example. A tells B of a surprise which he has in store for
his wife, and then B assures A that he will reveal this secret
to no one.

3. An *entrusted* secret is one which is confided to another on the condition that it be kept hidden. The agreement to maintain secrecy may be explicit or only implicit.

The secret that exists between the physician and his patient is called an entrusted or professional secret. A patient in consulting a physician may either expressly exact from him the promise that any knowledge obtained from the patient will be guarded as a secret, or he may merely take it for granted that the physician will keep all such information to himself. This latter is usually the case, and it should be noted that the physician's obligation in this event binds to secrecy just as strictly as in the former.

Example. In examining Mrs. A, a married woman, Dr. B learns that she has recently had a therapeutic abortion. This knowledge must be protected as a professional secret.

Prying into Secrets

Every person has a strict right to his secret. This right is founded either on the ownership that each one has over the fruits of his own thoughts, industry, and talent, or on the right that each one has to his good name. A secret belongs, then, to its owner, and one may not steal that secret. Hence, in order to learn the secrets of others one may not eavesdrop, bribe servants to communicate secret knowledge of family affairs, try to trick others into betraying secrets, or open the letters of others and read the contents.

The Obligation of Respecting Secrets

In the various types of secrets there is a difference regarding the binding force of the obligation imposed on those who share a secret.

1. A *natural* secret obliges its possessor, under pain of serious moral wrong, to keep the matter hidden if it is of grave importance. Justice would be violated if the unlawful revelation of the secret would cause damage to the party concerned.

Example 1. A, knowing of a secret crime of B, reveals it without a justifying reason and as a result B is discharged from his position.

Example 2. Out of mere spite A discloses the secret fact that B has committed adultery several times, and so B is deprived of his good name.

Charity only is violated if the revelation of the secret violates no right but merely causes sadness or embarrassment.

Example. Without a justifying reason A reveals to B's mother the secret fact that B on one occasion became drunk, though not through his own fault.

2. A *promised* secret obliges according to the wish of the one making the promise. Hence promised secrets may bind under pain of serious or of slight moral wrong, and either from justice or from fidelity only, the nature of the obligation depending upon what the promiser intended.

3. An *entrusted* secret always obliges in justice and the obligation in matters of grave importance is serious.

Example. Miss A, a social worker, in taking the case history of B discovers that B has committed a grave theft about which no one else knows. Miss A is not free to reveal this secret, which was entrusted to her in her professional capacity.

When Secrets in General May Be Revealed

In general, the obligation of any type of secret is ended:

1. If the guarded knowledge has already become public property. This holds good even though the manner in which the secret was disclosed was illicit.

Example. A, steaming open B's private letters, discovers that she committed an abortion and then openly publishes the matter. C, who knew about the crime under entrusted secrecy, may now speak of it with others. He must, however, guard against confirming what is known publicly by the use of knowledge which was entrusted to him secretly. He must also avoid scandal in the use of the knowledge committed to him.

2. If one may justly presume the permission of the party concerned to reveal the secret.

Example. A's father has entrusted C with the plans of a secret invention of his which he intended to sell later. A is now in great need of money, but his father will not return home for several months. C can reasonably suppose that A's father would consent to his selling the invention to help his son if money can be obtained in no other way.

It is lawful to discuss the above-mentioned secrets with anybody else who possesses the same secret knowledge. In case of a sacramental secret, however, this is not allowed. By a sacramental secret is understood a secret entrusted to a priest in confession.

Example. A, a physician, knows under secrecy that B has a venereal disease. He may discuss this fact with B's uncle, who has accidentally learned the secret.

When Natural and Promised Secrets May Be Revealed

With regard to natural or promised secrets, the obligation ceases when keeping the knowledge hidden would involve grave inconvenience:

1. To the one who owns the secret knowledge.

Example. A learns by chance that young B is nearly going out of his mind with secret worries, and he informs B's father so that he may help his son to get rid of these anxieties.

2. To the one who shares the secret.

Example. A, confined in the same cell in prison with B, discovers the secret fact that B has on two previous occasions, while imprisoned in a foreign country, killed his cell mates by administering to them a subtle poison. A reveals this knowledge in order to save his life.

3. To an innocent third party.

Example. A, the chum of B, learns that B is engaged to marry C, a good and wholesome girl. To protect C, A tells her about the hidden infectious disease with which B is afflicted.

48

4. To the state.

Example. A learned by accident that B intends to put poison in the soup at a banquet given for the nation's senators. He promised B that he would not divulge the secret; but, on thinking it over, he decides to make known the plan to murder these congressmen.

If the guarding of a secret will not result in injury to a third person, and if I expressly promised to guard the secret, even at the cost of grave inconvenience to myself alone, I am then bound to do so.

When Entrusted Secrets May Be Revealed

Ordinarily the physician experiences little difficulty with regard to keeping professional knowledge secret. Very extraordinary conditions may arise, however, which create a conflict between the rights of the patient and those of others. Hence a physician should bear in mind that the obligation of privileged communications ceases when revealing the knowledge is necessary to avert grave harm:

1. From the state or community. It has always been an accepted principle that the common good takes precedence over the good of the individual.

Example. Mr. A, examined by Dr. B, is found to have highly active pulmonary tuberculosis. Learning that Mr. A intends to sail on a steamship which is to leave the next day for an extended cruise and that he refuses to disclose the condition of his health to the ship's officials, Dr. B sends them word of the impending danger.

2. From an innocent third party.

Example. Dr. A discovers in his examination of B that the latter is infected with primary syphilis. B is to marry the following morning, and his fiancée is a healthy girl. Dr. A urges his patient either to postpone the wedding until a cure of the disease can be effected or to inform the girl of his condition. Since B refuses to follow either of these suggestions, Dr. A

49

himself sends a warning to the girl. Dr. A is justified in thus acting. He need not warn the girl, however, if he foresees grave inconvenience for himself or distrust of physicians on the part of others, since the obligation is one of charity only.[18]

3. From the one to whom the secret is entrusted or from the one whose secret it is.

Example 1. A tells Dr. B, as an entrusted secret, where he (A) was on October 10. Dr. B, by revealing this fact to C, can prevent C from shooting A. In order to safeguard A's life Dr. B may licitly reveal this entrusted secret to C.

Example 2. A, who has been entrusted with secret knowledge of B's act of murder, is falsely indicted for the same crime. If A can escape punishment in no other way, he may reveal the fact that B is the real culprit.

In the examples that have been given secrets need not be maintained at such a price; for if the obligation continued to exist even in such circumstances as these, then most persons, including physicians, would understandably refuse to accept such secrets and this attitude of theirs would redound to the great detriment of the whole community.

In all such circumstances secrets may be revealed insofar as is necessary, for the individual is clearly not obliged, either by the natural law or by a promise that he himself makes, to act in a manner opposed to any virtue or to violate the right of an innocent person to be protected against an unjust attack. For one who accepts a secret to bind himself to keep it at any cost whatsoever would be equivalent to his obligating himself to suffer even very serious personal injury or unjustly to

[18] "Sometimes, however, a physician must determine whether his duty to society requires him to employ knowledge, obtained through confidences entrusted to him as a physician, to protect a healthy person against a communicable disease to which he is about to be exposed. In such instance, the physician should act as he would desire another to act toward one of his own family in like circumstances. Before he determines his course, the physician should know the civil law of his commonwealth concerning privileged communications" ("Principles of Medical Ethics." In *Guide to Services*, chap. 2, sec. 2, pp. 104-05. Chicago: The American Medical Association, 1955).

permit grave wrong, if need be, to the state or to some third party. It would be unreasonable for another to look upon him as bound to secrecy that is so absolute. This principle is accepted by men in general, and hence it is commonly recognized that the inviolability of a secret, whether it be natural, promised, or entrusted, is not absolute. The one exception to this principle is the sacramental secret. One who confesses his sins to a priest does so because he believes that God has commanded him to confess them and that forgiveness is contingent upon his confessing them. God, when placing upon the sinner the obligation of confessing his sins, also placed upon the priest the absolute obligation of secrecy.

A physician must, according to the law of certain states, report individuals to the police if they come to him with gun or knife wounds. Though the physician often would not be bound in conscience to disclose this information, he may do so in order to avert grave harm which might otherwise be visited on him. If he failed to report, he would be liable to fine and perhaps imprisonment as accessory to a crime.

Reading Others' Letters, Case Histories, or Reports

Reading private documents which belong to others, such as letters, reports on patients, case histories, and the like is morally wrong unless (1) one has or can reasonably presume the permission of the owner of the secret communications, or (2) such an action is thought necessary for averting grave harm from the state, from an innocent third party, or from oneself. The degree of moral wrong which is involved will depend on the importance of the secret information which the reader prudently foresees he will unjustly acquire.

The Professional Secrets of Physicians

It may be said in general that professional secrets include everything of a secret nature concerning the patient's health which the physician learns from him during the performance of his professional duties. In this category are all confidential communications about himself or others which the patient makes to the physician to clarify his case and all knowledge of secret defects or ailments which the physician acquires while rendering medical services. He is, therefore, held to entrusted secrecy if during the examination of the patient he discovers, for example, that the latter had a syphilitic infection many years ago, or that she had attempted an abortion, or that she has cancer or epilepsy. The obligation to keep such information hidden does not expire when the patient has discontinued the services of the physician or when the patient dies; it lasts, as a rule, forever.

The obligation of respecting a professional secret affects, not only the physician who receives the secret, but others as well. All others to whom a physician entrusts as a professional secret the knowledge which he himself has are bound by the same obligation of strict secrecy, whether the knowledge was imparted to them rightly or wrongly, prudently or imprudently. A surgeon, for example, may deem it necessary to consult a pathologist or another surgeon about a vexing phase of a case which he is treating. These consultants then share in the professional secrets which have on that occasion been communicated to them and are under an obligation not to reveal them. When a physician seeks the advice of other physicians in regard to a case, he can usually present the case as a hypothetical one, without revealing the identity of his patient. Under such circumstances the physician would not be violating his obligation of secrecy. If there is danger, however, that the one whom he consults will know or suspect who the patient is, the physician should have the express consent of his patient or at least know that he can reasonably presume consent.

What is to be said of the medical secrets of patients who are minors or who are destitute of reason? May the physician freely communicate their secrets to their parents or legal guardians? In replying to this question one must distinguish between the case of infants and the case of children who have the use of reason. With regard to infants, those who are charged with their care (their parents or legal guardians) have a right to share in any secret knowledge which pertains to their child. In this same category belong adults who from birth have been unable to reason. Parents of children who have the use of reason, however, have the right only to that secret knowledge which the physician acquires by virtue of his medical examination of the patient. The parent has a right to this knowledge, for the physician is acting as the agent of the parent when he examines the child. The parent, moreover, has a right to know whatever is necessary in order to provide for the child's health and best interests. The personal revelations, however, which such children make to the examining physician may not be communicated to the parent without the child's consent. The child, even though he be a minor, owns his own thoughts; and when he imparts secret knowledge to his physician, he is presumed to wish to share that knowledge with him alone. Hence if a young patient reveals to the examining physician some immoral action of which he has been guilty, such as masturbation or theft, the physician must keep that knowledge hidden, even from the child's parents. With such children may be classified imbeciles, morons, old people who are suffering from senility, and adults who became insane after they had reached the age of reason. In the case of these patients the parents or nearest of kin have a right to those secrets only of which knowledge is required in order that they may be able to give proper care to those for whom they are responsible. They have no right to receive other secrets of the patient, especially such as are connected with morally imputable actions.

Since the physician is obliged to use due diligence in keeping hidden all professional secrets, he must see that the confidential reports, case histories, correspondence, medical prescriptions, and so forth regarding his patients be kept in a safe and secret place. In order to insure greater security in this matter, some physicians employ for the name and address of the patient a code which is known to themselves only. It is important that the physician make sure of the trustworthiness of his office assistants.

Case 11
Illicit Revelation during Surgery

Dr. A was operating on the patient for a genitourinary ailment. During the course of the operation, pointing out the inflamed condition of the os uteri, he remarked: "That cervical stem that she has been using caused this damage." (The patient during a consultation had mentioned to him that she used this instrument to prevent conception.) His words were overheard by four or five others who were in the operating room.

Solution. Dr. A was guilty of a violation of professional secrecy and at least of detraction.

Explanation. It can be taken for granted that some of those in the room would not have noticed the irritated organ and that, even if they did, they would not connect this morbid condition with the practice of artificial birth control. Hence the surgeon in making his remark was guilty of injuring the reputation of the patient in the eyes of others. It is understood in this case that the surgeon did not have the explicit or implicit permission of the patient to use the operation without restriction for purposes of demonstration or instruction.

Case 12
Revealing Remarks Made under Anesthesia

"Yes," said Dr. A to the wife of his patient, "your husband talked a good deal as he was coming out of the anesthetic and often pronounced the name Mary Lou. Was she some old girl friend of his?"

Solution. The surgeon acted illicitly.

Explanation. The surgeon's imprudent observation could cause grave evil, unless it was evident from the tone of his voice or from some other attendant circumstance that he was merely joking.

Case 13
Secret Wire Recordings

Dr. A, a psychiatrist, finds that the most effective method of studying his patient is to make a wire recording of all his interviews with him.

Note taking, he has found, if done in the presence of the patient, has a disturbing influence on him, and if making a written record is delayed until after the consultation, useful details may be entirely lost sight of. Dr. A as a rule informs his patient that a wire recording is desired and obtains his permission to make it. At times, however, he wishes to take the recording without the patient's being aware that it is being made.

Solution. In order that his action be licit Dr. A must have the patient's permission for the recording. This permission may be either explicit or implicit.

Explanation. We are not permitted to draw from another his secret thoughts without his permission. He alone has complete ownership of his secret knowledge, and it is not licit to make him impart this knowledge to another against his will. He has, moreover, the right to limit the extent to which the secret knowledge is communicated. If he wishes to converse with the physician alone and is opposed to having the conversation recorded, his wishes in the matter must be respected.

Experience proves, however, that the patient as a rule readily consents to the wire recording when it is explained to him that the recording merely replaces the less satisfactory practice of note taking and will be protected by professional secrecy.[19] Hence there is rarely any difficulty about obtaining the explicit consent of the patient for the use of this method. Sometimes, however, the physician foresees that the therapy will be endangered if the patient is aware that a recording is being made of the interview. In such cases, if the patient is mentally deranged, consent to using the method can be licitly given by his nearest of kin. If the patient is mentally sound, at least his implicit consent is required. This implicit consent may be looked upon as being present when the physician is reasonably certain that, if the matter could be fully explained to the patient, the latter would not object to the wire recording.

[19] See Frederick C. Redlich, M.D.; John Dollard, M.D.; and Richard Newman, M.D., "High Fidelity Recording of Psychotherapeutic Interviews." *American Journal of Psychiatry* 107:42-48, July 1950.

Such wire recordings afterward may be employed in clinics in teaching and research work if the patient consents to their use. Without the patient's consent the recording may not be employed for clinical purposes unless it is previously edited most carefully so that the patient could not possibly be identified by anyone in the audience.

THE AVOIDANCE OF UNNECESSARY SURGERY

THE natural law forbids unnecessary surgery, for such surgical operations are needless mutilations of the human body. In not a few instances, moreover, the unnecessary surgery places the patient in danger of death, and this without a justifying reason. A surgeon, therefore, who knowingly performs an operation which is not medically indicated violates the law of nature.[20] He increases his guilt if he exacts a fee from the patients who were not only not helped by the needless surgery but were perhaps positively injured.

It is a well-authenticated fact that in this country today not a few physicians resort to surgery that is not required for either the physical or mental well-being of the patient. There is altogether too much surgery and too much surgery that is unskillfully performed.[21] The caesarean section is too often resorted to without need and, not rarely, with unfortunate results.[22] At a meeting of the American Medical Association, Dr. Munger, a well-known urologist, stated that "in the surgical treatment of diseases of the kidney the fetish for nephrectomy comes near to being the surgical 'original sin.' "[23] Dr. Bennett informed the American Medical Association of the

1937
Reference

[20] See Gerald Kelly, S.J., *Medico-Moral Problems,* pt. 4, "Unnecessary Surgery," pp. 38-41. St. Louis: Catholic Hospital Association of the United States and Canada, 1952.

[21] See *American Medicine: Expert Testimony out of Court,* vol. I, pp. 472-82. New York: American Foundation, 1937.

[22] *Ibid.*

[23] Arbor D. Munger, M.D., "A Plea for a More Conservative Attitude in Renal Surgery." *Journal of the American Medical Association* 132:675-79, November 23, 1946.

astonishing and almost unbelievable fact that of a group of some hundred psychoneurotic patients whom he had studied, seventy-two had been <u>falsely</u> diagnosed as suffering from organic disease and about ninety surgical operations at least had been performed unnecessarily.[24]

[handwritten margin note: wrongly! should be proper word. Author uses to know the surgeons . . . intents of the . . .]

Since the layman is incapable of passing judgment on the necessity of surgery in any particular case and would not, as a rule, come to know of cases where the operation performed was medically inadvisable, the responsibility for eliminating these grave abuses in surgical practice lies with the medical profession. It is the collective duty of the members of the medical profession to take action. A mistaken interpretation of medical ethics should not prevent conscientious physicians from reporting cases of malpractice which come to their attention. The code of ethics of the American Medical Association outlines the duty of physicians in this regard: "A physician should expose, without fear or favor, incompetent or corrupt, dishonest or unethical conduct on the part of members of the profession."[25] Recently the American Medical Association through its Board of Trustees declared itself in favor of the establishment of various state and county grievance committees.[26] In case of alleged improper practices both the patient and the physician are given a fair hearing.

REFERENCES

Bonnar, Alphonsus, O.F.M. *Catholic Doctor.* London: Burns Oates and Washbourne, 1951.

Davis, Henry, S.J., *Moral and Pastoral Theology,* vol. II, pp. 141-99. London: Sheed and Ward, 1949.

[24] A. E. Bennett, M.D., "Faulty Management of Psychiatric Syndromes Simulating Organic Disease," *Journal of the American Medical Association* 130:1203-08, April 27, 1946. For a statement about unnecessary hysterectomies see Norman F. Miller, M.D., "Hysterectomy—Therapeutic Necessity or Surgical Racket?" *American Journal of Obstetrics and Gynecology* 51:804-10, June 1946.

[25] "Principles of Medical Ethics." In *Guide to Services,* chap. 3, sec. 4, p. 105. Chicago: The American Medical Association, 1955.

[26] *Journal of the American Medical Association* 142:573, February 25, 1950.

Finney, Patrick A., C.M. *Moral Problems in Hospital Practice.* St. Louis: B. Herder Book Company, 1942.

Fisher, J. Harding. "The Malice of a Lie." In J. F. Leibell, editor, *Readings in Ethics,* pp. 528-33. Chicago: Loyola University Press, 1926.

Hayt, Emanuel. *Some Aspects of the Confidential Character of the Hospital Medical Record.* St. Louis: Catholic Hospital Association of the United States and Canada, 1951.

Kelly, Gerald, S.J. "Unnecessary Surgery." *Linacre Quarterly* 18:99-103, November 1951.

La Rochelle, Stanislaus A., and C. T. Fink, C.M. *Handbook of Medical Ethics,* fourth edition. Westminster: Newman Bookshop, 1943.

McFadden, Charles J., O.S.A. *Medical Ethics,* second edition. Philadelphia: F. A. Davis Company, 1949.

Middleton, Reginald. "The Obligation of Veracity." In J. F. Leibell, editor, *Readings in Ethics,* pp. 555-64. Chicago: Loyola University Press, 1926.

Moore, Thomas Verner, O.S.B., M.D. *Principles of Ethics,* fourth edition. Philadelphia: J. B. Lippincott Company, 1943.

Newman, John Henry Cardinal. "Lying and Equivocation." In J. F. Leibell, editor, *Readings in Ethics,* pp. 543-54. Chicago: Loyola University Press, 1926.

Regan, Robert E., O.S.A., S.T.D. *Professional Surgery in the Light of Moral Principles,* chap. 10, "The Medical Secret," pp. 114-18. Washington: Augustinian Press; Catholic University of America, 1943.

Walsh, James J., M.D. "Medical Professional Secrecy." *America* 53:539-40, September 14, 1935.

———— "The Medical Secret: A Problem in Morals." *Homiletic and Pastoral Review* 29:466-74, February 1929.

FURTHER APPLICATIONS OF
GENERAL PRINCIPLES

THE preceding chapter discussed certain problems of ethical conduct of interest to physicians. Some of these problems are encountered constantly by every physician who is practicing his profession; others may occur less frequently. The present chapter is devoted to a discussion of five problems concerning which the physician needs to be informed: the means that must be used to preserve life, defense against unjust attack, the principle of the twofold effect, cooperation in evil, and scandal.

Everyone is obliged to take prudent care of his health. God created man and committed to him the care of his life. When the Creator brings men into this world, He intends that they continue to exist, to ward off death, to live on for a time at least. That this intention is present on God's part is obvious from the fact that He has implanted in man the very strong instinct of self-preservation. This natural instinct prompts man to shrink from death, to cling tenaciously to life. Since the instinct is natural, its origin can be traced to the Author of nature, to God Himself. God might have decreed that man be kept in existence quite independently of any cooperative act on man's own part. The Creator of all things has seen fit to cause the flowers, the fruits, and the trees to continue to exist and to grow, the planets to exist and to whirl through space, without their aiding one whit in accomplishing all this. But God endowed man with a free will. He has given him the power to cooperate in the task of surviving and He has imposed upon him the duty of doing so.

In this work on medical ethics the discussion of the obligation of using means for survival is limited to situations in which the individual will certainly or almost certainly die, suffer a complete nervous breakdown, or be rendered incapable of doing his ordinary work either permanently or for a long period of time unless medical measures of one kind or another are taken. Since all men have an obligation of taking reasonable care of their health, no one is free, without sufficient reason, to expose himself to the danger of contracting even a simple and more or less harmless disease, but the obligation of avoiding such diseases is ordinarily not grave. It is not our purpose, however, to discuss cases in which the danger to life or health is only slight; nor will we say anything concerning various questions commonly discussed by ethicians: the morality of granting oneself certain indulgences, such as smoking and moderate drinking, which may perhaps shorten life to some extent; the licitness of imposing upon oneself penances and austerities in the quest for spiritual perfection; the right of individuals to incur the danger of death in the service of humanity. Such questions are not considered to fall within the scope of the present work. On pages 259-62, however, will be found a brief discussion of the morality of exposing oneself to the danger of death in experimental work with new drugs.

MEANS THAT MUST BE USED TO PRESERVE LIFE

CONFINING ourselves, then, to situations in which medical measures are necessary if life or health is to be preserved, we ask to what extent one is obliged to ward off disease and death and whether one must employ all available means, no matter how unusual they may be or how painful they may prove. To this question the ethician replies that man is obliged to use only ordinary means to safeguard his health and that he may, but need not, employ extraordinary means. The term "ordinary means" is not always understood by physicians in the same sense in which it is used by ethicians. The physician may look upon certain medications or certain operations as ordinary procedure because, although they may involve great expense or very radical surgery, they are nevertheless the generally approved remedy for some particular ailment. This is not the ethician's meaning of ordinary procedure. Ordinary means of conserving life, as understood by the ethician, are those which are not extraordinary. The nature of extraordinary means is explained on pages 67-72.

That man is held to the use of ordinary means only is evident from an analysis of human nature. Men in general do not possess the energy or the fortitude to employ extraordinary measures to preserve their life. The obligation to preserve life by means that are very painful or very difficult to obtain would be regarded by the generality of mankind as an intolerable burden and as an exorbitant and unproportionate price to pay for the benefit gained. No one can be under the obligation of doing what is impossible. An act may be impossible in one of two ways, either physically or morally. It is physically impossible when one has not at his command the physical means of performing the action. It would, for example, be physically impossible for a blind man to read by using his eyes. An act is called morally impossible if its performance would overtax the will power and courage of the normal person. It is clear, therefore, that God does not oblige us to use such means in order to survive; but we are at liberty to use them if we can and if we so desire. There is nothing that forbids our using extraordinary measures to conserve or to regain our health.

As regards ordinary means, the obligation of using them is present only if the means in question are not wholly useless. If, for example, a patient who has carcinoma of the stomach can retain no food at all, then obviously food taken orally need not be given to him, though it certainly must be considered an ordinary means of preserving health. "No one is obliged to do what is useless" is an adage to which ethicians frequently refer and which finds fitting application here.

It should also be noted that ordinary means differ very much among themselves and that as a consequence the obligation of using them may be greater in some cases than it is in others. Ordinary means may be divided into three classes.

The first class of ordinary means includes those means that are in constant use by men in general, even though their health is perfect and no danger is present. All men, for example, use food daily and ordinarily control its use, at least to the extent of avoiding foods that make them violently ill. All men place some limit on the amount of work that they undertake. All men get a minimum of rest and sleep daily, take exercise occasionally, allow themselves a certain amount of sunshine and fresh air, and consider that they should have a yearly vacation of two or three weeks. In case of illness or impending illness it is very customary for physicians to insist upon the use of some or all of these means and to specify in detail their amount, quantity, or frequency.

A second class of ordinary means includes those that are unusual so far as men in general are concerned, though usual in the case of those who are ill, the employment of which is unaccompanied by severe pain or by danger. Here we have such things as complete physical examinations, with all the tests of various kinds that are included; the use of ordinary medicines; X-ray treatments; blood transfusions; intravenous feeding; the use of hormones; medical baths; massage; enemas; simple subcutaneous surgical operations; the extraction of teeth and the setting of bones; physical therapy; and other means of a similar kind. The educated adult of today, if he is ill or hospitalized, looks upon all such means as matters of routine. Thousands of individuals, however, some of whom are otherwise well educated, look upon all or some of these means with suspicion or aversion and declare that they will never use them.

In the third class of ordinary means we have means that are unusual so far as men in general are concerned, the employment of which is or may be accompanied by severe pain or by danger. Here we have such things as deep X-ray therapy and shock treatment, and in particular those surgical operations which, as we shall say on pages 74-75, must in some cases be looked upon as ordinary means.

If a means is an ordinary means, the patient has an obligation of using it; but this obligation is more binding for the first class than for the second and more binding for the second class than for the third. It is important to keep this fact in mind when considering cases involving the use of ordinary means. If the case is a difficult one and if the decision, so to speak, hangs in the balance, the nature of the ordinary means that the physician has recommended may have an influence on the final decision. There is indeed an obligation of using ordinary means, but this obligation is not the same for all types of ordinary means.

Greater and Lesser Lengthening of Life

We have spoken of the obligation resting upon the individual of using ordinary means for the preservation of his life. There are cases in which a surgical operation or the use of a certain treatment may give promise of preserving one's life for many years to come. If a man in his twenties who is otherwise in perfect health suffers a ruptured appendix, an appendectomy may be the means of preserving his life for fifty years or more. The same operation, in the case of a man in his eighties, could at best do no more than add a few years of life. Would the obligation of undergoing surgery be equally binding in both cases? We cannot speak of preserving life without thinking of the length of time for which life can be preserved by the use of a certain means. Our problem is to establish some reasonable norm concerning the minimum length of time that the proposed means must promise to add to the patient's life if the use of the means is to be considered obligatory.

It should be noted in the first place that the ethician depends upon the physician for a decision concerning the probable effects of the proposed means. The physician will be far less positive in statements that he makes immediately after the presence of a disease has been discovered than he will be when, in the later stages of the disease, serious bodily deterioration has taken place. Even in the beginning, however, the physician will not hesitate to set a probable minimum and a probable maximum number of months or years of life for the patient if he submits to the proposed treatment or operation and another minimum and maximum number of months or years if he refuses to submit to it. The ethician accepts the prediction with the same limitations; but so far as it is humanly possible to foresee the future, he forms a moral judgment of the *certain* life expectancy of the patient—whether, for example, this be six, twelve, or some other definite number of additional months of life. A judgment concerning the *certain* life expectancy usually enters into the evaluation of the patient's duty to use the proposed medical treatment or to submit to the surgery.

Let us particularize the above statements by describing the cases of three patients whom we shall call George, Henry, and Ignatius. All three are in need of the same surgical operation— for example, an appendectomy—for the saving of their lives, and the surgery is urgently needed and cannot be deferred. Let us suppose that the operation must be judged an ordinary means for the conservation of life because it would involve neither great hardship nor expense nor danger of death nor subjective horror (see pages 60-63). All three patients must have the surgery if they are to live, but the circumstances are quite different in each of the three cases. George is a young man, twenty-five years of age, who has enjoyed habitual good health and whose life expectancy after the appendectomy would be great. Henry is an old man of eighty, who very probably could not live more than two or three years after the operation. Ignatius, a married man of forty, is dying of cancer, and competent physicians have concluded that, even though there were no question of a necessary operation, he will certainly die within three months. We may now ask what the obligation of these three patients is in the matter of conserving life.

In attempting to answer this question we must keep in mind the fundamental principle that a patient in need of a certain treatment or operation for the conserving of his life is obliged to employ that means if it is considered to be what is called an ordinary means for conserving life. If, therefore, in any of the three cases that we have described the means is accounted ordinary, the patient is held to its use. This is true, however, only on the supposition that the means would be certainly effective in saving life. There is no obligation to employ a means which is at most only probably effective.

The problem arises, however, as to what constitutes in a particular case an ordinary means of preserving life. Before a strict obligation to employ certain measures can be said to exist, there must be present a just proportion between the good effects which presumably will follow and the inconveniences and difficulties attendant upon the use of the measures in question. If, for example, from the employment of certain measures no good effect or practically no good effect would result, the use of these measures is clearly not obligatory, for no one, as we noted above, has an obligation of doing what is either utterly useless or practically so. If, moreover, only slight good would be produced, a slight reason would excuse one from employing the means in question. If the good effect of an appendectomy would be to prolong life for not more than a month, would not the use of this means, which involves a number of inconveniences, be rightly termed nonobligatory? Even if the life expectancy following an operation were three months, would a patient such as Ignatius, who is dying of cancer, be obliged to submit to it?

We may conclude that, even though a certain means must in general be classified as an ordinary means of preserving life, there can be circumstances when its use is not obligatory. Before the use of any means is of obligation, there must be a reasonable proportion between the good effects which will follow and the inconvenience and hardship which its use would involve. A reasonable norm for guiding the physician is this: The more closely a certain measure which in general is classified as an ordinary means approaches, because of the particular circumstances of the patient, the category of extraordinary means, so much the less is there an obligation of employing it. Hence in regard to the three classes of ordinary means described above we may conclude that for everyone the use of the first class (food, drink, and the like) is obligatory. The use of the second class of ordinary means (ordinary medicines, examinations, treatments, and the like) is obligatory provided that in the case of the individual patient their use would not involve very grave inconvenience, very grave expense, or the like. The use of the third class of means (surgery, deep X-ray therapy, and the like) in certain cases and under certain circumstances would not be obligatory.

Let us now return to the cases of the three men described above. We begin by accepting the principle, as stated on pages 74-75, that an appendectomy performed by a competent surgeon in a modern and well-equipped hospital must be looked upon as an ordinary means. The use of this ordinary means, however, is not obligatory unless there is a reasonable proportion between the good effect, which is the prolongation of life, and the bad effects in terms of cost, pain, and inconvenience. We may conclude that, unless the life expectancy after surgery is at least three or four months, the operation is not obligatory from the viewpoint of the duty of warding off death imposed upon men by the Fifth Commandment. This remains true if the patient, who will *certainly* live after the operation for three or four months, will *probably* live for a much longer time. If the surgery would ensure the patient six or more months of life, it must be considered an ordinary means and one that is obligatory. Both George, a young man twenty-five years of age, and Henry, a man of eighty who might live for two or three years after the operation, are obliged to undergo the appendectomy. Ignatius, who in the judgment of competent physicians will certainly die of cancer within three months, need not submit to the appendectomy. It is assumed that in all three cases there are no unusual circumstances, such as extreme and uncontrollable horror of the operation, which might render surgery nonobligatory. Such circumstances must of course be weighed when there is question of the existence or nonexistence of an obligation.

Extraordinary Means and the Obligation of Using Them

The principle which serves as a guide in regard to the use of extraordinary means is this: *One may, but need not, use extraordinary means to preserve his life.* Obviously, the problem is to distinguish clearly between what may properly be considered extraordinary and what is ordinary. We may define as an extraordinary means whatever here and now is very *costly* or very *unusual* or very *painful* or very *difficult* or very *dangerous,* or if the good effects that can be expected from its use are not proportionate to the difficulty and inconvenience that are entailed.

If the operation, the treatment, the medicine, or the appliance necessary for conserving one's health were very expensive, one would not be obliged to purchase his well-being at such a price. For determining what would be considered extraordinary in the matter of expense we may view the case according to either the *relative* or the *absolute* norm. If, for example, a man were very poor and the medical care prescribed to save his life were to cost a sum which to the average man would not be prohibitive but to him would prove a very grave burden, he would not be obliged to go to the expense of obtaining this medical care. Here we apply the relative norm in gauging what is extraordinary in regard to cost, considering as extraordinary that which the individual could not bear without very grave inconvenience.

The absolute norm, on the other hand, establishes a maximum amount beyond which no one need go in spending money to care for his health. This norm is based on that which *people in general* would find very costly. The average person would experience very grave inconvenience in paying for medical care which cost a great sum of money. It is difficult to fix the amount exactly, but it seems that in normal times $2,000 or more would certainly constitute such a "great sum" for the average man. Hence if the treatment required for one's cure of a fatal disease would cost $2,000 or more, he would not be obliged to employ so costly a remedy.

Let us suppose that an individual whose health requires costly treatments is exceedingly wealthy. He could, without being caused any inconvenience by the expense, pay for such medical care. Despite his financial status, treatments costing $2,000 or more would be considered extraordinary means of preserving his life. He would, it is true, find those means easy which the average person would find hard, and therefore he is in a very unusual position. In his case the absolute rather than the relative norm should be applied.

Because of special circumstances the principle that one may, but need not, use extraordinary means to preserve his life may not apply in a specific case. Under certain conditions one might be obliged to use extraordinary means; under others he might have a duty of refraining from their use. This will become clear from an analysis of three imaginary cases.

Each of three patients, Robert, Samuel, and Thomas, has been told by a competent physician that only the immediate amputation of his right leg, which is in a gangrenous condition, can save his life. Because of the hardship and shame which each would experience in going through life with a prosthetic leg the amputation, as stated on page 75, is to be considered an extraordinary means. The general principle governing the use of extraordinary means would leave each patient free to submit or not to submit to the amputation, but because of special circumstances the general principle ceases to be applicable to the cases in question.

Robert, a thirty-year-old patient, is aware of the fact that his death would leave his wife practically helpless, for she would find it extremely difficult to earn a livelihood. His growing children, moveover, need his wholesome influence in the home. Samuel, a man sixty years of age, although reared a Catholic, has been living outside the Church for thirty-five years. Now at long last he has come to his senses, but he has difficulty in accepting the whole of Catholic doctrine. He feels that he needs a great deal of time for reflection on this matter and sincerely judges that he is not spiritually prepared for death. Thomas, a forty-year-old married man, is deformed and badly crippled. For many years he has been a grave burden to his wife; and he well realizes that the required surgery, by saving his life, will increase his wife's hardships and exact even greater sacrifices on her part in the future. Robert, it seems clear, because of the best interests of his wife and family, is required in conscience by the virtue of piety to submit to the amputation. Samuel too must have the operation, for he is obliged in charity toward himself to use those means that are necessary for the salvation of his soul. Thomas, on the other hand, has no obligation to submit to the surgery. Unless, however, his wife opposes such a decision, might not Thomas rightly judge that he is obliged to forgo the operation? Charity, it seems, in view of the circumstances of the case, might urge him to do so. Since, however, one as a rule clings tenaciously to life no matter how burdensome one's life may be, it would often be preferable not to insist unduly on the obligation in cases such as that of Thomas.

We note, therefore, that there are circumstances which can affect one's obligation to use or not to use extraordinary means of conserving life. Death resulting from the refusal to make use of extraordinary means could be the cause of grave loss or injury to the patient himself or to others. While the vast majority of men will use any means whatsoever rather than die, cases do occur in which patients say that they will submit to extraordinary means only if obliged in conscience to do so. In all such cases consideration must be given to the nature and gravity of the loss or injury; to the obligation, if any, that the patient has of preventing this loss or injury; and to the proportion existing between the good effects (the avoidance of loss or injury) and the evil effects (the suffering or inconvenience of the patient). It should be remembered that the success of the extraordinary means which are suggested must be assured before an obligation of using them can be said to be present.

Respirators, Oxygen Tents, and Other Special Means

The use of the iron lung, the respirator, or the oxygen tent is considered extraordinary means if any one of the following three conditions is verified: (1) if its use is very costly, (2) if the apparatus is very difficult to obtain, or (3) if it is a *permanent* adjunct required to keep the patient alive. In the case of the iron lung and the respirator, the expense involved in protracted use would ordinarily be very great. Moreover, they would often be very difficult to procure. Whenever either of these conditions is verified, such apparatus would be considered extraordinary means. The use of oxygen in the cities of America would not, as a rule, entail too great a cost, unless of course it were to extend over a very long period of time. Oxygen, moreover, is readily available in most hospitals in this country. In the United States the oxygen tent or mask should as a rule be looked upon as ordinary means. If, however, either the oxygen tent or the iron lung were permanently necessary to keep a person alive, it would for this reason be considered an extraordinary means. By "permanently necessary" we mean that it would be necessary for a long period; for example, for six months or more. On the other hand, when the use of oxygen or the iron lung is nonpermanent and merely *remedial*—that is, when the purpose in their use is to tide the patient over a temporary crisis, as in acute pulmonary edema—it must be deemed an ordinary means.

The incubator used for the purpose of keeping an infant alive is either an ordinary or an extraordinary means according to circumstances. An incubator may, in general, be defined as an enclosure whose air, humidity, and temperature are regulated to suit the needs of the infant. An enclosure of this kind can be made, with little cost and inconvenience, in any home. Such an enclosure is similar to a room in which the heat and the moisture are carefully regulated by the nurse to suit the delicate condition of a sick person; hence this procedure cannot be called an extraordinary means. The modern mechanical device, however, with its oxygen control, humidity regulator, and thermostat-controlled heating unit is often difficult to procure, and for this reason it will in many places be rightly termed an extraordinary means of preserving an infant's life.

X-ray treatments to be taken daily for a month would be regarded as ordinary means unless they were very costly or, as perhaps would be true in some sections of the country, very difficult to procure. Deep therapy by X ray can sometimes be very painful. Where this is true, such treatment can be classified as an extraordinary means of preserving one's health.

"Unless you remain in bed for six or eight months, you will die within the year," said a physician to one of his patients; "you need perfect rest for that length of time." Would such a patient have to consider this remedy an ordinary means of conserving his life? If a person is able to be up and around (for example, a tubercular patient), a six-month stay in bed

71

would for him be a very grave inconvenience. Hence there would be no strict obligation, on the score of conserving his health, for him to follow his physician's advice.

Taking injections of insulin, intravenous feeding, and the use of vitamins and medicine would, as a rule, be considered ordinary means. If, however, any of these is very expensive in a particular place, then in that locality it would be deemed an extraordinary means. Insulin can cause some patients extreme pain. For such patients its use would be an extraordinary means of averting death.

Surgical Operations as Ordinary and as Extraordinary Means

A surgical operation would be considered an extraordinary means of saving one's life if it involved very great expense, or a very grave inconvenience, or very severe pain, or if it could not be had without very great difficulty, or if the thought of such surgery would produce in the patient very grave and unconquerable horror. In many cases, perhaps in the great majority of cases, none of these conditions is present, and surgery would be considered an ordinary means of preserving one's life so far as the conditions that have been mentioned are concerned. There is another condition, however, which is clearly present in many cases and which some would maintain is at least remotely present in all cases, and that is the possibility that the surgery may result in death. Surgery must be considered an extraordinary means whenever its use entails very grave danger of death. Any surgical operation must be judged to be an extraordinary means when the very grave danger of death connected with it would constitute for the normal patient too great a price to pay for good health or for the prolongation of life.

In practice it is often difficult to determine whether a given surgical operation, because of the danger of death that is connected with it, should in a particular case be classified as an

extraordinary means of conserving life. Many surgical operations which in former times were as a rule considered extraordinary means because of the danger of death must today be
classified as ordinary means. In days gone by operations such
as a caesarean section, a hysterectomy, goiter surgery, and the
like entailed grave danger of death. Today, however, because
of the great progress of medicine, the danger involved in such
operations can be very slight. No data are available, however,
which would enable us to classify all types of surgical operations according to the amount of danger connected with them.
It may be known that a certain number of patients died after
certain operations, but it does not follow that they died chiefly
because of the operations. Moreover, it has never been decided
how soon after an operation a patient must die in order that
his death may be directly attributed to the surgery.

It rests with the physician to decide, on the basis of his
knowledge and experience, how much danger is involved in a
proposed operation. His judgment must be based upon a reasonable moral estimate. His judgment, moreover, must take
into account the age and condition of his patient. When a patient is in normal health except for the condition that makes
an operation necessary, the amount of danger present in his
case may be reasonably presumed to be no greater than the
amount usually present in the case of other patients whose
general condition is apparently similar to his. It is of course
true that, because of some weakness which remains hidden
from the expert eye of the examining physician, grave danger
may occur during the operation. It is also true that some altogether unforeseeable reaction may occur, even when the patient's health has been medically established as normal. These
remote possibilities, however, are very rare exceptions which
should not deter the physician from deciding the case on the
basis of what he is able to observe and discover.

It is difficult to express mathematically the degree of estimated danger which would place a particular type of surgery

in the classification of ordinary or extraordinary means. In order, however, that surgeons may have a safe rule to guide them in practice we venture to suggest the following approximate norms.

1. Apart from accidental circumstances (for example, old age, a weak heart, and the like) which in a particular case increase appreciably the danger, surgery in which the percentage of mortality is low must be considered ordinary means. A mortality rate of 10 per cent is judged a low percentage in regard to this matter.

2. If the percentage of mortality in a given type of operation is between 15 and 20 per cent, or higher, such surgery can clearly be classified as extraordinary means.

3. Any percentage between these two norms would indicate that the means are doubtfully ordinary, and therefore in practice their use is not obligatory.

We may note here that a certain operation may have a very low percentage of mortality when it is performed in a modern, well-equipped hospital, but a very high percentage of mortality when performed under less favorable circumstances. We should also remember that certain operations, which may not be judged dangerous in themselves, place the patient in grave danger when because of some unexpected event they must be greatly protracted. The general weakening effect of a long operation may increase the risk notably. Some operations, moreover, have a low percentage of mortality if the operating surgeon is highly skilled, but a high rate if the surgeon is not a specialist in that particular operation. Since no one knows a patient's condition and the accompanying circumstances better than his own physician, it is for the latter to weigh all such circumstances and to evaluate accordingly the nature of the means and the obligation involved of employing them.

Most physicians would agree today that, if we think only of the amount of danger involved, the following operations, performed in a well-equipped hospital by a sufficiently skilled surgeon, must be deemed ordinary means of saving one's life: (1) tonsillectomy; (2) appendectomy; (3) the removal of the gall bladder; (4) the removal of a female breast; (5) stomach surgery for ulcer; (6) a caesarean section; (7) a hysterectomy; (8) goiter surgery and like operations. Although in some of these operations a surgeon of skill is required, in the large cities of the United States of America today there is usually little difficulty in obtaining the aid of a qualified surgeon. Even surgery that brings grave danger of death may become obligatory if refusal to submit to the operation would certainly bring death within a few days, for the surgery would practically establish the only possible hope of conserving life. It would be unreasonable that a means which could save one's life should be spurned merely because it involved so slight an anticipation of danger. The obligation of submitting to an amputation such as that of a leg or a hand must be judged in the light of the hardship or shame which the patient would experience in going through life with such an affliction. The element of danger would not excuse one from submitting to such an amputation, for today such surgery does not involve grave danger of death.

Case 14
An Appendectomy as a Required Ordinary Means

The patient, a male 58 years of age, has inoperable carcinoma of the stomach and has been told that he will certainly die within two years. One evening he is hurried to the hospital in excruciating pain. A medical examination reveals that he has a ruptured appendix. His physician informs him that, without an operation, he cannot expect to live many days. Does the patient have an obligation of submitting to this surgery?

Solution. The patient must make use of this surgery to save his life.

Explanation. On the assumption that the appendectomy would not involve very grave danger, extraordinary suffering, or very great expense, the patient would be obliged to undergo the operation. In such circumstances an appendectomy must be viewed as an ordinary means of preserving life. Although the patient is doomed to die within two years, the use of a measure such as this would not be morally considered too great a price to pay in order to safeguard even that short span of life. Besides, it not infrequently happens that such patients live well beyond the time of their predicted death.

Case 15
Optional Removal of a Colostomy at the Risk of Life

The patient, a woman 70 years of age, has undergone surgery for the removal of an abdominal growth. In spite of her serious heart condition the operation was successful. Several weeks afterward the surgeon mentions the possibility of removing the temporary colostomy, but he warns her that danger to her life would be involved in this surgery. The patient, however, declares that, no matter how great the risk, she will have the operation.

Solution. In this case the colostomy in itself presumably involves merely moderate inconvenience and annoyance. If the danger of the proposed surgery is very great, a patient with a serious heart ailment would not be justified in permitting the operation. It may well be, however, that the temporary colostomy causes the patient so great repugnance and enduring discontent that this subjective reaction would constitute a sufficient reason for running the grave risk of the corrective surgery.

Explanation. Objectively considered, the good effect (the elimination of inconvenience) to be gained by the proposed surgery is not proportionate to the evil effect (the grave danger of death). If, therefore, the patient were psychologically normal in this matter, she would not desire (nor would she be allowed) to purchase so comparatively small a benefit at so great a price.

The Use of Artificial Means by the Dying

Must a dying person in whose case no medical care can cure or control the disease endeavor to prolong his life for a short time (for example, a week or two) by means which are ordinary but artificial? So far as any obligation arising from the Fifth Commandment is concerned, we answer that in such cases the dying person need not use artificial helps such as intravenous feeding, oxygen, blood transfusions, or chemical stimulants to prolong life. Such a patient for the conservation of life is held to the use of natural means only, such as food, drink, and the like. In the case of a patient, for example, who is in the last stages of cancer or of a very aged person who is dying, medication could do nothing either to effect a cure or even to halt the advance of the disease or ailment. Such medication, therefore, because it is genuinely useless, need not be employed.

The Obligations of Patients and Relatives

To summarize what has been said, a patient is obliged to use ordinary means to preserve his life but is not obliged to use extraordinary means. The position taken by some to the effect that a patient is guilty of suicide if he refuses to use extraordinary means is not tenable.

In refraining from the use of extraordinary means a patient is certainly not guilty of suicide nor of any other wrongdoing. He is not guilty of suicide, for (1) he is performing no prohibited action which is directly aimed at killing himself and (2) he is not failing to perform an obligatory action required to preserve his life. That he is performing no prohibited action is obvious. That he is not failing to perform any obligatory action is likewise clear, for the obligation to conserve one's life does not require that a man should employ *any and every possible* means to this end. His duty is limited to the employing of means that are morally possible. The means may be *physically* possible; but if they are not *morally* possible, one's obligation to use them to preserve life is at an end.

Let us suppose that an individual whose home is in Alaska falls ill, and that the attending physician assures him that he cannot avoid death unless he moves to distant California or Arizona, and there lives on expensive medicines. To carry out the physician's prescriptions will cost a fortune, and the individual in question is a poor man. Strictly speaking, his relatives could borrow the large sum of money required for his trip and continued medication, but they would have to slave for years to repay the loan. In such a case the means necessary to conserve health are *physically* possible; they are not, however, *morally* possible. They constitute so heavy a burden that one would be looked upon as unreasonable if he were to bind a person to use them. Such means of preserving health can justly be termed extraordinary. To purchase continued good health at the cost of these measures would be too great a price and one which a bountiful Creator would not demand that His creatures pay.

The near relatives who are responsible for the patient also have obligations in regard to the choice of means. The parents must make the decision as to whether extraordinary means are to be used in the case of the children under their care. The husband or the wife must decide the matter when their spouse is not able to pass judgment on the question because he or she is unconscious or mentally deficient. In the case of adults in general who are incapable of expressing their wishes, the nearest relative should make the decision. This decision should be based on the presumed preference of the patient.

The Duties of Physicians in Regard to Means

The physician's obligations in regard to the choice of means are not identical with those of the patient, for the physician must use not only ordinary means to keep his patient alive, but he is obliged to employ extraordinary means also whenever his patient wishes him to do so. The patient is obliged to use the ordinary means of cure, and the physician who has assumed the care of the sick person shares in this obligation. The patient is perfectly free, though not obliged, to use means that are obviously extraordinary. By virtue of his contract with the patient the physician must follow his patient's wishes in this regard. Hence if the sick person desires the use of extraordinary means, the physician must make use of them insofar as they are available.

In a particular case the physician must make it clear to the patient that there are means (though these are extraordinary) of saving his life. In complicated cases it may not be feasible for the physician to lay before the patient all the medical factors involved in order that the sick man may decide whether extraordinary means are to be employed or not. This is particularly true when the patient is not too intelligent or is perhaps befuddled from the effects of his illness. Hence it can happen that the physician will have to make the decision for the patient. Moreover, in proposing to the patient the question of using extraordinary means, the physician, by his tone of voice and the phrasing of his words, can greatly influence the patient's answer. In speaking of means which are extraordinary the physician can say to the patient, for example: "This procedure will give you the only chance you have of saving your life," or he can say, "Your case is hopeless. I can *try* this procedure if you wish, but the chances of success are slight and it will be costly." Both statements might be truthful under the circumstances, but the first would encourage the patient to use the proposed means while the second would tend to discourage him from doing so. If the physician does seek to discourage the patient from using every possible means, he should have sound and good reasons for his action.

Oftentimes the physician himself must decide whether extraordinary means of preserving or prolonging life should be used. The patient himself may be unconscious, and his relatives may either be absent or unable or unwilling to make a decision. The general ideal of the medical profession today is to fight for the preservation of life to the last moment, and to this ideal the ethician gives his heartiest approval. The only regret of the ethician is that there are certain misconceptions concerning the preservation of life in two cases: in the case of the unborn child and in the case of the incurably ill for whom euthanasia is sometimes thought to be indicated. If the ethician exempts the patient from the obligation of using extraordinary means, it does not follow that he wishes to discourage their use. The ethician is not free to declare that a certain action is a grave moral wrong unless it is in truth a grave moral wrong. In solving cases involving the use of extraordinary means the ethician confines himself to stating what is permitted and what is forbidden, saying nothing about what he thinks the ideal character might be expected to do.

Case 16
The Use of Extraordinary Means for a Patient in Coma

The patient is in the state of coma because of a very grave blow on the head and it is altogether impossible that he be saved. The physician is certain that, because of severe cerebral lacerations, he can never regain consciousness. The patient's wife wishes the physician to use only ordinary means to keep him alive. Must intravenous feeding and oxygen be employed in order to prolong his life for a few weeks?

Solution. In this case there is no obligation to use intravenous feeding or an oxygen tent.

Explanation. Medication which gives no hope at all of curing, or at least of arresting the progress of, a bodily ailment may in general be considered a useless means for preserving life. No one is obliged to do what is useless. In the present case oxygen and intravenous feeding would, it is true, prolong life briefly, but the mere prolonging of life for so short a time in the present circumstances would, as a rule, be entirely fruitless. An exception to this rule would be the case where the patient has not as yet been given all the spiritual aid which can be administered to one in this state. If, for example, the patient is a Catholic and has not been given the last sacraments, every means available should be employed in order to keep him alive until he is visited by a priest.

Extraordinary Means and Minors

All will undoubtedly concede that a man's right to life is a strictly personal right and that, since one has a right to achieve the end, he also has a right to the use of the ordinary means by which this end may be accomplished. Mere children, too, no matter what their age may be, have as human beings the right not only to life and health but to the ordinary means for conserving them. This right of theirs to *ordinary* means must be respected by their parents. The right of a minor to *extraordinary* measures for conserving his life is subject to a very definite limitation.

If a minor is living at home and is being supported by his parents, whatever he may earn by doing the work of which young persons are capable and in which they often engage, such as serving as clerks in stores, running errands, and so forth, becomes the property of his parents. Parents may wisely permit their children to keep and use all or part of the money thus earned, but they are not obliged to do so. It is a different matter if the minor has received money as a gift or legacy. In this case the money belongs strictly to the minor, since parents have no right to set at naught the wishes of the donor. Whatever was given was given to the minor, not to them. Since minors might only too easily squander money thus given to them or permit themselves to be fleeced, parents do have the obligation of acting as its custodians and of supervising its use, yet the money remains the possession of the minor.

It follows that, if a minor possesses in his own name funds sufficient for providing extraordinary means of preserving his life, he has the right to use the funds for that purpose. The question of the advisability of using or not using extraordinary means to preserve life will involve, in a particular case, a degree of considered reflection of which a very young child is incapable and which for an infant or a child who has not as yet become able to reason is of course quite impossible. In such cases the parents or guardians must make the decision for him. It is their obligation to do whatever they prudently think the child would reasonably request if he were actually able to pass judgment on the matter. On the other hand, a fifteen-year-old boy or girl, unless notably retarded mentally, would be capable of making a decision for himself.

If the child's case calls for the use of means which are extremely costly and if he in his own right is very wealthy, he may rightly require the use of these extraordinary measures for preserving his life. The same is true in the case where a rich friend or relative of the child offers to defray all the expenses involved in the extraordinary care of the child. But let us suppose that the case does not require a great outlay of money but that it does involve very grave pain or very grave danger to life and may therefore rightly be classified as an extraordinary means of preserving life. In this event the child himself has the right to make the decision to use or to reject such measures, for it is his life which is in jeopardy and it is he who will have to undergo the pain or run the grave risk which the operation or the treatment involves. The presumption is, of course, that the child is old enough to be able to form a reasonable judgment. If his parents in such a case refuse to permit him to make the choice, they err gravely.

If a child has no source of revenue other than that which the parents provide for him, he has no right to the use of very expensive means for the care of his health. Parents may refrain from using such means if the child is so young that they must decide the matter for him and may refuse to permit their use if the child is old enough to request or demand them. In such cases, however, charity could impose upon parents the obligation of using extraordinary means if they are able to do so without proportionate inconvenience.

In making this statement we have in mind the principle, already explained, of the absolute norm as opposed to the relative norm. A treatment may be so costly as to exceed the maximum required under the absolute norm and yet not cause serious inconvenience to parents who are very wealthy. In these circumstances the parents would be obliged in charity to employ the necessary extraordinary means of conserving the child's life. An obligation in charity could arise also in case the young patient's companionship would in a few years greatly benefit his brother, the only other child in the family, especially if the latter, because for example of the remoteness of the home, has no playmates in his age group. We have confined our analysis principally to a study of the obligations of strict justice, for these usually involve far greater difficulty than duties arising from the virtue of charity. (See pages 18-19.)

The following cases, illustrating conditions under which ordinary or extraordinary means may be necessary, include cases involving adults and cases involving minors.

Case 17
Appendectomies as Ordinary Means

The physician has diagnosed the patient's ailment as acute appendicitis. The patient tells the physician that he wishes the operation only if he is morally obliged to have it. The physician informs him that, since every appendectomy involves some danger of grave complications, this means of preserving life is extraordinary and therefore not obligatory.

Solution. The physician is in error. An appendectomy must in general be regarded as an ordinary means of preserving life.

Explanation. In modern American hospitals which provide the usual hygienic facilities for surgical operations, appendectomies involve little risk to life and are not very costly. Hence they must be classified as ordinary means of conserving life. If, however, the surgery had to be performed in primitive circumstances where the danger of further infection was great, it would be looked upon as extraordinary means of conserving life.

Case 18
An Application of the Relative and of the Absolute Norm

Mr. A, a very poor man, is told by his physician that in order to save his life he must undergo an operation which, together with the required hospitalization, will cost over $1,000. Because of his great poverty Mr. A considers the expense so great that the operation would be an extraordinary means of preserving his life. He does not mention to his physician that he is a veteran and therefore entitled to hospitalization in the veterans' hospital in the city where he resides.

Solution. Mr. A is not obliged to undergo the operation at his own expense, but he is obliged to make use of the free services that are available to him.

Explanation. If Mr. A himself would have to pay the bill, he need not have the operation, since under the principle of the relative norm the operation would be considered an extraordinary means. If, however, the government would defray all expenses because he is a veteran, the money consideration would not release him from the obligation of using this means to conserve his health. An operation costing over $1,000 would not be considered an extraordinary means so far as the absolute norm is concerned. It should be noted, moreover, that a patient is not free to appeal to the principle of the absolute norm if the state, county, city, or Federal Government is ready to provide without cost to him all the medical services that may be necessary.

Case 19
Caesarean Sections as Extraordinary Means

Mrs. D is told by her physician that the child she is carrying in utero is viable and that its life can be saved only by a caesarean section. Mrs. D informs him that she will not submit to this operation, because she considers it an extraordinary means of safeguarding the infant's life.

Solution. Under normal circumstances Mrs. D would be obliged to submit to the caesarean section.

Explanation. A caesarean section today usually involves little danger to the mother when the surgery is performed in a modern, well-equipped hospital. Provided Mrs. D's general health is normal, she would therefore be obliged in charity to use this means of saving the infant in her womb. If, moreover, the child would die without baptism unless the mother permitted the caesarean section, the child would be in extreme spiritual necessity. In that event Mrs. D would be obliged to expose herself to grave risk of death in order to provide for the spiritual welfare of her offspring. The physician must beware, however, of mentioning the mother's obligation in this case if he prudently judges that she would in any event refuse to permit the surgery. In such circumstances the physician's warning would do more harm than good, for it would not help the child, since the operation would not be performed, and it would put the mother in bad faith, since she will refuse to do what she has been told is of grave obligation.

Case 20
Medication To Prevent Threatened Miscarriage

Mrs. T, pregnant for 4 months, has begun to suffer uterine bleeding. Her physician warns her that she will very probably have a spontaneous abortion unless he continues to give her medication. "In cases such as this," he says, "it has been found that, when nature tends to abort, the child will be physically or mentally defective if saved through medication. Hence I advise you to let me stop medication so that nature may take its course."

Solution. Unless the proposed medication is very costly or very painful, the patient is obliged in charity to use it.

Explanation. The usual therapy for the condition described is not notably costly nor notably painful, and the results are reasonably good. The therapy is therefore an ordinary means of preserving the fetal life. The physician would undoubtedly judge that this type of treatment constituted ordinary care of a child's health if the child were two or three years of age. The fact that the person concerned is but a four-month fetus would not change the classification of the means, which must still be considered ordinary. The incidence of monsters under the conditions described does not appear to be greater than the incidence of monsters in so-called normal pregnancies. The ill-advised warning of the physician does not have sound medical foundation.

Case 21

Corpus Luteum Therapy as an Ordinary Means

A woman 12 weeks pregnant has been operated on for an ovarian cyst. After the surgery it is discovered that the corpus luteum of pregnancy is enclosed in the excised cyst. The physician can prevent a possible abortion by the use of progesterone and estrogen. Since the patient does not wish to have the child, the physician will refrain from this therapy if morally permitted to do so.

Solution. The physician may not in this case licitly refrain from the use of the therapy.

Explanation. The only justification for refraining from using the indicated therapy would be the fact that the drugs are so costly as to constitute an extraordinary means for the mother. Progesterones and estrogens have been chemically synthesized and are not so costly as to be considered an extraordinary means. If because of unusual conditions of time or place the therapy would be very expensive, the physician would not be obliged to use it, for the mother obviously wishes him to use only ordinary means to preserve the pregnancy.

Case 22

Costly Blood Transfusions as Extraordinary Means

The patient, a 22-year-old hemophiliac, is hemorrhaging because of traumata resulting from an automobile accident. His physician informs him that blood transfusions are necessary if his life is to be saved and that, insofar as he is able to foresee, these will probably have to be given several times a week for two or three months. Since each transfusion would cost $25 and the patient is very poor, he feels justified in refusing to permit this treatment if it proves impossible to obtain free blood from a blood bank or to find donors.

Solution. The patient acts licitly in this case.

Explanation. In the present case the relative norm may be employed in order to judge what means may be considered extraordinary. Since the patient cannot pay for so many blood transfusions, he rightly concludes that these are a relatively extraordinary means and that he is not obliged to go in debt in order to pay for them.

Case 23

Travel as an Extraordinary Means

A 15-year-old boy is told by the family physician that, in order to recover his health, he must go to Mexico and remain there for six months or more. The boy's parents, however, refuse to permit him to leave their home in Pittsburgh.

Solution. The physician's recommendation involves the use of extraordinary means of preserving life. If the parents are the ones who would be called upon to defray the expenses connected with the costly journey and sojourn in Mexico, they may refuse to finance the plan.

Explanation. One may, but need not, use extraordinary means to preserve his life. The cost of procuring the remedy for a disease can be so great that it constitutes an extraordinary means of conserving one's health. Such measures a parent is not obliged to employ in order to conserve his own life, nor is he bound to do so in order to safeguard the life of his child if he himself must provide the very large sum of money which would be necessary. If, however, the child, independently of his parents, can furnish the necessary funds, his parents may not, because of the expenses required, refuse him permission for the trip. Apart from the question of the money involved, other circumstances (for example, the lack of necessary supervision) may alter the case. Because of the moral weakness of the boy such a sojourn in a foreign country where he would be removed from the wholesome restraints of the home might prove exceedingly dangerous.

Case 24

Surgery in the Case of a Minor

The patient, a boy aged 11 years, is suffering from a malignant tumor. Unless the growth is excised, the boy will certainly die within a year.

The parents, however, refuse to permit the operation. What should the physician do?

Solution. It is the father as a rule who should decide whether the surgery is to be performed or not. If the physician believes that the operation would serve the best interests of the child, he should try to persuade the parents to permit it.

Explanation. If the operation is an ordinary means of conserving life, the parents are obliged to permit the surgery. In order to force them to yield to his request in the matter, the physician may invoke the help of civil authorities. If, however, because of its cost, the operation would be rightly considered an extraordinary measure for preserving life, and if the parents are the ones who would be compelled to defray this very grave expense, they would have the right to refuse permission for surgery. If, on the contrary, either the boy himself or some friend will pay for the surgery and hospitalization, the parents may not rightly prevent the operation. In the event, moreover, that the expenses involved would not constitute too great a burden for the parents in question, they would be obliged in virtue of the law of charity to have the surgery performed. See page 82.

Case 25
Leg Amputation in a Minor

A girl 8 years of age is afflicted with osteogenic sarcoma of the thigh. Unless her leg is amputated, she will die within about a year. An operation would give her one chance in ten of living; but if saved, she would be a cripple. Her father refuses to permit the amputation. Is he justified in his action?

Solution. If the father sincerely judges that in these circumstances his decision serves the best interest of the child, his refusal is licit.

Explanation. Without the operation the child will certainly die within about one year. The amputation of the leg would not certainly prolong her life beyond that time, but it does give solid hope of prolonging her life for many years. Because the suggested amputation would constitute only a *probably effective* remedy, it would not be obligatory for the parent to employ it. It is within the competence of the father to give the final decision in this matter, for he is the one who has the responsibility for the care of the child and he it is who has the authority for permitting the use of such doubtful means for conserving his daughter's life. A child of eight would hardly be qualified to weigh the advantages and the disadvantages of the suggested surgery. Hence the parent, viewing on the one hand the possible saving of the girl's life and on the other the grave danger of the operation, the necessity of going through life encumbered by a prosthetic leg, and the small probability of the success of such an amputation, might judge that, all things considered, it is preferable to forgo the surgery.

Case 26
Costly Throat Surgery on a Minor

A baby is born with a single head and two bodies. In order to keep the baby alive a very delicate throat operation is necessary. The operation and protracted hospitalization will cost several thousand dollars. Must the parents have this operation performed?

Solution. The parents need not take upon themselves the very grave financial burden of so costly an operation.

Explanation. The operation and the necessary hospitalization would be very expensive and they would therefore constitute an extraordinary means of conserving life. Since it is here assumed that the money to cover the cost of the surgery would have to be provided by the parents, they are not obliged to use such measures in order to save the child's life.

"But," one might object, "if the child were a normal one, the parents would use every available means to keep it alive, no matter how costly this might be. Hence, even in the present case, must they not use such means?" If the child were normal, the average parent would, it is true, take upon himself almost any burden, however great it be, to insure the child's survival, but he would nevertheless be going beyond what is of strict obligation. If, then, in the case of an abnormal baby he wishes to limit himself to his duty, he may licitly do so.

Case 27
Artificial Respiration as an Ordinary Means

An infant is born with a hydrocephalic condition and requires artificial respiration at once. The infant, if it lives, can never be normal and will be a very grave burden to his parents. Must the attending physician use artificial respiration to bring about in the infant normal breathing or may he refrain from this procedure? If he does nothing, the infant will soon die.

Solution. The physician must apply artificial respiration to this infant.

Explanation. Artificial respiration of a temporary nature is an ordinary means of tiding a person over a crisis, and therefore it is obligatory.

88

The fact that this young patient is horribly abnormal does not alter the solution of the case. Every infant, no matter how grossly deformed he may be, is a human being and as such has the same right to life as that which is enjoyed by a perfectly normal child. Whatever a physician would be obliged to do for a normal child, he must do for this hydrocephalic.

Case 28
Gavage as a Means of Preserving Life

The infant can neither suck nor swallow. He must be fed through a stomach tube, and gavage will be permanently necessary to keep him alive. There are also indications that he may be an imbecile. The physician judges that the circumstances are such that gavage may be considered an extraordinary means of preserving life, and informs the parents that they may licitly have the gavage discontinued.

Solution. If gavage is *permanently* necessary to keep the child alive, it may rightly be deemed an extraordinary means, and because this care would involve such exceptionally grave inconvenience to the parents, there is no obligation on their part to continue this type of feeding.

Explanation. If gavage is required over a long period of time, say six months, this care would clearly prove very burdensome for the parents, and therefore they need not undertake such care for the prolongation of the life of their child, just as they would under ordinary conditions have no obligation of prolonging their own lives by such means. The fact that in the present case the patient is probably an imbecile does not enter directly into the moral problem involved, for an infant, whether normal or subnormal, must be given the benefit of what are considered ordinary means for the preservation of health and life. The parents are free to use extraordinary means to preserve the child's life, and those who counsel them would ordinarily not think of suggesting that they refrain from doing so. It is one thing, however, to praise as noble and truly Christian the determination to preserve an infant's life at any cost, and quite another thing to declare that failure to use even extraordinary means will make the parents guilty of very serious wrongdoing in the eyes of God. Reason tells us that there must be limits to what is of strict obligation. So far as the medical aspects of the case are concerned, it may be noted that an infant unable because of brain injury to suck or swallow at birth ordinarily either learns to do so or expires within a relatively short time.

Case **29**

An Infant Requiring the Services of a Trained Nurse

An infant is born blind and with a double cleft palate and harelip. He cannot be fed in the normal way but must receive nourishment through a tube. Since because of circumstances no member of the family can undertake to feed the child, the services of a trained nurse or of a practical nurse will be necessary. Are the parents obliged to provide the services of a nurse?

Solution. If the services of a trained nurse are required over so long a period that the expense would constitute a most grave burden for the parents, the parents need not assume this great expense for the preservation of the child's life.

Explanation. In some cases of cleft palate the baby may be fed by means of a special nursing nipple; but if the child's condition is such that a trained nurse must be in constant attendance, the great expense to be defrayed by the parents in providing such care over a long period would release them from the obligation of employing this procedure. See Case 28 for our comment on the reasons for distinguishing between what a high ideal suggests and what the natural law requires. The fact that parents ask an ethician whether they are obliged in conscience to undergo a certain expense does not necessarily indicate that they are callous or selfish. It often happens that the money which might be spent for the care of one child is urgently needed for the care or education of another child.

SELF-DEFENSE AGAINST UNJUST ATTACK

CLOSELY related to the question of our obligation to use ordinary means for the preservation of life is the question of the lengths to which we may go to protect our life against the attack of an unjust aggressor. One very important reason for including a discussion of this question in a work on medical ethics is the fact that the right of an individual to defend himself against an unjust attack has sometimes been alleged as an argument for therapeutic abortion. The unborn child has been represented as an aggressor against the life of the mother. He is threatening her life; and therefore, it has sometimes been argued, she may procure or consent to his death in order to preserve her own life. In order to provide a basis for a judgment upon this argument we may present very briefly the principles accepted by ethicians as applying to cases in which there is question of one's right to self-defense against an aggressor.

When Force May Be Used against an Unjust Aggressor

We have at times the right to use force, even a deathblow, against an unjust aggressor. Our right to life involves the right to use the means necessary to protect our life, provided such means do not violate the rights of others. In the case of unjust aggression the use of force and even of a deathblow may be the only means of saving our life. The rights of others are not thereby violated, for the assailant's right to live is suspended during his unjust attack. Moreover, he can easily protect his life by merely ceasing from the attack. The right to use force against an unjust aggressor is present if the following conditions are verified.

1. Recourse to civil authority must be impossible. The common good demands that as a rule the state alone use physical compulsion, for if any private citizen could at will employ force in defending his rights, the peace and order of the community would be disturbed.

2. The attack must be actual or immediately imminent. It is wrong to kill before the attack, for if this were permitted, there is danger that timorous, suspicious, and evil-minded persons would use force against many purely imaginary attacks. To allow the use of force against merely prospective attacks would inevitably lead to grave abuses. It is not permissible to kill after the attack is over, for then defense is too late and the act of killing would constitute revenge.

3. The attack must be unjust. A robber, justly fired upon by police officers, may not kill them to protect his own life.

4. The force employed must be proportionate to the loss threatened and must not exceed what is necessary. Killing is not allowed if wounding would suffice for proper defense;

wounding is not permitted if disarming the adversary or summoning help would be enough.

When Killing an Unjust Aggressor Is Licit

In order to justify killing an unjust aggressor the loss threatened must be one's life, a grave mutilation, or an object of great value. The sum threatened could be either of great value in itself or of great value to the owner because of his poverty or need. If the stolen property can be recovered later by recourse to civil authority or in some other manner, killing would not be permitted. Chastity, as a precious possession, may also be defended by these extreme measures against the attack of an unjust aggressor.

Even if the unjust assailant is intoxicated or insane, it is permissible to use proportionate force against him, for one's right to defend himself remains the same under these conditions. Even though the assailant attacks inculpably, as happens when he does not realize what he is doing, one may justly defend oneself against him.

Ordinarily an individual would not be obliged to use his right to employ force in repelling an unjust attack, for he is bound merely to use ordinary means to preserve his life, and the use of violence is considered an extraordinary means. If, however, one is needed by one's family or by one's fellow citizens, one would have an obligation in piety to protect oneself.

Defending Others against Unjust Attack

What one may do for his own self-defense he may also do in safeguarding the rights of others. At times one must go to another's defense. We are obliged by charity to go to the assistance of one in danger of death, even at the cost of grave inconvenience to ourselves. (See pages 18-19.) Hence we may use whatever force is necessary to save an innocent man from one who is attempting to murder him. At other times one must in justice protect another who is being unjustly attacked. A policeman, for example, must defend a citizen against high-waymen. He is bound in justice rather than merely in charity because of the position which he has voluntarily accepted.

The Unborn Child Not an Unjust Aggressor

In 1852 the Academy of Medicine of Paris declared that therapeutic abortions were licit in desperate cases. This decision marked the beginning of the practice of therapeutic abortion. It is immediately evident that the licitness of the practice cannot be defended save on the ground that the unborn child is an unjust aggressor. The principle that a completely innocent person—in the present connection, one who is engaged in no unjust attack—may be wantonly killed in order to save the life of another is demonstrably false. Men starving on a life raft at sea, for example, have no right to kill one member of the group in order to eat his flesh and thus save their own lives. If it is licit to kill an unborn child, the only reason can be that he is an unjust aggressor. The fact that he is not an unjust aggressor is evident from the following considerations.

1. The unborn child is doing nothing directly to attack the life of the mother. He is merely growing and developing according to the laws of nature. He possesses a right to life. If he loses his life, as perhaps he may, it must be through natural causes and not through a direct attack upon him.

2. The unborn child finds himself where he is, not because of any act of his own, but because of the free act of one or both of his parents.

3. If the unborn child is a threat to the life of the mother, this is due as a rule, not to the fetus itself, but rather to the mother, who because of anatomical or physiological conditions is having difficulty in bringing her pregnancy to term. But even though the unborn child were himself the sole source of peril, he would still not be an unjust aggressor.

The question of therapeutic abortions is discussed in greater detail on pages 189-205. Our purpose here is to establish the fact that the unborn child cannot be looked upon as an unjust aggressor. We might remark in passing that, if an unborn child could rightfully be considered an unjust aggressor because the mother might die if she continued to carry him, he could just as rightfully be considered an unjust aggressor under other circumstances. We consider as an unjust aggressor one who attacks, not only our life, but also possessions of great value. Now, honor and good name are possessions of great value, and it would follow that unmarried mothers could licitly obtain abortions in order to avoid public shame. Admit the licitness of abortion for this reason, and it is only a short step to defending abortion when another child would impose a severe financial burden. Those members of the medical profession who defend therapeutic abortion are therefore implicitly defending principles leading to evils and abuses which they themselves would oftentimes be the first to condemn.

Case 30
Physician Attacked by Insane Patient

Dr. A, a resident physician in a mental hospital, is attacked in the corridor by a violently insane patient who has succeeded in escaping from his room. May Dr. A use force against this unjust aggressor?

Solution. Dr. A is justified in using force, even though in subduing the patient he inflicts a deathblow.

Explanation. Dr. A has a right to defend himself against unjust attack. He should endeavor to subdue the patient without inflicting injury, but he need not refrain from action which may possibly result in the patient's death, provided this action appears to him to be the only effective means of protecting himself.

THE PRINCIPLE OF THE TWOFOLD EFFECT

WE HAVE just given reasons for the fact that a therapeutic abortion is morally wrong. Later we will defend the thesis that a uterus may sometimes be removed despite the fact that a living fetus is present. Physicians sometimes have difficulty in seeing the difference between the two cases, in both of which death results for the unborn child. The difference lies in this, that in the second case the principle of the twofold effect can be rightly applied, while in the first case it cannot be rightly applied. The principle of the twofold effect is applicable in many medical situations and should therefore be clearly understood.

It very frequently happens that an action results in more than one effect with moral implications. A city board of health, for example, permanently hospitalized a woman known to be a carrier of typhoid, and the action was sustained by the courts. This action produced two effects with moral implications. One effect was to protect the public against disease and death. Another effect was to deprive a morally innocent individual of her liberty.

If one pauses for a moment to think of events that occur constantly in his daily life, he will realize that innumerable actions have two effects with moral implications. To take but one example, if a physician answers an emergency call at two o'clock in the morning, he is on the one hand rendering a service to a patient in need and is thus performing a virtuous act, but his action may on the other hand have certain undesirable consequences. By rising when he does he may cause inconvenience, worry, and loss of sleep to members of his family. If he himself has been somewhat unwell, he may retard his recovery. If he is to operate early in the morning, he may do the surgery with less than his usual efficiency and thus expose his second patient to some danger. Any one of these consequences, if sought deliberately, directly, and without adequate reason, would be morally wrong, though usually not seriously wrong. It is necessary for us to have a precise knowledge of the conditions under which we may perform an action one effect of which would be morally wrong if the required conditions were not observed. Before laying down the principle and showing its application, we will explain certain concepts that should be clearly understood.

First, we must note that an action may be willed or intended in either one of two ways. It may be willed or intended either *directly* or *indirectly*.

To will or intend directly is to will or intend a certain action either as a means to a certain end which one has in view or as the end itself.

Example 1. The wife of Dr. A is slowly and painfully dying of cancer. With her consent Dr. A administers to her a death-dealing drug. Dr. A directly wills and intends the death of his wife.

Example 2. Dr. B performs a craniotomy as a means of saving a young pregnant woman's life. Dr. B directly wills and intends the destruction of the fetus as a means of safeguarding the mother.

In cases in which an action is willed or intended indirectly, the one who is acting does not will or intend a certain action in itself, but wills or intends some other action, knowing that the action which he does not directly will or intend will follow. By directly willing Action X, which is the cause of Action Y, he indirectly wills Action Y.

Example 1. Dr. C performs an appendectomy, knowing that his patient, because of the circumstances of the case, will suffer acutely after the operation. Dr. C directly wills the removal of the appendix. He indirectly wills the suffering for the patient that will follow.

Example 2. Dr. D is finding it increasingly difficult to support his family as he would wish to do. He therefore keeps in his office a supply of contraceptives which he sells at a good profit to patients in order, as he says, to save them the embarrassment of asking for contraceptives in drugstores. Dr. D is himself somewhat opposed to the use of contraceptives and does not urge his patients to use them, but he realizes that patients would not spend money for contraceptives only to throw them away. Dr. D directly wills the selling of contraceptives as a means and the making of money as the end or purpose. He indirectly wills the illicit use of the contraceptives by his patients.

Second, we must note that an action viewed in itself may be either good, bad, or indifferent. The act of praising God is in itself morally good. The act of blaspheming is in itself morally bad or evil. Very many acts, such as those of walking, eating, writing, studying, and so forth, are indifferent in themselves; that is, in the abstract or apart from concrete circumstances. When we say that they are indifferent we mean that they may become either good or bad according to the circumstances under which they are performed and the purpose or intention of the one performing them.

For a surgeon to cut human flesh with a scalpel is an act which may be either morally good or morally wrong. If he plunges the scalpel into the heart of an enemy, the act is morally wrong. If, desirous of saving a human life by removing a malignant tumor, he uses the scalpel in surgery, the act is morally good. In discussing the twofold effect of an action we do not look upon the action as a mere physical act. We take the action considered morally; that is, viewed in its conformity with or difformity from the norm of morality.

As regards actions that are evil in themselves, we may divide them into two classes.

1. There are actions that are evil as regards the very substance of the act. Such actions under all circumstances, if knowingly and deliberately performed, are evil. The morality of such actions is absolute, for they are substantially bad. They do not depend on any particular condition for their evil. An example of an action that is substantially bad is hatred of God. No circumstance imaginable could make this action other than objectively evil.

2. There are actions that are evil because of the lack of the right to perform them in the one acting. In these actions the substance of the act is indifferent, but since the one acting has not the right to perform them, they become evil. An example of such an action is the taking of another's property. The substance of this action is indifferent, for to treat as one's own the property of another can be either morally good or morally evil. The act is illicit if the one taking another's property has no right to do so. In some cases taking another's property is licit; for example, a destitute, starving man may take from another's goods what he needs to survive.

When considering the morality of an act, we must take into consideration the nature or substance of the act, the circumstances under which it is performed, and the purpose or intention of the one performing it.

The Principle of the Twofold Effect Explained

The principle of the twofold effect may be stated as follows. It is allowable to perform an action that will produce a good effect and a bad effect provided (1) the good effect and not the evil effect is *directly intended,* (2) the action itself is good, or at least indifferent, (3) the good effect is not produced *by means of* the evil effect, and (4) there is a proportionate reason for permitting the foreseen evil effect to occur. Let us comment briefly on each of these four conditions.

1. The good effect and not the evil one must be directly intended, for if the one acting directly intends the evil effect, the act becomes morally wrong because of his evil intention. An evil intention corrupts any action.

2. The action itself must be good, or at least indifferent. If the action itself is evil, evidently it is forbidden. This second condition is verified if the contemplated action is not included in either class of actions that are evil in themselves. (See nos. 1 and 2, page 97.)

3. The good effect must not be produced by means of the evil effect. If the evil effect causes the good effect, then the evil effect is *directly intended,* at least as a means of producing the good effect. But directly to intend evil is always forbidden, for we are always bound to avoid what is morally bad. If we

directly intend evil in our action, then an essential part (the intention) of the action is evil. It may be that one's ultimate purpose in performing the action is very praiseworthy, but that ultimate purpose cannot change the evil nature of the substantially bad action which one is now placing. Evil may never be done, even in order that good may come of it. One may never tell a lie, even in order to save one's life or to prevent injury to one's own or to another's good name.

4. There must be a proportionate reason for permitting the foreseen evil effect to occur. The law of charity forbids us to risk injuring ourselves or others without necessity. Hence if we had no proportionate reason for allowing the foreseen evil effect to follow from our action, we would be unnecessarily causing injury to our neighbor. When we say that the reason must be proportionate we mean that, if the evil effect is slight, a slight reason would suffice for allowing it to occur; and that, if the evil effect is grave, the reason for placing the action in question must also be weighty.

In the following examples we note how these four conditions are fulfilled.

Example 1. N, trapped by fire on the top floor of a forty-story building, hurls himself out the window in order to avoid the excruciating torture of death by fire. He is dashed to pieces on the pavement below. N clearly realized that a fall from such a height would certainly be fatal.

CONDITION 1. N does not wish to be dashed to pieces. He intends merely the avoiding of death by fire.

CONDITION 2. Flinging himself out the window is in itself an indifferent action. It is merely the act of withdrawing from a place fraught with agonizing torture. N intends only the jumping away from the fire and not jumping to death. He does not wish to be killed. His act is that of fleeing from the present danger with which he is threatened.

CONDITION 3. The good effect (the accomplished escape from the flames) is not produced by the evil effect (being dashed to pieces), for even though he were not killed (because, for instance, he landed in a deep pool of water or on the thirty-eighth floor offset), the good effect would still follow. Hence the evil effect is not the cause of the good effect.

CONDITION 4. There is a proportionate reason, for N is not putting his life in greater or more immediate jeopardy and he is escaping horrible agony.

Example 2. A submarine captain in time of war torpedoes an armed merchant ship of the enemy, although he foresees that several innocent passengers on board will be killed as a result of the explosion.

CONDITION 1. The captain intends merely to lessen the power of the enemy by destroying an armed merchant ship. He does not wish to kill the innocent.

CONDITION 2. The captain's action of torpedoing an armed merchant ship in time of war is not evil in itself.

CONDITION 3. The evil effect (the death of the innocent passengers) is not the cause of the good effect (the lessening of the enemy's strength).

CONDITION 4. There is sufficient reason for permitting the evil effect to follow, and this reason is the administering of a damaging blow to those who are unjustly attacking the captain's country.

On the contrary, the principle of the twofold effect could not be cited to justify the following case, for all the conditions necessary are *not* verified.

Example 3. Miss N, an unmarried woman, finds herself pregnant. In order to avoid the disgrace of giving birth to an illegitimate child she takes an abortifacient medicine, justifying her action by this, that the potion will have two effects: a good effect (the saving of her reputation) and an evil effect (the death of the child).

CONDITION 1. Miss N's purpose in bringing about an abortion is to rid herself of the danger of losing her reputation. Her intention is good.

CONDITION 2. The act which Miss N sets out to accomplish is that of emptying the uterus of its contents. This is the act of directly inflicting a fatal blow on an innocent human being, the fetus. Obviously the fetus is innocent; it has done no wrong; and, because it is nonviable, to remove it from the uterus is to remove it from the only place where it can continue to live. Hence Miss N's act of taking the abortifacient is intrinsically evil; it is the crime of murder.

Case 31
Hormonal Treatment and Erotic Stimulation

The patient, a 64-year-old male, is suffering from severe senile osteoporosis of the spine, and his physician is treating him with estrogen and testosterone. The patient informs the physician that his erotic desires are being strongly aroused. Must the physician desist from the treatment?

Solution. If the treatment is medically indicated, it is morally justifiable provided there is not immediate danger that the patient will desire or approve the erotic reactions.

Explanation. Treatments of this nature, and others such as the application of ointment to the genital area, are permitted when they are medically indicated. If in the course of a medical examination or of necessary medication the genital organs are strongly stimulated, this is but the unwelcome and unintended effect of an action which in itself is indifferent. In all such cases the intention of both the patient and the physician is good, for they are but endeavoring to restore sound health to the body. The evil effect (the erotic stimulation) does not produce the good effect (the cure of the body). There is, moreover, a proportionate reason for permitting the evil effect to follow if it should happen to occur.

COOPERATION

COOPERATION, as we use the word here, means concurrence with another person in an act that is morally wrong. This concurrence may be accomplished in either one of two ways: by acting together with another in doing something that is morally wrong or by supplying another with what is helpful to him in doing something that is morally wrong. The question of cooperation is a very practical one for physicians. Men in other walks of life may perhaps never find themselves in a position in which they must decide whether it is permissible for them to cooperate in one way or another in an act which they themselves consider morally wrong. Physicians, on the contrary, do frequently find themselves in such a position. This is particularly true in the case of interns, resident physicians, and anesthesiologists.

We must make a careful distinction between formal cooperation in an act that is morally wrong and merely material cooperation. Formal cooperation always renders one guilty of wrongdoing. This is not true, however, of material cooperation, which may or may not be wrong according to the circumstances in each case.

Formal Cooperation

Formal cooperation is that in which either of the two following occurs.

1. One acts with another in performing an external act that is morally wrong in itself.

Example. Dr. X, a married man, is convinced that Y is having illicit relations with X's wife. In revenge, and to put a stop to these relations, he determines to abduct Y and to castrate him. Dr. N, a friend of Dr. X, accompanies him and participates in the surgery. Dr. N is guilty of formal cooperation.

2. One helps another in performing an act that is morally wrong, but he helps by doing something that is not in itself morally wrong. He thoroughly approves what the other is doing, however, and is willing to do whatever he can to assist in its execution. Because of his will and intention in the matter he is guilty of formal cooperation.

Example. In the case just given of the castration of an enemy, Dr. X's chauffeur drives the car used to abduct Y and to take him to the place where the castration is performed. The chauffeur is entirely in sympathy with Dr. X's action and would do more to help if he could. He is guilty of formal cooperation despite the fact that the mere driving of a car, considered in itself, has no moral implications.

Formal cooperation in an act that is morally wrong is always morally wrong. It is opposed to charity and to any other virtue which the action of the principal agent violates. Adultery, for example, is a cooperative act that is opposed to charity, justice, and chastity.

Material Cooperation

Material cooperation is that in which, without approving another's wrongdoing, one helps him perform his evil action by an act which is not of its nature morally wrong.

Example. In the case of the man unjustly castrated, already described, someone who knew the purpose for which they were to be used provided Dr. X with surgical instruments necessary for the castration. He does not approve of the castration and is under some form of compulsion to act as he does. His cooperation is what is called material cooperation.

Material cooperation in another's evil act is allowed when one has a proportionate reason for so acting. "When one has a proportionate reason" means that, in the case under discussion, good effects occur that balance the evil effects that result from the cooperation.

Cooperation in such circumstances is licit for two reasons. First of all, the action of the one who cooperates is not in itself morally wrong. It is not morally wrong in itself, for example, to give surgical instruments to a physician. Second, the one who cooperates materially by providing instruments does not desire nor approve the illicit use to which the instruments are to be put. He foresees that, through his material cooperation, an evil act will be performed; but his obligation of preventing this act is an obligation of charity, not an obligation of justice. Now, charity does not oblige one to love another more than one loves himself. It does not oblige him, therefore, to prevent harm from coming to another if in so doing he would suffer an equivalent harm himself. It follows, then, that there do occur circumstances in which material cooperation is permissible.

Principles Applying to Material Cooperation

The following principles apply to material cooperation under the several conditions that may exist.

PRINCIPLE 1. Material cooperation is never licit when it would appreciably help on an action that is gravely injurious to the common good. The reason is that the lesser good (the private good of an individual) must yield to the greater good (the common good).

Example. There have been very numerous cases of typhoid in the city, and the city health commissioner has traced the source of infection to the water supply. The mayor, who previously opposed the building of a filtration plant and who must soon run for re-election, demands that the health commissioner conceal the evidence from the newspapers and that he destroy all the documents that bear on the case. The mayor threatens reprisals if the health commissioner does not cooperate with him. In such a case the common good of the people would take precedence over the private good of the health commissioner, who would not be free to cooperate materially with the mayor. By releasing the evidence he would save many lives, for the people would take steps to purify their water supply.

PRINCIPLE 2. When cooperative action would contribute toward the performance of an action that is gravely injurious to an innocent third party, material and necessary cooperation is allowed only when exacted through fear that refusal on the part of the one who is asked to cooperate will bring him injury equal to that of the third party. The cooperation is called "necessary" when the cooperator's aid is such that, without it, the evil deed would not be committed. A synonym sometimes used for necessary cooperation is indispensable cooperation.

The reason for this principle has already been given: that charity does not require one to love another more than one loves oneself and that in consequence one is not obliged to prevent harm from coming to another if in doing so one would suffer equivalent harm oneself. Necessary or indispensable material cooperation in an action resulting in the death of another may sometimes be permissible if refusal to cooperate would result in death to oneself. If the cooperation is not necessary or indispensable—that is, if the evil deed would be committed even if cooperation is refused—then the evil that one escapes by cooperating need not be equivalent to the evil that will come to the innocent third party. The evil that one escapes must, however, be a grave evil and not one out of all proportion to the evil suffered by the innocent third party.

Example. N, a druggist, is about to close his store late at night when a man walks in and points a gun at his head. "I told her I would kill her if she kept on lying to me, and I am going to do it. Give me some arsenic or I'll blow your brains out." If N cannot dissuade the intruder from carrying out his plan and if he cannot avoid providing the arsenic or another poison by using some subterfuge, he may licitly give the intruder the poison. Under the circumstances he is not obliged to sacrifice his own life in order to save the life of another.

PRINCIPLE 3. In cases in which material cooperation is neither clearly illicit because of serious injury to the common good nor clearly illicit because of injury to an innocent third party, but where the action involved is gravely wrong, it is necessary to consider how closely the cooperative act is connected with the principal act. We may distinguish in the following manner.

1. If the cooperative action is very proximate, only a *very grave* reason makes cooperation permissible. Charity forbids cooperation of this kind without a proportionate reason.

Example. A, a druggist, has developed an effective contraceptive which he compounds and packages in his own store.

B, a registered pharmacist, compounds the contraceptive. Only a *very grave* reason would permit B to act as he does.

2. If the cooperation is less proximate, a *grave* reason would allow one to cooperate.

Example. C, a clerk in the same drugstore, sells the contraceptives to those who call for them. If C is in real need of the money he earns as a clerk and cannot obtain other employment, he may remain in his present position. He should, however, find if possible another position in which he would not have to sell such articles.

3. If the cooperation is remote, a *slight* reason would suffice to permit one to cooperate.

Example. In the same drugstore Miss D has charge of the cash register and receives the payments made by customers. She may continue in this position even though she is not in special need of the money that she earns.

In all such cases the ethician would urge individuals to dissociate themselves entirely from activities that are morally wrong, and he would praise the one who suffers severe hardship and inconvenience rather than cooperate in a grave matter with an evildoer. If asked, however, whether in a particular case an individual has an obligation in conscience of refraining from any kind of cooperation, the ethician must answer the question according to sound and accepted principles.

Case 32
Serving as Assistant at an Illicit Operation

Dr. N has been asked to assist at a tubal ligation on a mentally defective woman, the purpose of the operation being to prevent her from bearing defective progeny. Dr. N would find it extremely difficult to avoid lending his assistance at this operation, and refusal might cost him his position. May he, as first assistant to the main surgeon, sponge, suture, and so forth?

Solution. Dr. N may not of course do the actual cutting or ligating of the tubes; but, given a weighty reason, he may as first assistant perform at this operation the actions mentioned above, provided scandal is avoided.

Explanation. Dr. N may never licitly perform the actual sterilization of this patient, for this is intrinsically evil. The actions of sponging and suturing which as first assistant he is called upon to perform are not evil in themselves. Dr. N's help merely facilitates the act of the main surgeon, and this material cooperation on his part may be permitted for a proportionate reason. He does not intend the evil act of sterilization; but because he cannot without grave difficulty avoid performing the services of first assistant, he lends his material cooperation. If Dr. N is not independent but is obliged by his position in the hospital to serve as assistant, it would often happen that there would be no question of scandal if, given a grave reason, he lent his assistance. See "The Avoidance of Scandal," pages 112-13.

Case 33
Avoiding Formal Cooperation in an Abortion

An unmarried girl, 2 months pregnant, comes to Dr. N and tells him that, if her father discovers her condition, he will disown her and drive her from home. Asked to perform an abortion, Dr. N refuses. "If you won't do it," the girl says, "I'll go to Mrs. H, the midwife across the street." Dr. N knows that Mrs. H is very slovenly and that very probably she would cause the girl serious infection and perhaps even bring about her death. Nevertheless he remains adamant in his refusal.

Solution. Dr. N must refuse to perform the abortion.

Explanation. Abortion is a direct and fatal attack on an innocent living human being and must always be looked upon as murder. In the case as described, Dr. N's cooperation would be formal, for it would consist in performing an intrinsically evil action; namely, directly emptying the uterus of a living nonviable fetus. Hence he could under no circumstances be permitted to accede to the girl's request.

Case 34
Cooperating When in a State of Doubt

Dr. B, an intern, is assisting Dr. T, a surgeon, in an operation. During the course of the operation Dr. B begins to doubt about the licitness of the surgery being performed. What should Dr. B do?

Solution. It may be said, in general, that Dr. B may in a case such as this continue without scruple to lend his material cooperation.

Explanation. Material cooperation is licit provided the one who lends his assistance has an upright intention and provided there is present a weighty reason for thus acting. Dr. B's intention in this case is good; and even though the operation were certainly illicit, there would be a weighty reason for his not withdrawing once the surgery has been begun. Besides, it is here doubtful whether the surgical procedure is actually illicit. If Dr. T is a surgeon of sound principles, the presumption would be that he is acting licitly in the present instance. Dr. B should in such circumstances take it for granted that Dr. T is doing nothing irregular.

Case 35
Calling Attention to a Mistake in Surgery

Dr. X, an intern, is assisting Dr. Z, a well-known surgeon, in the operating room. Dr. X notices Dr. Z make a serious mistake during the surgery. Should Dr. X call Dr. Z's attention to the mistake or should he maintain silence?

Solution. Dr. X is obliged in charity to call Dr. Z's attention to the mistake only if all of the three following conditions are verified: (1) if he is certain that Dr. Z's action is a mistake which is gravely injurious to the patient, (2) if calling attention to the incident would save the patient, and (3) if Dr. Z would not resent the intervention and refuse to be guided by what Dr. X says.

Explanation. Dr. X in many cases would not be sure that a mistake had been made, for Dr. Z might have serious reasons for a procedure of which Dr. X could be ignorant. In some cases, too, Dr. X's intervention would not save the patient, for the operating surgeon would merely ignore the interruption. Moreover, it might well be that the mistake could not be remedied, and hence calling the surgeon's attention to it would not undo the wrong. If, moreover, the interruption would cause Dr. X grave harm or other serious evil effects, his obligation to intervene, which is one of charity, would cease to exist. But even though the circumstances of the case may not oblige Dr. X to act, he is nevertheless free to do so.

Case 36
Signing for a Therapeutic Abortion

Dr. D is an attending physician in a hospital which will not permit a therapeutic abortion unless three physicians sign a statement to the effect that the abortion is medically necessary. Dr. D is opposed on moral grounds to therapeutic abortions. May he licitly sign a statement if asked to do so?

Solution. This is a difficult case involving material cooperation to which only a conditional answer can be given. Dr. D may licitly sign the statement if each one of four conditions is verified: (1) that his cooperation is not necessary or indispensable (see page 104); (2) that the statement which he signs is merely a declaration to the effect that the conditions prescribed by the hospital for therapeutic abortions are known to exist in the case in question and not a declaration to the effect that the abortion ought, medically or morally, to be performed; (3) that Dr. D has a well-founded fear that refusal to sign would result in some grave injury to himself, such as the loss of his position as a member of the staff or a serious setback to his professional career; and (4) that his act of signing will not be a cause of scandal.

Explanation. Since Dr. D is opposed on moral grounds to therapeutic abortions, his cooperation would be material and not formal. The act of declaring that certain conditions prescribed by a hospital actually exist in a given case is not evil in itself. Since Dr. D's cooperation is not necessary or indispensable, the injury to himself which he seeks to avert need not be equivalent to the evil to the unborn child, the innocent third party in the case. It is assumed that Dr. D knows that a therapeutic abortion can never be looked upon as medically indicated (see pages 188-205); hence he could not conscientiously sign a statement affirming that the abortion is either medically necessary or morally permissible. The seriousness of the injury to himself, the probability that it will occur, and the certainty that scandal will not result will need careful investigation. Hence we do not by any means wish to affirm that the statement in question could licitly be signed in all cases, nor do we wish to discourage any physician from being faithful to his highest ideals, even at heavy cost to himself. As a matter of fact, it seldom happens today that a physician must suffer for following his conscience. It nevertheless remains true that material cooperation of the kind here described is sometimes licit, and the ethician must admit the possibility that all the necessary conditions might in a rare and unusual case be found to have been fulfilled.

Case 37

Inserting a Diaphragm in a Patient

Dr. B is asked to measure Mrs. K for a diaphragm and to insert this contraceptive device in her vagina. Since Dr. B knows that Mrs. K considers contraceptive measures not only licit but under some circumstances almost mandatory, he is not sure that he may not licitly accede to her request. If he does not do so, he will lose Mrs. K as a patient, and no doubt a few others also.

Solution. Dr. B may not licitly accede to this patient's request.

Explanation. This case involves an application of the doctrine expounded above concerning the act of cooperating in another person's evil action. The evil action of the other person is in the present case the use by Mrs. K of a contraceptive. We know that artificial birth control is of its very nature evil. Fitting a patient with a contraceptive device would be to facilitate her practice of artificial birth control, and therefore it would constitute cooperation in an action evil of its nature. The patient obviously intends to have sexual relations and at the same time to frustrate their natural purpose. If a physician inserted a contraceptive diaphragm, he would be helping the patient to frustrate the law of nature. The fact that Mrs. K has incorrect ideas does not alter Dr. B's duty to avoid cooperating in the objectively evil conduct of another.

Case 38
Instructing a Patient in the Use of Contraceptive Measures

Dr. G, a Catholic physician, is asked by Mrs. C to give her instructions on the best methods of contraception and to supply her with the necessary materials or instruments for this practice. "I am sorry," Dr. G tells her, "but I cannot do this for you. Why not see Dr. T? He and I have different ideas on the subject of contraceptives and I feel sure that he will fix you up."

Solution. Dr. G is guilty of gravely illicit cooperation.

Explanation. The problem in this case pertains to cooperating actually with another in that person's use of contraceptive devices in her marital relations. Dr. G is not permitted to impart to his patients information on the manner of practicing artificial birth control, for this act would be one of cooperation in actions which are intrinsically evil (namely, the patient's contraceptive coitions). It is, moreover, equally true that he is forbidden to recommend the patient to another who will readily give the requested instruction, for so to act would generally involve the desire or the hope on Dr. G's part that the other physician will do what is forbidden, or it would at least facilitate his patient's receiving birth-control instructions. Dr. G should refuse to help on in any manner the spreading of the vice of artificial birth control. He should realize, too, that he can give grave scandal by making suggestions such as the one given in this case, for he would thus lead others to entertain the false idea that the prohibition against artificial birth control is merely an ecclesiastical law binding on Catholics alone.

110

Case 39

Medical Partnership with an Unethical Physician

Dr. B has invited Dr. A to form with him a medical partnership for operating a private clinic. Dr. B is a physician of considerable skill, but he is known to use without hesitation unethical procedures. From a financial point of view Dr. A would gain much from his association with Dr. B, but he wonders whether he would be morally justified in entering into this partnership.

Solution. Assuming that Dr. A could not avoid cooperating with Dr. B's evil actions and that general scandal would be given by his business connections with Dr. B, this medical partnership would not be permissible for him.

Explanation. Let us assume that Dr. B makes it a practice to perform criminal or therapeutic abortions, or to perform contraceptive sterilization, or to fit contraceptive instruments for female patients, but that Dr. A, a religious-minded physician, refuses to engage in such practices. In spite of Dr. A's attitude, is it not likely that Dr. B would demand that, if Dr. A refuses to perform these services, he should at least refer the patients to his legal partner for such help? Dr. A could not do this without being guilty of moral wrong, for he would be persuading the patient to go to one who would undoubtedly perform the illicit operation or action. Thus Dr. A would implicitly approve the evil to be done, and this is never permitted.

If, moreover, Dr. B were known to be one who performs actions that offend against the natural law, Dr. A, his legal partner, would be placed by many in the same category. If Dr. A, a physician who was thought to have a high standard of morality, were thus apparently to give his approval to the evil practices of Dr. B, public scandal would follow. People would conclude that if Dr. A, whom they esteem as a man of sound ethical principles, approved such actions, these actions must be licit. These and other reasons would, in practice, make it almost impossible for Dr. A to become Dr. B's medical partner in the clinic without moral fault.[1]

Case 40

Summoning a Clergyman for a Dying Patient

Dr. V, a Catholic, is asked by his patient, X, to summon a Lutheran minister to his bedside. "I wish him to give me the last rites of the

[1] On the subject of medical partnerships see John J. Lynch, S.J., "A Doctor Wants To Know about Medical Partnerships," *Linacre Quarterly* 21:4-11, February 1954.

church," X explains. Dr. V wonders whether he as a Catholic may do this.

Solution. Dr. V may ask the Lutheran minister to visit X.

Explanation. When a non-Catholic patient asks a Catholic physician to summon for him his minister, the physician may accede to this request. In calling the minister he should merely mention to him the fact that his patient has asked that he be summoned. A Lutheran physician, or a physician of any other faith, is equally permitted to summon a priest for a Catholic patient, even though he is convinced that Catholicism is a form of false worship. While it would be morally wrong for one to participate himself in worship which he is convinced is false, it is not morally wrong for him to summon a minister of that worship to the bedside of a patient in spiritual need who under the circumstances will accept religious assistance only from a minister of his own faith.

THE AVOIDANCE OF SCANDAL

SCANDAL is a sinful or seemingly sinful word, action, or omission which tends to incite or tempt another to sin. It is sufficient if the word, act, or omission *may* induce others to sin, even though the sin does not follow. If one realizes that he is giving scandal, he is accountable for it, even though the scandal does not actually occasion a sin.

Direct Scandal and Indirect Scandal

1. *Direct scandal* is that in which the sin of the other is intended. All those are guilty of direct scandal who seek to corrupt others, to teach them the ways of evil, and to lead them into sin. Direct scandal involves a twofold sin: a sin against charity and a sin against that virtue which the scandalizer attacks. It is a malicious act for which there can never be an excuse.

2. *Indirect scandal* is that in which the other's sin is foreseen but not wished. It may be either illicit or licit.

Indirect scandal is illicit under two circumstances: first if the act giving scandal is in itself morally wrong, and second if the act is in itself good or indifferent but if the one who performs it does not have sufficient reason for acting as he does in circumstances in which he foresees that others will be incited to evil.

Indirect scandal is licit if the act is in itself good or indifferent and if the one performing it has a sufficient reason for acting as he does despite the fact that he foresees others will be incited to evil. It is licit to perform a good or indifferent act if a sufficient reason exists, even though it is foreseen that some will be scandalized. Life would be intolerable if we were obliged to avoid even virtuous actions because of the malice, ignorance, or weakness of others. So far as his own good name is concerned, it is possible for a physician to make himself so well known as a man of high principles that all but the malicious will take it for granted that he has a good reason for everything he does. So far as the weak are concerned, the physician will remember that he cannot safely talk and act in the presence of adolescents as he might talk and act in the presence of his colleagues. Good judgment must govern the physician when there is question of indirect scandal. Direct scandal is an evil thing that can never be condoned.

Case 41
Irreligious and Immoral Magazines in a Reception Room

Dr. M, as is ordinarily done, provides magazines that patients may read while waiting in his reception room. Among these magazines are some that are irreligious, atheistic, or highly suggestive in tone. Dr. M defends his action by saying that his patients include Catholics and non-Catholics, believers and unbelievers.

Solution. Dr. M's practice must be condemned.

Explanation. Reading may be fruitful of good or evil, for the printed word can either help or harm the reader. The law of charity bids us not only to avoid injuring our neighbor, but also to avoid running the risk of doing so. To provide others indiscriminately with reading matter which is obscene, blasphemous, bigoted, or mendacious violates the law of charity. It can be reasonably assumed that, if a physician's waiting room contains dangerous or tainted publications, some of his patients will undoubtedly be harmed by them.

113

Case 42

Referring a Patient to an Abortionist

The patient, 4 months pregnant, is suffering from rheumatic carditis. There had already been a considerable amount of cardiac damage at the time of conception. Dr. N believes that the only way to save her life is to empty the uterus. "I do not perform these operations myself," he informs the patient's husband, "but you could let Dr. X take over the case." Dr. X, he knows, will not hesitate to perform an abortion.

Solution. Dr. N's action is gravely illicit.

Explanation. Dr. N is implicitly inviting the husband to have the abortion performed by Dr. X, for his purpose in suggesting that the husband have Dr. X take over the case is clearly to have this physician empty the uterus. He thus wills the evil act of directly killing the fetus and therefore, objectively, he is guilty of murder.

Case 43

Giving a Harmless Drug as an Abortifacient

The patient asks Dr. J for some drug to produce an abortion. In order to thwart the patient's purpose of killing the fetus Dr. J gives her a harmless medicine and dismisses her. Is his action blameworthy?

Solution. Dr. J may not licitly act in this manner.

Explanation. The patient has made plain to Dr. J her evil intention of killing the fetus. To all appearances the physician approves of her intention, for he does not try to dissuade her from pursuing her plans and he actually gives her a drug which apparently is an abortifacient. The virtue of charity would not permit him to act in this way. The physician is violating his obligation to the human fetus, which is in grave peril. He should make a better effort to prevent death from overtaking the child. He is, moreover, violating his obligation to the patient, for charity demands that he do whatever he reasonably can to persuade her not to procure an abortion. Scandal on the part of others, also, will no doubt arise when the patient tells her friends how Dr. J "helped" her.[2]

Case 44

Instructions on Means of Avoiding Venereal Infection

The physician is asked that he give a 21-year-old male patient complete instructions about the best safeguards against venereal infection. It

[2] See Joseph P. Donovan, C.M., "Doctor Fakes Abortion." *Homiletic and Pastoral Review* 44:213, December 1943.

is evident that the young man intends to engage in illicit and pro-
miscuous sex relations. The physician is in a quandary as to whether
he may impart such information to this individual and give him
· appliances for protecting the genital area.

Solution. The physician in revealing to the young man the preventives
of disease must beware of thus encouraging him to sin. If, however,
he would give no scandal in so acting, the physician may inform the
patient of means which may licitly be used in lawful marital relations
to prevent infection. He must not provide the patient with contraceptive devices. If he can do so without grave inconvenience, the
physician is obliged in charity to endeavor to dissuade the patient
from performing his proposed sinful actions. He could endeavor to
convince him of the fact that illicit sex relations constitute a grave
moral evil and that they militate against future marital happiness, for
those marriages are happiest in which neither party has been guilty
of illicit sexual intercourse.[3]

Explanation. Although the imparting of information about licit means of
avoiding infection is a morally indifferent action, in some cases it
would be interpreted as giving approval to the patient's sinful intention. The physician must guard against such scandal, which would
perhaps be more likely to occur if the physician were known as a
Catholic or a religious-minded non-Catholic. The physician may not
provide the young man with contraceptive instruments, for he would
thus be cooperating materially in sins against nature.

Case 45
Advising Masturbation

The patient is suffering from intense nervous strain. In order to relieve
his nervous tension the physician advises him to practice masturbation at least once a week.

Solution. The physician's advice is gravely illicit.

Explanation. Masturbation is of its very nature evil, and therefore it is
never permitted even though the purpose of the masturbator be
good. Even if the physician judges (without sound medical authority) that self-abuse will relieve a severe nervous condition of the

[3] For a brief but scholarly study of various problems relating to imparting
information about, and distributing means of, preventing venereal infection, see
E. J. Mahoney, *Questions and Answers*, vol. II, *Precepts*, pp. 79-81, n. 407,
"V. D. Prophylactics" (London: Burns Oates and Washbourne, 1949); Donald
A. McGowan, "V. D. a Matter of Moral Conduct," *Linacre Quarterly* 14:1-4,
July 1947.

patient, he may never licitly counsel him to practice masturbation. The intention is good, but the means are evil.

Case 46
Advising Illicit Sexual Intercourse

A young man in his twenties consults Dr. N about his pending marriage. "I am afraid," the patient confides, "that my fiancée and I may not be sexually compatible. I would hate to marry her only to discover that we are not compatible." "Why not test yourself out with her now?" asks Dr. N. "That is the only way in which you can be certain before marriage that you are compatible."

Solution. Dr. N's advice is gravely illicit.

Explanation. The act of marital intercourse is licit only between two persons who are duly married to each other. The fact that a man and woman are engaged to be married gives them no right to the privileges of the married. Hence this patient would be guilty of grave wrong if before marriage he indulged in sexual intercourse with his fiancée. Dr. N, in suggesting that his patient perform this evil action, incurs grave guilt.

Case 47
Discouraging a Patient from Practicing Continence

Dr. Z has carefully examined the patient, a 25-year-old male, and has found nothing organically wrong. "You are extremely nervous," he tells the young man, "and, as your physician, my advice to you is that you have sexual intercourse at least once a week. You need these sexual relations and you can't wait until you get married. Sexual abstinence, you know, is injurious to your general health."[4]

Solution. Dr. Z's advice is gravely illicit.

Explanation. According to the law of nature sexual intercourse is licit between those persons only who are married to each other. The natural law forbids extramarital sex relations, for such conduct is directly opposed to the orderly propagation of the human race. In marriage alone can effective provision be made for the orderly propagation of the race.[5] For one to have the marital act with a person

[4] A case of this type is described in Winfred Overholser, M.D., and Winifred V. Richmond, *Handbook of Psychiatry*, pp. 18-19 (Philadelphia: J. B. Lippincott Company, 1947).

[5] See Edwin F. Healy, S.J., *Marriage Guidance*, pp. 133-35. Chicago: Loyola University Press, 1948.

116

to whom he is not married is a grave wrong against nature. "But," one might ask, "is not fornication a perfectly natural act if it is performed without contraceptive devices? Nature has made the sexual organs for this use." In reply to this question we point out the fact that human beings are made up of both body and soul, of an animal element and of a rational element. The act of fornication does not go counter to the merely animal element in man, it is true, but it does offend, and offend gravely, against man's rational nature. Sexual relations between a man and woman are natural to rational animals (that is, to human beings) only in the married state. Coitus indulged in outside marriage frustrates nature's purpose in endowing human beings with the sex faculty. If a physician advises an unmarried person to engage in an act which nature reserves for the married alone, he is guilty of an attempt to seduce into sin.

No evidence can be adduced in support of the assertion of Dr. Z in Case 47 that sexual abstinence is injurious to one's general health. Authorities of the very highest standing in the field of medicine have testified repeatedly to the fact that sexual continence is in no wise detrimental either to physical or to mental health. We give here the statements of a few well-known physicians.

James Foster Scott, M.D.: ". . . there is yet comfort for the unmarried man in those pages which show that perfect continence is quite compatible with perfect health; and thus a great load is at once lifted from the mind of him who wishes to be conscientious as well as virile and in health, with all the organs of the body performing their proper functions. . . . There is an erroneous and widespread belief that exercise of the sexual functions is necessary to maintain health. . . . It is a pernicious pseudo-physiology which teaches that exercise of the generative functions is necessary in order to maintain one's physical and mental vigor of manhood."[6]

W. R. Gowers, M.D.: "With all the force that any knowledge that I possess can give, and with any authority I may

[6] James Foster Scott, M.D., *The Sexual Instinct*, pp. 39, 95-96, 99. New York: E. B. Treat and Company, 1899.

have, I assert, as the result of long observation and consideration of facts of every kind, that no man ever yet was in the
slightest degree or way better for incontinence; and I am sure,
further, that no man was ever yet anything but better for perfect continence."[7]

William Acton, M.D.: "One argument in favor of incontinence deserves special notice, as it purports to be founded on
physiology. . . . No continent man need be deterred by this
apocryphal fear of atrophy of the testes from living a chaste
life."[8]

Max Huhner, M.D.: "In the following pages I shall endeavor to prove that continence is not detrimental to health,
considered either from a physiological or a psychological standpoint. . . . The sexual organs are constructed upon entirely
different principles than most of the other organs of the body.
They are constructed for intermittent action and their functions may be suspended indefinitely without harm to either
their anatomy or physiology. . . . I sent a circular letter in
1910 to many of the most prominent neurologists in the United
States, asking them if they had ever seen cases of nervous disease which could be attributed to continence. In practically
every case I received the answer that not only did they consider continence physiological, but that they did not believe,
from their experience, that continence ever leads to nervous
disease."[9]

For further quotations which confirm this stand of the
medical authorities cited see Raoul de Guchteneere, *Judgment
on Birth Control*, Chapter 5, "The Medical Aspect of Birth
Control," pages 169-72 (New York: The Macmillan Company,
1931); Edward Roberts Moore, M.D., *The Case against Birth
Control*, pages 43-46 (New York: Century Company, 1931). In

[7] Quoted in Max Huhner, M.D., *Diagnosis and Treatment of Sexual Disorders
in the Male and Female*, p. 344. Philadelphia: F. A. Davis Company, 1945.

[8] *Ibid.*, p. 336.

[9] Max Huhner, M.D., *Diagnosis and Treatment of Sexual Disorders in the
Male and Female*, p. 334. Philadelphia: F. A. Davis Company, 1945.

a comparatively recent (1949) publication Dr. Luigi Scremin records the testimony of some prominent physicians from many different countries who agree that perfect continence or chastity is not detrimental either to mental or to bodily health. Among those quoted are A. Stefani, University of Padua, professor of physiology; H. W. Knipping, Düsseldorf, director of the Medical Polyclinic of the Academy; L. Klotz, Cologne, medical director of the Evangelical Hospital; F. Volhard, Frankfort-on-the-Main, professor of the Medical Clinic of the University; A. Buchholz, Hamburg, professor of psychiatry at the University; M. Weinberger and A. Luger, Vienna, professors of the Medical Clinic of the University; J. Froment, Lyons, professor of the Medical Clinic of the University; A. Chauffard, Paris, professor of the Medical Clinic of the University; J. Pelnar, Prague, professor of the Medical Clinic of the Czech University; K. H. Bouman, Amsterdam, professor of psychiatry at the University; N. M. Popov, Sofia, Bulgaria, professor of psychiatry at the University; R. Vogt, Oslo, professor of psychiatry at the University; D. K. Henderson, Edinburgh, professor of the Psychiatric Clinic of the University; E. Farquhar Buzzard, Oxford, professor of medicine at the University; B. Sachs, New York, professor of the Clinic for Nervous Diseases of Columbia University; Stanley Cobb, Boston, professor of psychiatry at Harvard University.[10]

REFERENCES

Banning, Margaret Culkin. "Case for Chastity." *Reader's Digest* 31:1-10, August 1937.

Bourke, Vernon J. *Ethics*, pt. 2, chap. 11, "Justice and the Persons of Others," pp. 351-65. New York: The Macmillan Company, 1951.

Bouscaren, T. Lincoln, S.J. *Ethics of Ectopic Operations*, "Principle of the Double Effect," pp. 30-38. Milwaukee: Bruce Publishing Company, 1944.

[10] Luigi Scremin, M.D., *Il vizio solitario*, pp. 139-51. Milan: Istituto di Propaganda Libraria, 1949.

Kelly, Gerald, S.J. "The Duty To Preserve Life." *Theological Studies* 12:550-56, December 1951.

—— *Medico-Moral Problems,* pt. 5, "Ordinary Means of Preserving Life," pp. 6-10; "Extraordinary Means of Prolonging Life," pp. 11-15. St. Louis: Catholic Hospital Association of the United States and Canada, 1954.

McFadden, Charles J., O.S.A. *Medical Ethics,* chap. 2, "The Foundations of Morality," pp. 13-45. Philadelphia: F. A. Davis Company, 1951.

O'Donnell, Thomas J., S.J. "Modern Medical and Surgical Means for the Preservation of Life." *Linacre Quarterly* 18:22-31, February 1951.

PROBLEMS CONNECTED WITH SURGERY

S URGERY has already been discussed in Chapter Two, pages 25-26, where we spoke of ghost surgery, and in Chapter Three, pages 72-75, where we spoke of surgical operations as ordinary and as extraordinary means of preserving life. The present chapter discusses the licitness of surgery in general and the moral problems that arise when surgery is used for different purposes. We include all problems except those connected with pregnancy, delivery, and psychiatry, to each of which a separate chapter is devoted.

Oftentimes surgery does not involve the removal of any part of the human body. This is the case, for example, in some operations for hernia or in operations for fractured bones. In many other operations, however, some part of the body is removed, and for this reason we will begin our treatment of the morality of surgical operations with a brief discussion of the ethics of mutilation.

THE ETHICS OF MUTILATION

MUTILATION IS AN ACTION (an excision or the equivalent) by which an organic function or the use of a member of the body is intentionally destroyed either partially or wholly. The action consists of cutting out, crushing, burning, X-raying, or in some such manner directly destroying a part of the human body or of rendering an organ permanently inoperative. The

mutilation may result in the suppression of an organic function—for example, the destruction of one's vision or power of
procreation—or it may consist in the amputation of an arm or
a leg. To strip off skin from the body to use for grafting is not
a mutilation, for in this operation no organic function or member of the body is destroyed. Neither would a blood transfusion, nor a face-lifting operation, nor dental extraction be
considered mutilations in the technical sense of the term. Even
procedures such as these, however, which are not mutilations
in the strict sense of the term, may not be licitly used without
a justifying reason.

The general rule regarding mutilation is this, that mutilation is licit only when necessary for preserving the health of
the whole body. The reason that the scope of justifiable mutilations is thus limited is that man has the supreme ownership
neither of the whole body nor of its various parts, and that he
is therefore not permitted to treat them as though he were the
supreme owner.[1] Man is merely the custodian of his body and
its parts. Directly to destroy the body or one of its parts is to
exercise over that object supreme ownership. One cannot act
more clearly in a manner that implies ownership over a thing
than by destroying it, for by so doing he puts an end to its
very existence.

Mutilation is, however, licit if it is required to conserve the
health of the whole body. To save one's life even at the expense of losing part of the body is the act of a wise adminis-
trator. The whole obviously is better than any single part; and
since God has made us stewards of our bodies, we may presume that He desires that we sacrifice a part of the body if
that is necessary to conserve the rest.

Example. Dr. J, finding that T's foot is gangrenous, orders
him to the hospital in order that he may amputate the foot.
Dr. J's action is perfectly licit.

[1] For proof of the fact that God is the supreme owner of man see *Catholic
Encyclopedia,* article "Suicide."

It is not always necessary, in order that a mutilation be licit, that the part which is excised should be in a pathological condition. If the present state of the body is such that some part of it threatens the life of the whole, that portion of the body may be sacrificed.

Example. Dr. Q is called to the scene of a railroad wreck. The locomotive has overturned and the engineer has suffered severe head and chest injuries. The engineer's foot has been so pinned under part of the locomotive that it will be hours before a crew with acetylene torches can release it. Dr. Q, convinced that the engineer will die unless rushed to a hospital at once, amputates the foot. Dr. Q's action is licit.

THE ETHICS OF SURGERY IN GENERAL

I F AN operation is to be justified morally, it must be necessary, or at least proportionately useful, for the physical well-being of the patient. The graver the danger involved, the greater must be the surgeon's reason for operating. Hence if surgery endangers the life of the patient, it may be performed for a grave reason only. A grave reason would be present if the operation were required to cure a serious ailment or to relieve severe chronic pain. Every major surgical operation must be considered potentially dangerous. In desperate cases a very dangerous operation is licit if there is a genuine (though slight) chance of success, for it is preferable to risk hastening the patient's death than to withhold this last possible remedy.

The physician should as a rule acquaint the patient and his responsible relatives with the degree of danger involved in the proposed surgery and must obtain his consent before proceeding. This consent should be had explicitly when possible; but when this is not feasible, implicit permission will suffice.

The ethician accepts the judgment of the physician to the effect that a certain operation is medically necessary or advisable under given conditions. The only task of the ethician is to decide whether the operation is licit. If there is a conflict of opinion, however, the ethician may adduce evidence to show that the operation is not as necessary as some claim it to be.

Case 48
Dysmenorrhea and Presacral Neurectomy

The patient, a 35-year-old female, is suffering from primary dysmenorrhea. Her physician recommends that presacral neurectomy be done.

Solution. If presacral neurectomy in this case is medically indicated, it is morally permissible.

Explanation. In most cases of dysmenorrhea conservative measures would suffice aɪ l the physician would have no reason for the resection of the presacral nerves. If in severe cases presacral neurectomy is judged to be the most effective remedy, there is no moral objection to its use.

Case 49
Needless Surgery

Miss E, a novelist, plans to write a story about a woman confined to a hospital after surgery. She therefore requests a surgeon to schedule her for an appendectomy and to go through all the steps of the operation except the actual removal of the appendix.

Solution. A reputable surgeon would refuse to be party to such an operation; his action would be illicit if he did perform it.

Explanation. Although this operation would not involve mutilation in the strict sense of the term, there would be something in it approaching mutilation, and also the danger that always accompanies a major operation. Miss E could obtain by means of interviews the information she seeks. Adequate justification for the operation would be lacking.

ALLEVIATIVE SURGERY

WE HAVE said (page 123) that surgery is permissible for the purpose of relieving severe chronic pain. It is also permissible for the purpose of lessening such pain, even in cases in which an organ must be sacrificed.

Case 50
Bilateral Orchiectomy To Alleviate Pain

The patient, 45 years of age, has cancer of the prostate gland. It is certain that he cannot be cured, but the physician requests permission to perform a bilateral orchiectomy for the purpose of relieving the patient's constant suffering.

Solution. This operation is licit if medically indicated.

Explanation. This is a case of remedial sterilization. The purpose of the bilateral orchiectomy is to retard the growth of the malignancy and to alleviate pain.

PREVENTIVE SURGERY

I**T IS** licit to remove an organ or some other part of the body if there is sound reason for believing that the organ or the part is making or can be expected to make the patient's condition notably worse. The application of this principle is illustrated in the following cases.

Case 51

Removal of a Normal Appendix

Dr. T has just removed the patient's infected gall bladder. He would like to remove her appendix also. The latter is in healthy condition but may cause trouble later. May Dr. T do an appendectomy?

Solution. Dr. T may excise the healthy appendix.

Explanation. In removing this organ Dr. T is ridding the body of a probable source of danger. The appendix is relatively unimportant and the threat which its presence involves justifies its removal.

When the abdomen is already open for other surgery the removal of the normal appendix is accomplished with little risk to the patient. If the removal would mean a notable risk to the patient, neither the physician nor the ethician would, ordinarily speaking, approve of it. In cases in which the abdomen is not opened for some other necessary operation, would a surgeon be justified in performing an appendectomy if he is convinced that the appendix is completely healthy? As a rule, there would not be due proportion between the risk incurred and the good hoped for, and therefore the surgery would not be justified. Special circumstances, however, might provide a justifying reason for such an operation. A military leader or a missionary, for example, may be about to leave for a foreign

125

land where medical aid is very difficult to obtain. If he were to be taken down with an acute attack of appendicitis in that country, he would probably die. This unusual circumstance would constitute a sufficient reason for having an appendectomy before his departure abroad, even though the abdomen had to be opened for this surgery only.[2]

Case 52
Orchiectomy in Carcinoma of the Prostate

A young man is suffering from carcinoma of the prostate gland. His testes are in a healthy condition. Because it is known, however, that the androgen secretions of the testes can stimulate further growth of a malignancy, the surgeon, after excising the prostate, wishes to do a bilateral orchiectomy. May he licitly do so?

Solution. He may licitly perform a bilateral orchiectomy if the operation will probably benefit the patient and if it is the most effective therapy available. If less drastic means (for example, treatment by hormones) are available and would be equally effective, bilateral orchiectomy would not be licit.

Explanation. This case is very similar to that of an oophorectomy performed to prevent metastasis. (See Case 79, Preventive Oophorectomy.) Here the continued functioning of the testes would help to spread the cancer and would therefore increase the danger to the life of the patient. Although a complete cure cannot be effected, the patient is helped greatly by the cessation of the endocrine functioning of the testes. In cases where the physician judges that bilateral orchiectomy is indicated, the operation may be licitly performed. The fact that the patient's testes are in a healthy condition does not alter the licitness of the operation. These organs are judged to be a present source of danger to the body, and therefore they may be sacrificed for the good of the whole.[3]

[2] See Gerald Kelly, S.J., *Medico-Moral Problems*, pt. 1, pp. 35-39, and pt. 4, pp. 38-41. St. Louis: Catholic Hospital Association of the United States and Canada, 1948-1949, 1952.

[3] Pius XII, in an address to the delegates present at an Italian urology congress, declared that the removal of the testes is licit when this is necessary to cure a grave ailment or to prevent metastasis. See *Acta Apostolicae Sedis* 45:674-75, October 8, 1953. See also John J. Clifford, S.J., "The Morality of Castration for Carcinoma of the Prostate," *Theological Studies* 5:439-52, December 1944.

Case 53
Bilateral Vasectomy To Prevent Epididymitis

The patient, a male 75 years of age, has been subjected to a prostatectomy. In conjunction with the operation on the prostate gland the
surgeon wishes to do a bilateral vasectomy. His reason for the bilateral vasectomy is to prevent danger of epididymitis. May the surgeon
perform the bilateral vasectomy in order to prevent epididymitis?

Solution. The bilateral vasectomy may in this case be licitly performed.

Explanation. The infection of the epididymis which is termed epididymitis is not in itself dangerous, but it is quite painful and would
necessitate several weeks of confinement in bed. The bilateral vasectomy in this case has as its object, not rendering the man incapable
of producing offspring, but rather cutting off the path by which infection might travel down to the epididymis. The purpose of the operation, then, is not contraceptive, nor is the operation in itself evil.
Whether or not it is licit in a particular case will depend upon
whether or not there is present a reason which is grave enough to
compensate for the actual loss of fertility in the patient. Hence we
must distinguish various types of patients, for the loss experienced
would not be as great in an old man who is probably sterile as in a
young man who is probably fertile. The operation, then, is licit if
the physician judges that the consequences of not operating would
be sufficiently grave. It rests with him to decide whether in a particular case there is due proportion between the patient's loss of
potency and the danger of epididymitis. The physician's intention
in performing the bilateral vasectomy must of course never be to
render the patient incapable of producing offspring. In all cases,
where possible, the consent of the patient should be had before the
vasectomy is performed.

Case 54
Bilateral Vasectomy for Benign Prostatic Hypertrophy

The patient, a man of 60, has a benign prostatic hypertrophy. After
doing a prostatectomy the surgeon wishes to perform in addition a
bilateral vasectomy.

Solution. If the bilateral vasectomy is necessary to prevent epididymitis
and there is no less drastic means of prophylaxis, the surgeon may
perform this operation.

Explanation. The averting of epididymitis is a sufficiently grave reason
for permitting this patient to be deprived of the capacity to generate

offspring. The patient is no longer in the younger age group; consequently there seems to be a due proportion between the loss suffered and the danger averted.[4]

Case 55
Circumcision of Newborn Males

Dr. J makes it a practice to circumcise all male infants shortly after birth. He says that this is merely routine procedure and that it is recommended by most competent physicians.

Solution. Unless there is a positive indication for circumcision, the operation should be omitted.

Explanation. It has been said that too many physicians practice routine circumcision and give little thought to the complications that can result.[5] In by far the majority of the operations, it is true, there have been no serious complications, but in some cases severe hemorrhage and infection have developed from the surgery. Unsightly scars, too, have at times resulted. To expose an infant to such dangers, though they be remote, would not be justified unless there were present a compensating reason. If the prepuce cannot be retracted, there would of course in most cases be a sufficient reason for operating. In premature babies, or in those not gaining weight as they should, or in

---

[4] During the year 1949 twenty-five physicians, mostly urologists, were consulted on the question of permitting routine vasectomy with prostatectomy. The conclusions drawn from the survey were: "(1) *Routine* vasectomy should not be done with prostatectomy when the subject is in the younger age group (e.g., the early fifties). With men in this group, the vasectomy should be limited to cases in which there is some special reason for it, e.g., general debilitated condition, previous history of infection, etc. (2) In other cases, despite the availability of the new drugs, routine vasectomy on the occasion of prostatectomy is not clearly wrong, but limitation of the practice should be encouraged." See Gerald Kelly, S.J., "Notes on Moral Theology. Fifth Commandment," *Theological Studies* 11:43-44, March 1950; *Hospital Progress* 30:218-20, July 1949; Gerald Kelly, S.J., *Medico-Moral Problems*, pt. 2, "Vasectomy with Prostatectomy," pp. 35-41 (St. Louis: Catholic Hospital Association of the United States and Canada, 1950).

[5] "Large percentage of cases are done unnecessarily—some harmfully. If no real redundancy of prepuce, and only simple adhesions, best handled by daily retraction (at bath time) for 10 to 14 days following birth" (Charles O. McCormick, M.D., *A Textbook on Pathology of Labor, the Puerperium and the Newborn*, second edition, pp. 351-52. St. Louis: C. V. Mosby Company, 1947). See also Henricus J. Stander, M.D., *Williams Obstetrics*, eighth edition, p. 800 (New York: D. Appleton-Century Company, 1941); H. Close Hesseltine, M.D., "Circumcision," *Journal of the American Medical Association* 140:368, May 21, 1949.

those suffering from a blood disease or some infection, there would hardly be sufficient reason to run the risks involved. Some physicians, it seems, circumcise all male infants, and their motive appears to be mercenary. Such physicians act in a manner unworthy of their high calling.

CORRECTIVE SURGERY

B Y CORRECTIVE surgery we understand in this place sur- gery directed toward correcting the defects of nature or surgery rendered necessary by defects of nature. The cases include the removal of superfluous or distorted members, oper- ations on Siamese twins, operations for hermaphroditism, and the production of an artificial vagina.

Case 56
Removal of a Second Pair of Legs

A baby girl is born with an extra pair of legs growing from her epigas- trium. In order to rid the girl of this abnormality the surgeon excises the extra members.

Solution. The excision of the extra legs is licit.

Explanation. A parasitic member or form, which is certainly not a sep- arate human person, has no right to life in itself. If it notably inter- feres with the good of the individual upon whom it has fastened itself, it may be sacrificed without scruple.

Case 57
Amputation of a Distorted Leg

A girl, 10 years of age, has been crippled from birth. Her right leg is badly shrunken and twisted, so that she requires the use of crutches habitually. The surgeon wishes to amputate the leg just above the knee, so that she may, with the help of a prosthetic leg, lead a more normal life.[6]

Solution. The amputation of the right leg is justified.

Explanation. In amputating the leg the surgeon is cutting off a part of the body which is not only useless but a positive hindrance to the girl's leading a normal life. As it is at present, the leg cannot fulfill its primary purpose. The distorted limb prevents the girl from joining

[6] A case somewhat similar to the present one is described in "Improvised Bone Bank," *Time* 58:71, October 15, 1951.

129

her playmates in their recreational activities. With the aid of a prosthetic leg the girl can walk without crutches, dance, and play some games. Thus the surgeon's act is aimed at supplying for a defect, or at remedying nature, and is rightly regarded as licit.

Case 58
Separation of Twins United at Vertebral Column

At birth twins were normal except that they were united at the vertebral column. All their vital organs were completely separated. The surgeon suggested an operation that would sever the connecting link and let them live individual lives. This surgery, however, might kill one or both twins. Would the surgeon be justified in performing such an operation?

Solution. If there is good reason for judging that the operation will be successful, it may be licitly performed.

Explanation. The surgeon's purpose in performing this operation is certainly beyond reproach. He wishes to separate these two persons so that each will not be a constant and very grave burden to the other. Without surgical intervention their lives cannot be normal. The surgeon's action is not intrinsically evil, for the operation is aimed at remedying a defect of nature. The good result envisioned by the surgeon (the separation of the bodies) is not caused by the evil result (the exposing of the twins to the danger of death). There is, finally, a proportionate reason for thus exposing the twins to the danger involved.

Case 59
Separation of Siamese Twins To Prevent Infection

A and B are Siamese twins who are obviously distinct individuals but whose bodies are united at the sternum. Twin A becomes infected with a fulminating bacteremia which will almost certainly prove fatal. Unless the twins are separated by surgery before the death of Twin A, Twin B will also die. May the surgeon now perform the necessary operation?

Solution. If the operation would kill Twin A, it may not be licitly performed. If the operation would not be fatal to A but would merely put his life in graver danger than is now present, the surgery may licitly be performed. A's consent to the operation should if possible be obtained beforehand.

Explanation. If the operation is of such a nature that it would kill Twin A, it would be equivalently murder, and murder, an act evil in itself, may never licitly be employed even though the purpose for which it is committed is most noble. In the event that the operation to sever the twins unexpectedly proved fatal to Twin A, the surgeon, in order to save Twin B, would have to wait until Twin A died and then separate his body from that of Twin B. If, however, the operation of severing the two bodies would not prove fatal to Twin A but would merely expose him to very grave danger of death, it would be justified by the application of the principle of the twofold effect. In such circumstances the surgery is not directly destructive of life and the good effect, the saving of Twin B, fully compensates for the added danger to which Twin A is exposed. It is assumed in this case that antibiotics have proved ineffective or that they are for some reason unobtainable.

Case 60
Craniopagus Parietalis

Siamese twins, 5 months old, were united at the top of the head. They clearly acted independently in eating, in sleeping, in bowel and bladder functions, and had individual body temperatures. The state of their health was good. The surgeons, at the parents' request, undertook to separate the heads. Most painstaking preparations were made and preliminary surgery of an exploratory character was performed. In the final operation, however, it was found that the infants shared a common sagittal sinus. In order to accomplish the separation this sagittal sinus would have to be given either to one or to the other. The superior sagittal sinus is a major vein through which blood flows from the brain to the heart. The surgeons completed the separation of the heads, the superior sagittal sinus being given to the stronger twin. Was the complete separation of these twins licit?

Solution. Insofar as the surgeons judged that there were sound medical reasons for assuming that the twin who was deprived of this venous channel could survive, the surgery can be justified.

Explanation. The surgery from the beginning was intended to aid the twins; for if they were to lead normal lives, the heads had to be separated. The intention of the surgeons, therefore, was most praiseworthy and they proceeded most carefully with the exploratory surgery. When the surgeons, explicitly authorized by the parents to make the choice, decided to give the superior sagittal sinus to the stronger twin, they had very sound medical reasons for concluding that the other blood vessels in the other twin would suffice to perform the work of the absent sagittal sinus. The separation involved merely the danger that one of the twins would die, and therefore, given a proportionately grave reason for permitting such risk (and a proportionate reason was surely present in this case), the surgery was licit. As has been explained in the treatise on the twofold effect (see pages 94-101), where the action itself is not evil, where the evil effect is neither intended nor directly produced, and where the good effect compensates for the evil one, the operation may be licitly performed. In the case of Siamese twins the great physical good which separation would effect compensates for even a grave risk to life.[7]

Let us alter the circumstances of Case 60. Let us suppose that medical research has established, by means of animal experimentation, the fact that it is impossible to live without a certain organ which Siamese twins share in common. If one twin is deprived of it, he cannot possibly survive. In that event the surgeon is not permitted to deprive one twin of this essential part or organ so that the other may live a separate life. He may not even begin the surgery, for it is illicit to inflict a fatal blow on one person, even to save the life of another. The fact that the "donor" twin is weaker and therefore less likely to grow to maturity would not alter the application of this principle, for the weaker twin possesses a right equal to that of the stronger one to the ownership of that common part or organ. If an exploratory operation is being made, surgery should go no further when it becomes known that complete separation would directly cause the death of one of the twins and the surgeon can only suture the incisions and leave the twins joined.

Let us assume that the physicians are convinced that the weaker twin cannot live long in any event. If separation is not effected within a few weeks, the risk to the stronger will be greatly increased. A physician may find it difficult to understand why it would not be licit, or even preferable, to sacrifice the weaker twin (whose life would thus be but slightly shortened), in order to save the life of the stronger. Thus at least one life would be safeguarded. All that can be said is this, that such surgery would violate the right of the weaker twin. Both have an equal right to the essential organ or part, which cannot be taken away from either one without inflicting a deathblow. There are circumstances in which it is not morally wrong to permit death by refraining from doing what might be done to

[7] For the description of a case of surgery of this kind see Herbert J. Grossman, M.D., and others, "Surgical Separation in Craniopagus," *Journal of the American Medical Association* 153:201-07, September 19, 1953.

prevent it, but there are no circumstances in which it is permissible to take positive measures to inflict death upon an innocent person. Once admit the principle that individuals are free to decide when an innocent person may be deprived of his right to life, and no one's life will be safe. The observance of the natural law oftentimes involves sacrifices, but these are insignificant in comparison with the suffering that mankind would be forced to endure if justice were abandoned as a norm of conduct and supplanted by expediency.

Case 61
Surgery To Correct Hermaphroditism

A 5-year-old patient was found to be an hermaphrodite. The characteristics of both sexes seemed to be equally developed. The surgeon consulted the parents about the case, and when they expressed a preference that the child be a girl, he removed its male organs.[8] Was his action licit?

Solution. If the male sex organs were but rudimentary and the child was very probably female, the surgeon acted licitly. He did well in consulting the parents to ascertain their wishes in the matter, for it was their right to make the choice.

Explanation. In this case the surgeon's act was merely that of remedying nature's defect in giving the child both male and female sex organs.[9]

Now possible To Accurately determine Sex by one Test,

There are various types of hermaphroditism which can present moral problems, and the surgeon should understand clearly what is permitted in each case. We shall, then, define and analyze the morality of corrective surgery in four distinct types of hermaphroditism.

1. *Complex hermaphroditism* is the existence in the same individual of the internal and external organs of both sexes.[10]

[8] An interesting study of the medical aspects of such cases was made by Frank Hinman, Jr., M.D. See "Advisability of Surgical Reversal of Sex in Female Pseudohermaphroditism," *Journal of the American Medical Association* 146:423-29, June 2, 1951.

[9] Dr. Ombredanne of the French Academy of Medicine presents some interesting cases of this in Peter Flood, O.S.B., M.D., editor, *New Problems in Medical Ethics,* Second Study, "The Marriage of Hermaphrodites," pp. 50-57 (Cork: Mercier Press, 1953).

[10] The definitions are taken from W. A. Newman Dorland, M.D., *The American Illustrated Medical Dictionary,* twenty-second edition, p. 671 (Philadelphia: W. B. Saunders Company, 1951).

There seems to be no well-authenticated record of any person who possessed both male and female internal and external organs of sex which were fully and normally developed. There have been of course some cases where an additional set of sex organs was present in a rudimentary state. Given, however, such a case as that of complex hermaphroditism, the subject may licitly have removed all the sex organs of the sex which he is rejecting. He has the right to place himself definitely in one of the two categories in which all human beings are as a rule placed by nature. He has the right to be either male or female. Once, however, his choice is made and he has been relieved of the supernumerary structure, he must adhere to that sex in his way of living.

2. *Dimidiate or lateral hermaphroditism* is that in which the organs of one side are male and of the other female. If in this case both the female and the male sex organs are normally developed, the hermaphrodite may reject the one sex and choose the other, as was said in no. 1. If, however, one side (for example, the female) is undeveloped and the other (the male) developed, he must choose the developed sex.

3. *Transverse hermaphroditism* is that in which the outward organs appear to be of one sex and the internal ones of the other. Sex is determined essentially by the presence of the ovaries or the testes. Hence in this type of hermaphroditism the sex of the individual must be looked upon as determined by the fact that there are present healthy, normal ovaries or healthy, normal testes. A female outlook, for example, in one who is anatomically male, as may occur in the case of transvestism, would not give the individual the right to have surgery employed to make him resemble anatomically a female.

4. *Unilateral hermaphroditism* occurs when one side has an ovary or a testis and the other has both an ovary and a testis, or an ovotestis. In this case the hermaphrodite must retain, on the abnormally endowed side, the corresponding ovary or testis which matches the one on the other side, though the super-

134

numerary organ of the other sex may be removed. If, for example, the person has on one side an ovary and a testis and on the other side an ovary, the testis may be removed, but the matching ovaries must be left intact, for they indicate that the prevailing sex of the patient is female.

Case 62
Psychic Hermaphroditism or Transvestism

John, 29 years of age, is married and the father of two children, but he nevertheless requests his physician to perform the surgery and prescribe the medications required "for making him a female." John asserts that, although his genitalia are undoubtedly male and of normal development, his outlook is entirely female. He now wishes, as he says, "to be changed into a woman." The physician, whose examination of the patient convinces him that John is a transvestite, wonders about the ethics of such "corrective" surgery.

Solution. Such surgery would be gravely illicit from the moral viewpoint and in some countries it would be illegal as well.

Explanation. John clearly belongs to the male sex, for his genitalia are certainly masculine and he is the father of children. Excising the testes and the penis would constitute a grave mutilation of the human body. As was said above (see page 122), mutilation is licit only when it is necessary to preserve the body's health or integrity or when the conditions required for the licit transplantation of organs, as explained on pages 139-41, are verified. In the present case there is no question of diseased organs; hence such surgery would be gravely wrong.

A further interesting question arises in connection with Case 62, just discussed. If a surgeon did remove John's genitalia, would John, who contends that he has a female mind or soul, be justified in comporting himself as a female? If, moreover, he were not married, could he licitly enter the state of matrimony with a man? First of all, we may observe that one whom nature clearly places in the category of male or female cannot alter this fact. He or she will always remain a member of his or her natural sex. In the case of a natural male such as John, it is true that the sex organs can be excised, an artificial vagina can be created by means of surgery, and the breasts can be somewhat altered by means of a female sex hormone. These alterations in the body, however, do not change a male into a female. Such an emasculated man should not then masquerade as a woman. Like other adult male transvestites, John is a man and has no right to mingle with others in a woman's disguise. To do so would no doubt create for John occasions of sinning and would be a source of constant scandal to others who knew the facts. After such surgery, moreover, he would be able to marry no one. He could not marry a woman, for he would be impotent because he cannot perform the natural functions of the husband in the marital act; nor could he marry a man, for he himself is still a member of the male sex.

Some cases such as this one have recently come to the attention of surgeons. "One leading London endocrinologist whom we have consulted has told our Special Correspondent that, within a few days of the publication of the recent so-called change from a man into a woman, he received twelve requests from men who want to be changed into women. Some of his colleagues have received similar requests. All have, as far as we know, been refused.

"A Danish surgeon who has performed some of these operations received no less than 465 demands for his assistance, after the details of one of his cases were published in the lay Press."[11]

Case 63
Surgery To Produce an Artificial Vagina

During the course of a premarital physical examination Ann is found to lack a vagina. An exploratory operation discloses the fact that she has no ovaries, tubes, or uterus. Deprived of a vagina, Ann obviously cannot validly marry, for she is incapable of performing the marriage act. Her physician offers to create a vagina in her by means of sur-

---

[11] "The Facts about Sex Changes," *Intelligence Digest Supplement*, p. 10, May 1954. See also Frederic G. Worden, M.D., and James T. Marsh, Ph.D., "Psychological Factors in Men Seeking Sex Transformation," *Journal of the American Medical Association* 157:1292-98, April 9, 1955.

gery. In the place where the vagina should be he would make an incision of sufficient length and width. To prevent the walls of the opening from growing together again after the operation he would use an obturator. When the walls of the wound were completely healed the obturator would be withdrawn, and the opening would have the form and appearance of a vagina. May the surgeon perform this operation? Once the operation is performed, may Ann marry?

Solution. This operation may be licitly performed. Once it is performed, it seems that Ann may licitly marry. She is obliged in charity, however, to notify her fiancé of her abnormality.[12]

Explanation. This operation may rightly be regarded as the act of remedying nature. Nature failed to give Ann a vagina. In order to make up for this deficiency, the surgeon supplies her with as close an imitation of the natural organ as is possible. The channel is of the same size as those produced by nature and it is located in the same place in the body as are natural vaginas. Moreover, it can perform, though imperfectly, the function of a vagina in regard to the marital act, and a woman is considered impotent only if she is unable to have sexual intercourse.

It is of course not certain that a woman with a surgically created vagina is not impotent. In spite of what was said in Case 63 about this operation's being a remedying of nature, the new opening is not a natural vagina. Hence it is doubtful whether the woman may be considered potent. Certainly she can never conceive, for the new vaginal passageway is entirely closed off at the inner end. The semen can go no further than where it was discharged. Since, however, only impotency which is certain is a barrier to marriage, Ann's condition seems to be no impediment to her marrying. Because, however, some may consider such a woman certainly impotent, Ann's pastor may feel obliged to consult the local bishop before assisting at the marriage.[13]

[12] For some interesting observations on the artificial vagina see John C. Ford, S.J., "Notes on Moral Theology. Marriage," *Theological Studies* 5:533-34, December 1944; Peter Flood, O.S.B., M.D., editor, *New Problems in Medical Ethics*, pp. 58-60 (Cork: Mercier Press, 1953).

[13] See *Codex juris canonici,* Canon 1031, 1, n. 3. Roma: Typis Polyglottis Vaticanis, 1936.

There are cases where the vagina is very rudimentary or where the woman has an infantile vagina. An operation to remedy such conditions would not differ, morally speaking, from the one which we have discussed in the case of Ann.

SURGERY TO IMPROVE PERSONAL APPEARANCE

THERE are no moral objections to plastic surgery in general. In some cases it is not only permissible but almost a necessity. A man whose nose has been badly damaged in an accident would be offensive to others, would live in a state of constant embarrassment, and would be handicapped in making a living if he did not have his nose reconstructed. Moral issues can arise, however, if the defect or blemish is not serious and if the operation involves danger.

Case 64
Removal of a Mole

The patient, a 16-year-old girl, has a very ugly mole on her neck. Her physician tells her that it can very easily be removed, but she doubts whether it is permissible for her to undergo such an operation merely for the sake of her personal appearance.

Solution. If the operation would appreciably increase the attractiveness of the girl, there would be sufficient reason for any risk involved, and hence the operation would be licit.

Explanation. Removing from the facial area a blemish that appreciably detracts from her beauty is for a woman a matter of no little importance. Hence the good which is sought would compensate for the risk of the evil effect which might result. There is some danger in even so simple an operation.

Case 65
Removal of a Healthy Breast

The physician finds that the patient's left breast had, for some reason unknown to him, already been excised. The patient, an unmarried woman 23 years of age, asks that the other breast be removed. Her reason for desiring this operation is in order that the upper portion of her body may be symmetrical. Would the physician be justified in operating for this reason?

Solution. The reason here given would not justify the surgery desired.

Explanation. In this case it is assumed that the right breast is in healthy
condition. The removal of the breast is not necessary for the good of
the body. To excise this organ would mean the suppression of a
function which nature intends for nourishing babies. Hence this
operation would be a mutilation. Merely to make the woman's body
more attractive in appearance would not constitute a proportionately
grave reason for destroying this organ.

THE TRANSPLANTATION OF ORGANS

BECAUSE of the rapid advances in surgical practice within
recent years, work has been accomplished in the transplantation of organs that would have been considered impossible a century ago. The most notable success has probably
been achieved in the transplantation of corneas from dead
bodies to living persons. When there is question of transplanting to a living person the healthy kidney of a person who has
just died or transplanting an ovary from a living woman to the
body of a friend whose ovaries are diseased and must be removed, the medical profession seems in general to be skeptical
concerning the results that can be expected. The ethician,
however, is not concerned with the success of such transplantations. Successful or not, they are being undertaken, and it
may be anticipated that they will be undertaken more and
more frequently in the future. It is therefore the responsibility
of the ethician to define the conditions under which transplantations are licit.

Man is a social being destined to live, not as a hermit, but
as a member of society. In order to perfect his nature man
stands in need of his fellow men. He requires their cooperation
to provide for his physical, intellectual, and spiritual needs.
Since such is his nature, it is evident that man has an obligation to assist his fellow men in their needs. He can render such
assistance in very many ways, one of which might be to sacrifice a part of his own body for the sake of another. Ethically,
the question is how far the individual may go in this respect.

To answer this question some theologians have distinguished between what they term the primary purpose and the secondary purpose for which man was given a body. The primary purpose of man's body and of all the parts of his body, they say, is to aid the individual in the prosecution of the end for which he was created. The secondary purpose is to aid other individuals in the prosecution of the same end. The existence of this secondary purpose is immediately evident. If man has an obligation of helping others, he may use his body in doing so.

The first way in which one can use his body to help others is by working for them. This of course presents no moral difficulty. One can then go further by giving a blood transfusion or by sacrificing some of his skin if skin is needed for grafting. Blood transfusions, skin grafting, and bone grafting present no difficulty. Finally, one can go to the length of giving one of his organs to another. This involves mutilation, or the impairment of bodily integrity. Some ethicians have indicated two general principles by which they judge the morality of the transplantation of an organ from one living person to another. Their first principle states no one may sacrifice the substantial integrity of his body to help another. Their second principle permits the loss of nonsubstantial integrity if there is present a proportionately grave reason. Let us examine the morality of these two principles.

When these ethicians state that the substantial integrity of man's body may not be sacrificed, they mean that no organic function may be suppressed entirely. When they say that nonsubstantial integrity may be sacrificed, they mean that the partial curtailment of a function is licit. The loss of nonsubstantial integrity can occur only in the case of double organs such as the eyes and the ovaries; for if a single organ such as the liver were sacrificed, there would be a complete cessation of function and a loss of substantial integrity. There would also be a loss of substantial integrity if *both* of two double organs such as the ovaries were excised for a transplantation, since the result would be a complete suppression of the organic function of these organs.

All moralists concede that transplantations which cost the donor his substantial integrity are illicit, for they directly and completely frustrate the purpose for which the organs in question were given. Certainly nature primarily intended that these organs should function for the benefit of the one to whom she gave them. The complete suppression of an organic function would go directly counter to its natural destiny. Are transplantations licit when they do not cost the donor his substantial integrity? Recently Pius XII spoke to a group of oculists about corneal transplants, and in this address he denied the validity of one of the arguments which some ethicians had used to prove the licitness of certain transplantations.[14] Because of the pope's words one may judge that the opinion which would permit transplants from a living person, even though they did not cost the donor substantial integrity, is in disfavor.[15]

The transplanting of organs from the body of a dead person to a living man or woman offers no moral difficulty. Obviously the natural primary purpose of all the organs of a dead person has been achieved during his life. After his death they can no longer serve that individual. They may, however, still be capable of serving the secondary purpose for which nature destined them; namely, to benefit other human beings. It is therefore licit to transplant any organs, double or single, from a corpse to a living body. The practice of removing the cornea from a person immediately after his death and grafting it to the organ of a blind man is highly commendable. The work

[14] *L'Osservatore Romano*, 14-15 Maggio 1956, p. 1, num. 112 (29.174).
[15] For discussions of the morality of transplantations see Bert J. Cunningham, *The Morality of Organic Transplantation* (Washington: Catholic University of America, 1944); Gerald Kelly, S.J., "Current Theology," *Theological Studies* 8:97-101, March 1947; Gerald Kelly, S.J., *Medico-Moral Problems*, pt. 3, "Organic Transplantation," pp. 22-28 (St. Louis: Catholic Hospital Association of the United States and Canada, 1951); John McCarthy, "The Morality of Organic Transplantation," *Irish Ecclesiastical Record* 67:192-98, March 1946.

that is being done by the Eye-Bank for Sight Restoration is therefore praiseworthy. Moreover, a living person may donate for transplantation the healthy cornea of an eye which is already blind because of some other incurably defective part of the organ, for this surgery would not destroy nor even diminish the function of vision in the donor.

Case 66
Ovarian Transplant

M, a married woman 25 years of age, had an oophorectomy several years ago but is now very eager to have children. Her physician assures her that it is possible to transplant an ovary from another woman's body into her own and that she would then probably be able to bear children.[16] Before beginning to look for a possible donor, M wonders whether such a mutilation would be licit.

Solution. An ovary obtained from a recently deceased person may be licitly transplanted.

Explanation. The act of excising the ovary or ovaries from a recently deceased woman is obviously licit, for the organs of that person have already fully completed their primary purpose of serving the one who owned them.

What was said in Case 66 of the morality of the gonadal transplant in the female may be applied to the transplantation of a testis from a male. The removal for this purpose of both testes from a deceased person may be permitted.

AUTOPSIES

A N AUTOPSY is the surgical examination of a human body after death in order to determine the exact cause of the death and to increase medical knowledge. If one is to succeed in discovering hidden diseases or sources of infection, post-

---

[16] Medical records apparently show only one case in which an ovary was transplanted from A to B and in which B became pregnant with an ovum from the transplanted organ and gave birth to a living child. See Robert T. Morris, M.D., "A Case of Heteroplastic Ovarian Grafting, Followed by Pregnancy, and the Delivery of a Living Child," *Medical Record* 69:697, May 5, 1906. See also "Transplantation of Ovaries," *Journal of the American Medical Association* 137:756, June 19, 1948.

[handwritten margin note: Morally ok but not possible medically at present]

mortem examinations are necessary. Even highly skilled physicians who have at their disposal the best in modern scientific equipment at times err in their diagnoses or are unable to determine the cause of death, and only an autopsy discloses the true cause of the patient's death. There is no doubt that much of the progress made in the field of medicine has been due to post-mortem examinations.

There is no law of the Catholic Church which prohibits autopsies. Catholics should, in general, permit an autopsy if the physician asks that it be done. A physician will not be inclined to request permission to perform an autopsy unless he has a very good reason for doing so. Post-mortem examinations, in addition to increasing medical knowledge in general, often give the family of the deceased the comfort of knowing that everything possible was done for him.

A post-mortem examination may not be begun until the patient is certainly dead. Care must be taken to avoid disfiguring the face and head of the corpse in any manner. Moreover, undue delay in returning the corpse to the home for the wake must be guarded against. In these delicate matters the feelings of the mourning relatives should not be overlooked. Physicians in general show themselves most prudent and considerate in this matter.

ANIMAL EXPERIMENTATION OR VIVISECTION

ANIMAL experimentation or, as it is more commonly called, vivisection, may be defined as experimentation on living animals, for the advancement of medical sciences, by means of drugs, ligatures, surgery, and so forth. "The methods of vivisection vary almost infinitely in severity: they include momentary and almost painless inoculations with a needle-syringe; serious surgical operations for the study of internal organs like the heart, lungs, or other viscera; experiments involving nothing but variations in environmental temperature; verification of the physiological effects of drugs; feeding experiments in

143

controlled conditions; and many others."[17] Is there any moral objection to the use of such experimentation?

Brute beasts have no rights. They were created by God merely for man's use. Their lives are completely at the disposal of man. They were brought into existence in order to help man to achieve his ultimate end in life. If, when dead, they accomplish this purpose more effectively, man may kill them. Man, then, is perfectly free to use them to provide for his pleasure (for example, through horseback riding, in circus performances, in hunting), to furnish food and clothing, to ease the burden of his labors (for example, through watchdogs). One of man's most destructive enemies is disease, and the medical research laboratories are ever seeking preventives against and remedies for this enemy. To this end much experimentation is required. Tests of new drugs and surgical methods must be made. If human beings are not to be needlessly endangered, these tests must first be made on animals. Most of the modern therapies, which have proved to be so great an improvement on the old methods, were developed and evaluated through experimentation on animals. Insulin, used in the treatment of diabetes, and adrenal cortical extracts, used to treat Addison's disease, were discovered by experiments on dogs. It was animal experimentation that led to today's effective treatment of tetanus and rabies, of pneumonia and scarlet fever, of anemia and syphilis. It was animal experimentation that aided so greatly in teaching us how to prevent smallpox, yellow fever, cholera, and bubonic plague.

Vivisection is therefore in itself licit. It uses animals for one of the purposes for which they were created. There are, however, occasional abuses which accompany the practice of vivisection. It sometimes happens, for example, that, although an anesthesia is indicated, this means is not employed to deaden the animal's pain. Other forms of cruelty, too, have been manifested in the treatment of the animals used for experimenta-

---

[17] *British Universities Encyclopedia,* vol. X, p. 452.

tion. Cruelty toward animals has a brutalizing effect on the offender, for it tends to make him less sensitive to human suffering and may lead him to indulge in cruelty toward his neighbor. The torturing of animals is at times motivated by sadism. It can happen, too, that those who make use of vivisection encourage, wittingly or unwittingly, sins of theft. Because they purchase dogs and cats for laboratory work without questioning the seller, they may as a result receive animals which have been stolen from their owners by children who are eager to make a little pocket money. To preclude such unwitting cooperation in thefts of this kind, reputable laboratories make it a practice to examine, insofar as possible, the title of ownership of those who offer animals for sale. Apart from the possible abuses here described, vivisection involves no moral problem and may be freely practiced without fault.[18]

REFERENCES

Ficarra, Bernard J., M.D. *Newer Ethical Problems in Medicine and Surgery,* chap. 11, "Autopsies," pp. 117-27. Westminster: Newman Press, 1951.

Kelly, Gerald, S.J. "Pope Pius XII and the Principle of Totality." *Theological Studies* 16:373-96, September 1955.

---

[18] For material on the morality of vivisection see John McCarthy, "The Morality of Vivisection," *Irish Ecclesiastical Record* 71:266-68, March 1949.

Chapter FIVE

Moral problems connected with pregnancy and delivery are discussed in the two following chapters. We are here concerned with certain other medical problems with moral implications. In some cases there is question of what the physician himself may licitly do; in other cases there is question of the extent to which he is free to cooperate by suggestion, advice, or instruction.

STERILITY TESTS

It HAPPENS TODAY quite frequently that a husband and wife who earnestly desire to have children find their marital relations unfruitful. The cause of the sterility may be a condition existing either in the husband or in the wife or in both.[1] Medical authorities recommend that the husband's semen be examined before the wife is given a sterility test, since this

---

[1] For a scholarly presentation of the standard procedures used in modern infertility studies see Joseph B. Doyle, M.D., "The Role of the Gynecologist," *Linacre Quarterly* 21:40-44, May 1954. Dr. Doyle, director of the Infertility Clinic of St. Elizabeth's Hospital, Boston, states: "It has been estimated that there are three million childless couples in the United States. If they would persevere with medical planning for parenthood, five hundred thousand of these couples would find their heart's desire." Concrete data on cases in which fertility was restored or spermatogenesis improved are found in S. J. Glass, M.D., and M. L. Lazarus, M.D., "Improved Fertility and Prevention of Abortion after Nutritional-Hormonal Therapy," *Journal of the American Medical Association* 154:908-10, March 13, 1954.

procedure is easier as a rule and less expensive. In a large proportion of the cases, moreover, it has been found that the male semen was the offending factor. The question therefore arises as to whether the methods of obtaining a sample of the male semen accord with the principles of the natural law. Some ways in which the semen sample is obtained are illicit, some are licit.

Illicit Methods of Obtaining Semen Samples

1. *Masturbation.* The sex organs are intended by nature to be used in placing acts which are directly conducive to the orderly propagation of the human race. The natural receptacle for the husband's seed is the vagina of his wife. Nature forbids his deliberately spilling the semen outside this organ. Self-abuse, therefore, even though it be indulged in for a good purpose, violates the law of nature. It is of its substance evil and in no set of circumstances is it ever permissible.[2]

2. *Contraceptive Devices.* The use of an imperforated condom or the equivalent during sexual intercourse is a direct frustration of the act of coitus, and therefore directly violates the natural law.

3. *Withdrawal.* For the husband to engage in sexual union with his wife until he is on the verge of orgasm and then to withdraw the penis from the vagina so that he may discharge the semen into a glass receptacle is, like masturbation, a direct frustration of nature and is gravely illicit.

Licit Methods of Obtaining Semen Samples

1. *Stripping the Seminal Vesicles of Their Contents by Massaging These Organs.* In this process of causing the fluid

---

[2] The following decision will be of interest to Catholic physicians: "The Holy Office was asked: Whether direct masturbation is permitted for the purpose of obtaining semen for the scientific detection of the contagious disease 'blenorragia,' and its cure. *Reply.* In the negative" (T. Lincoln Bouscaren, S.J., *The Canon Law Digest*, vol. I, p. 156. Milwaukee: Bruce Publishing Company, 1934).

of the vesicle to ooze out into the urethral canal so that the semen can be collected at the urethral meatus, the generative faculty is not set in motion, and hence there is no direct frustration of nature. Removing the fluid is equivalent to removing, for a good reason, other fluids of the body (for example, blood or bile) in a measure that causes no physical harm.

2. *After Coitus, Removing from the Vagina a Part of the Semen.* The portion of the deposit which is removed must be such as not to interfere substantially with the purpose intended by nature in the act of sexual intercourse.

It would not be permissible to remove from the vagina the whole deposit of semen immediately after coitus, for this would apparently constitute a direct and substantial frustration of nature. Some of the semen probably enters the uterus during coitus, but as a rule the quantity would be small. It is now thought by some physicians that a generous quantity of semen is required properly to condition and prepare the ovum for impregnation.[3] This opinion, though solidly probable, cannot be looked upon as certain, and therefore physicians are not obliged to be governed by the opinion in making their moral judgments. Precisely how much of the semen would suffice to fertilize an ovum if the required conditions are present is a medical question, and therefore one that the physician himself must answer.

---

[3] "Whether nature has been needlessly abundant in producing so many million sperm per ejaculate to fertilize but one egg is still a philosophic question. However, more and more evidence seems to indicate that a fairly large number of sperm are required to reach the egg before fertilization will occur. The work of Rowlands and others on hyaluronidase gives support to the view that some enzyme such as hyaluronidase is transported by the sperm to the egg, and must be present at the site of fertilization in adequate amounts to facilitate penetration of the egg. There is support of this view in observations on lower animals, in which a large excess of sperm is known to be needed for fertilization" (Edward T. Tyler, M.D., and Sheldon Payne, M.D., "Spermatogenesis and the Therapy of Infertility," *Journal of the American Medical Association* 134:770-74, June 28, 1947). See also I. W. Rowlands, "Capacity of Hyaluronidase To Increase the Fertilizing Power of Sperm," *Nature* 154:332, September 9, 1944.

3. *The Use of a Perforated Condom during Coitus.* The perforation must be large enough to permit the greater part of the ejaculation to reach the female genital tract, for otherwise the coitus would be substantially contraceptive and unnatural. After intercourse the semen which remains in the condom is collected. This semen, together with that clinging to the penis and the remnant extracted from the urethral canal, should provide enough for the test. Because the chemicals present in the processed rubber may exert a deleterious effect on the semen, some physicians do not favor the use of the perforated condom. To obviate this difficulty the perforated caecum of an animal (for example, a sheep) might be used.

4. *The Vaginal Cup.* The vaginal cup is used after normal coitus to cover the os vaginae so as to prevent the semen from leaving the female organ. After a time this cup is removed and the seed which has collected in it serves as a specimen.

5. *Testicular Biopsy.* A small fleck of tissue is removed from the testis and is examined for live sperm. The removal of semen from the testis or epididymis, though perhaps medically less satisfactory, is morally unobjectionable.

6. *The Cervical Spoon.* Before normal coitus the cervical spoon is inserted in the vagina so that the cup of the instrument lies immediately under the os uteri. After one hour the spoon is withdrawn and its contents examined. The remnants of the seed which are thus removed from the vagina would not appreciably increase the probability of fertilization were they left in the organ; and therefore the removal, which does not substantially interfere with nature's purpose in the coitus, is permitted for a good reason.[4]

[4] For material on this subject see John J. Clifford, S.J., "Sterility Tests and Their Morality," *Ecclesiastical Review* 107:358-67, November 1942; Joseph B. Doyle, M.D., "The Cervical Spoon: An Aid to Spermigration and Semen Sampling," *Bulletin of the New England Medical Center* 10:225-31, October 1948; William Kevin Glover, S.M., *Artificial Insemination among Human Beings* (Washington: Catholic University of America, 1948); John McCarthy, "A Lawful Method of Procuring Seminal Specimens for Sterility Tests," *Irish Ecclesiastical Record* 70:533-36, June 1948.

As regards the morality of medically analyzing a specimen of semen which was probably obtained by means of a gravely immoral action, it may be stated that a physician or a technician of a clinic is free to disregard the manner in which the semen was procured from the patient and that he need make no inquiry about the manner in which the semen specimen was obtained. Provided the analysis does not implicitly approve an immoral method of procuring the seminal specimen (for example, by means of masturbation) or does not incite another to such methods, the action of the physician or technician is licit. If he requests a semen specimen for a patient, he should indicate licit methods of obtaining the sample.

The Female and Infertility

The more common sterility tests which are currently employed on female patients involve no moral problem. Cervical and vaginal smears and their analysis, insufflation of the Fallopian tubes, and biopsy (where there is no danger of interfering with probable pregnancy)—none of these measures need be discussed by the moralist. If a physician judges that culdotomy or culdoscopy involves no appreciable risk of surgical damage, he is free to employ these measures. If, moreover, there is danger that this surgery will injure an internal organ and there is no other method of obtaining equally satisfactory results, the physician may with the patient's consent do a culdotomy or culdoscopy.[5]

ARTIFICIAL INSEMINATION

WHAT is to be said of the morality of artificially inseminating a woman? Must one distinguish between the case of a married woman and that of the unmarried? May a wife be licitly impregnated artificially by the seed of a man who is not

[5] See Joseph B. Doyle, M.D., "Exploratory Culdotomy for Observation of Tubo-Ovarian Physiology at Ovulation Time," *Fertility and Sterility* 2:475-86, November-December 1951; John J. Lynch, S.J., "Some Moral Phases of Infertility Problems," *Linacre Quarterly* 21:53-63, May 1954.

her husband? These are questions which, in the light of modern practice, assume not a little importance. In all the following cases let us assume that the semen has been obtained in a manner that is not in itself evil.

Donor Insemination

There is no reason which could be adduced to justify the artificial insemination of a married woman with the semen of one who is not her husband. The following considerations indicate the evil nature of such an act.

1. By virtue of the matrimonial contract a wife has the right to sexual intercourse with her husband. This right is exclusive and inalienable. Neither she nor her husband may confer upon another man a share in that right. Hence, even with her husband's consent, she is not permitted to have coitus with another man.

The act of artificially inseminating a woman partakes of the nature of a generative act. The wife has not the right to indulge in the generative act except with her own husband. Hence a wife may not permit herself to be inseminated artificially with the semen of one who is not her husband. The semen, moreover, is of its nature an integral part of coitus. A wife has no right at all to coitus with one who is not her husband, and therefore she has no right to receive into her genital tract another's semen, an integral part of coitus.

2. The practice of artificial insemination would be opposed to the good of marriage. Once conceded the right, even by their own husbands, to be inseminated artificially by the seed of some other man, wives would in many cases conclude that it would be preferable to receive the seed into their body in the natural way; namely, by normal sexual intercourse. Thus adulteries would be multiplied immeasurably.

3. Because husband and wife see a reflection of themselves and of each other in their own child, the child who is the fruit of normal marital intercourse forms a loving bond between

151

father and mother which unites their hearts very strongly. The child born of artificial insemination by the semen of a man not the mother's husband might easily become a source of discord in the home. This danger would be present even though the husband had consented to the process, for he would look upon it as another man's child.

4. Legal difficulties might arise in regard to legacies. "Technically, a child born as the result of artificial insemination is no more legitimate than one born following adultery of the wife consented to by the husband. It is always possible that at some future date a relative aware of the circumstances may attack the child's right to an inheritance from the foster father."[6] The *Journal of the American Medical Association* declared in an editorial: "The fact that the husband has freely consented to the artificial insemination does not have a bearing on the question of the child's legitimacy. If it did, by similar reasoning it might be urged that the fact that a husband had consented to the commission of adultery by his wife would legitimatize the issue resulting from the adulterous connection."[7] In the past, cases have occurred where the mother of the "test-tube" baby claimed part of the legacy of the deceased man who had provided the semen. Today, because the donor's identity is most carefully hidden from the wife and husband and because, occasionally at least, the semen of two donors is mixed together prior to the insemination, the danger of such civil suits is slight.

On December 12, 1954, Judge Gibson E. Gorman of the Superior Court, Chicago, Illinois, ruled that if the semen used in the artificial insemination of a married woman is not that of her husband, from the legal point of view the woman is guilty of adultery and the child thus begotten is illegitimate. The decree reads, in part, as follows:

[6] James R. Rosen, M.D., "Artificial Insemination." *Medical Economics* 20:51, January 1943.

[7] "Artificial Insemination and Illegitimacy." *Journal of the American Medical Association* 112:1832-33, May 6, 1939.

"Heterologous Artificial Insemination (when the specimen of semen used is obtained from a third party or donor) with or without the consent of the husband, is contrary to public policy and good morals, and constitutes adultery on the part of the mother. A child so conceived is not a child born in wedlock and is therefore illegitimate."[8]

5. Artificial insemination by the same donors in the same region gives rise to the danger that half-brothers and half-sisters will marry one another without their being aware of the blood relationship which exists between them. Mrs. X, for example, is artificially inseminated with the semen of Q and bears a boy. Mrs. Y, artificially impregnated with Q's semen, bears a girl. If Mrs. X's boy one day marries Mrs. Y's girl, it will be a marriage of half-brother with half-sister, for both children have the same father.

It is illicit, also, for an unmarried woman to permit herself to be artificially inseminated. An unmarried woman has no right to engage in sexual intercourse with anyone, and consequently she has no right to receive into her genital tract the male sperm. All artificial insemination, then, which is performed on an unmarried woman is immoral.

Husband Insemination

It is illicit for a wife to permit herself to be artificially inseminated by the semen of her own husband. By virtue of the matrimonial contract the wife has a right to sexual relations with her husband and with him alone. She has a right to those

[8] Quoted from the declaratory judgment of the judge of the Superior Court of Cook County in the case of Mary B. Doornbos *vs.* George Doornbos, No. 54S.14981. Reference to the case will be found in *New World* 72:1, December 17, 1954. It should be noted that this court decision does not settle the question with absolute finality. Edwin J. Holman, himself a member of the bar, speaks as follows: "There is little that can be said with any degree of assurance concerning the medicolegal aspects of artificial insemination, for such aspects have not been explored satisfactorily by any court of appellate jurisdiction in the United States" (Edwin J. Holman, "Medicolegal Aspects of Sterilization, Artificial Insemination, and Abortion." *Journal of the American Medical Association* 156:1309-11, December 4, 1954).

acts which of their nature are directed toward the begetting of offspring. These acts are sexual intercourse and the preparatory love play which precedes sexual intercourse. Artificial insemination is an act which takes place outside natural coitus and is in no way directed toward the sexual union of the husband and wife. Hence the wife has no right to permit herself to be the object of such an act. This type of artificial insemination was condemned by Pope Pius XII as objectionable.[9]

From an analysis of human nature we may with reason judge that God intended that children come into the world as the expression of love of two individuals for each other. He wished the human, not the scientific, reproduction of human beings. Science might be an aid to the human act of sexual congress; it was not intended, however, to be a substitute for the act. Marriage was to be a human, not an industrial, society. Although the primary purpose of marriage is procreation, that procreation must always be the result of a human act. Artificial insemination would dehumanize the family society and reduce it to the level of an industrial society.

It is permissible for a physician, however, after husband and wife have rightly performed the marital act, artificially to propel the semen deposited in the vagina into the uterus and Fallopian tubes, for the physician's act in this case would consist merely in aiding nature. To accomplish this he may use a syringe, syphon the semen from the vagina, and at once project it into the uterus and tubes. There is in the action momentary interference with the ordinary process of nature, it is true; but the interference is directly aimed at rendering that particular intercourse fruitful and in no sense may it be viewed as a frustration of nature. This process is rightly called, not artificial, but assistant, insemination.

Another mode of aiding the insemination of the wife is the use of the cervical spoon. (See page 149, no. 6.) The use of

[9] Pius XII, "Address to the Fourth International Convention of Catholic Doctors, September 29, 1949." *Catholic Mind* 48:250-53, April 1950.

the cervical spoon is intended to facilitate the passage of the semen into the uterus after sexual intercourse. There is no objection on moral grounds to the use of this method.

The Use of Douches after Coitus

Physicians are asked at times by married women about the use of a vaginal douche after sexual intercourse. Frequent douching of the vagina after the marital act destroys the protective secretions in the vaginal tract and tends to cause the tissues to dry up and become irritated. Hence, unless there is present some pathological discharge, vaginal douching is as a rule not indicated.

Some wives, however, "for hygienic reasons," as they say, wish to make use of douching after intercourse. May they licitly do so? The first point that must be stressed in reply to this question is that the woman must not make use of douching in order to endeavor to prevent conception, even though the douche consists merely of plain water. In such an action the wife's intention would be to frustrate nature, and this evil intention would render her action sinful. Let us suppose, however, that the wife's purpose is not contraceptive but solely one of cleanliness. Even in that event, she may not wash out the vagina immediately after the marital act. Such a douche would be gravely illicit. In the marital act there are three phases to consider: (1) the injecting of the semen into the vagina (and perhaps into the uterus), (2) the passage of the deposited semen into the uterus and into the uterine tubes, and (3) possible impregnation of an ovum by a spermatozoon. It is the first phase only which depends upon man's activity. The second and third phases take place independently of man's cooperation; they are the work of nature alone. When a wife uses a vaginal douche immediately after intercourse, she interferes with phases two and three. Even though her intention in so acting were not evil, she may not licitly use the douche unless, in accordance with the doctrine of the principle of the twofold effect, there is a proportionately grave reason which would compensate for the permitted (but not directly intended) frustration of nature. An illustration of such licit use of the douche is the case in which the vagina is gravely diseased or is causing great pain and requires constant douching. In this event, if there is no equally effective treatment available which would not destroy the semen, the wife is justified in employing the douche as usual. She may even do so, if necessary, immediately after sexual intercourse. Her intention in employing the douche must of course be, not to destroy the semen, but to heal the vaginal infection.

It does not follow, however, that a wife, after allowing a certain length of time to elapse, may never licitly wash out a healthy vagina after she has indulged in the marital act. After nature has been accorded sufficient time to accomplish her task, the vagina may be licitly cleansed of all remnants of the deposited semen. It is morally permissible to wash out the wife's vagina one hour after the sexual act has been performed, for the remnants of the male ejaculation which are then present, if left in the vagina, would not appreciably increase the probability of impregnation. Hence, for a reasonable cause, these remnants may be licitly removed. Hygienic reasons would justify their removal.

The morality of the use of douches when a woman has been raped is discussed in Chapter Eight, pages 275-78.

ARTIFICIAL BIRTH CONTROL

ARTIFICIAL birth control is the attempt by the use of unnatural means to prevent conception from resulting from the marital act. The means employed to achieve this end are either the voluntary interruption of the act or the use of contraceptive jellies, tablets, powders, or germicidal douches; mechanical devices such as condoms, diaphragms, and cervical caps; spermatoxin and hormonal injections; X-raying of the ovaries or testes; the cauterization, ligature, and cutting of the

Fallopian tubes or the vasa deferentia, and other such measures. The purpose of all such measures is to make it possible for individuals to enjoy the pleasure of sexual intercourse without exposing themselves to the risk of suffering any of the inconvenience that may result from the conception and birth of children.[10]

Artificial birth control is of its very nature evil, for it consists in performing a natural act (sexual intercourse) and at the same time attempting to destroy the natural effect of that act. For this reason artificial birth control is a practice which is opposed to nature. It is evil because it perverts the natural faculty. It must be judged to be gravely evil because it perverts the natural faculty on which depends the survival of the human race. On the reproductive faculty depends the procreation of human beings. There is no other way of peopling the world than through the use of this God-given power. To claim that God has left men free to prevent the natural consequences of the marriage act is to represent Him as willing to set aside His desire that the human race survive. Artificial birth control prevents the procreation of children and is therefore directly and seriously opposed to the purposes that God had in creating man, in making man male and female, and in making the family the foundation of social life. To permit artificial birth control would be to threaten the human race with extinction. If there are any acts which reason tells us must be gravely displeasing to God because they are opposed to the natural law, artificial birth control must be placed in this category because it is so direct a frustration of the purposes of God in a matter of the greatest moment.

[10] For the views of some physicians see Bernard J. Ficarra, M.D., *Newer Ethical Problems in Medicine and Surgery,* chap. 7, "Contraception," pp. 31-46 (Westminster: Newman Press, 1951); Joseph L. McGoldrick, M.D., "The A.M.A. and Birth Control," *Linacre Quarterly* 15:9-12, April 1948; Frederick W. Rice, M.D., "A Catholic Physician's Views on Family Limitation," *Ecclesiastical Review* 103:60-67, July 1940; Charles Leavitt Sullivan, M.D., "The Case against Birth Control," *Linacre Quarterly* 16:16-27, July 1949.

If there were any doubt about the matter, it would be resolved, for Catholics at least, by the statement of Pope Pius XI, who says:

"Any use whatsoever of matrimony exercised in such a way that the act is deliberately frustrated in its natural power to generate life is an offense against the law of God and of nature, and those who indulge in such are branded with the guilt of a grave sin."[11]

It is clear, therefore, that one who indulges in artificial birth control commits a grave sin against nature. Even a very grave reason would not justify this practice, whether followed regularly or only for a time. Even if the physician were to judge that marital intercourse would renew an infection of the wife's genital area (for example, in a case of trichomonal vaginitis), the use of the condom would still be gravely wrong. Hence neither extreme poverty, nor certain danger of death to the wife if she bears another child, nor any other consideration could ever make the practice licit.

"No reason, however grave, may be put forward by which anything intrinsically against nature may become conformable to nature and morally good. Since, therefore, the conjugal act is destined primarily by nature for the begetting of children, those who in exercising it deliberately frustrate its natural power and purpose sin against nature and commit a deed which is shameful and intrinsically vicious."[12]

Moral theologians unanimously agree that artificial birth control gravely offends God, and that it can in no circumstances be indulged in without grave sin.

Answers to Arguments in Defense of Birth Control

"But artificial birth control," one may object, "is no more unnatural than walking on one's hands, cutting one's nails, or

[11] Pius XI, *Christian Marriage*. In *Five Great Encyclicals*, p. 93. New York: Paulist Press, 1939.
[12] *Ibid.*, p. 92.

giving a person a haircut. Surely no one would contend that such actions as these are an abuse of nature. To be logical, then, one must admit that birth control is not an abuse of nature." To this objection we reply that abusing a natural faculty means to use it in a manner which destroys or directly hinders the purpose which nature intended that faculty to accomplish. Walking on the hands is merely putting the hands to a use in addition to the one for which they were primarily created. This operation is in no way frustrating nature. Paring one's fingernails or trimming one's hair in no wise interferes with the accomplishment of the purpose assigned by nature to these parts. None of these operations, therefore, may be reasonably called a frustration of nature.

"But," one may object, "the mutual happiness of husband and wife is one of the purposes of the matrimonial contract. Why, then, may they not practice birth control if their happiness could not otherwise be assured?" In reply we point out that some of the ends of the matrimonial contract are primary, some secondary. The secondary purposes must, in the order of nature, be essentially subordinated to the primary purposes of marriage. To act in such a way that the secondary purpose takes precedence over the primary purpose is obviously an abuse of nature. The primary purposes of marriage are the generation and the education of offspring. The secondary purposes of marriage are the allaying of concupiscence and the mutual help and love and happiness of both parties. To frustrate the primary purpose by engaging in artificial birth control in order to secure one of the secondary purposes of marriage is directly opposed to the dictates of the natural law.

Some social workers endeavor to justify the practice of artificial birth control on economic grounds. This practice will, they contend, greatly benefit the poor by helping them to avoid bringing into the world more children than they can afford to rear. But this argument in favor of birth control is based on obviously false reasoning, for the standard by which we judge whether or not an action is morally good does not consist in this, that it produces or fails to produce materially beneficial results. If this were to be the norm of a virtuous action, then perjury, suicide, and murder would at times be accounted virtuous.

Ever since the latter part of the eighteenth century, and especially within recent years, there have been those who contended that the time is not distant when the world will be unable to produce and to permit the distribution of enough food to provide the ever-increasing population with adequate diet. "Famine, disease, late marriages, and war," they assert, "will not check the population sufficiently; the true solution to this vexing problem is the artificial limitation of offspring through contraceptive practices." The Planned Parenthood Federation of America has been active in disseminating publications which foster this attitude.[13]

The arguments of these alarmists, however, regarding the world's alleged inability to provide adequately for its inhabitants are scientifically incorrect. It has been demonstrated that this earth is indeed physically able to feed the estimated population of many years to come.[14] In order to do this present waste in food will have to be avoided, the land which is now being farmed will have to be cultivated more efficiently, and new areas of arable land must be farmed. In *The World's Hunger* Frank Pearson and Floyd Harper say: "The requirements of nature for food production are so rigid that thus far

---

[13] Some of the publications at one time distributed by Planned Parenthood Federation of America are: *Too Many People*, by C. Lester Walker (New York: Harper and Brothers, 1948), who proposes birth control as a solution to overpopulation; *The Road to Survival*, by William Vogt (New York: William Sloane, Associates, 1948), which explains Planned Parenthood's role in meeting the threat of overpopulation; *The World Has Too Many People*, by Guy Irving Burch (*American Magazine* 141:38-39, 103-04, May 1946), who claims to know why so many in the world at present go hungry.

[14] See Clarence Enzler and the Subcommittee on Agriculture, *Can the World Feed Itself?* Washington: The Catholic Association for International Peace, 1950.

man has been able to use only a small proportion of the earth's land surface and has been defeated in most of his attempts to extend his boundaries."[15] To this claim Dr. Robert M. Salter, chief of the Bureau of Plant Industry, Soils and Agricultural Engineering of the United States Department of Agriculture, replies as follows: "At present only 7-10 per cent of the total world land area is cultivated. Except for some desert areas, perpetual snow and ice, tundra, and the most rugged mountains, there is virtually no limit to the acreage that can be brought into cultivation."[16]

Case 67
Refraining from Admonishing Patient Practicing Birth Control

Dr. X discovers that his patient in good faith has been practicing birth control. Must he inform her of its intrinsic evil?

Solution. Unless his silence in the matter would under the circumstances cause scandal because, for example, it can be foreseen that silence will be interpreted as approval, Dr. X need not inform the patient of the true nature of birth control.

Explanation. In this case we have the question of the possible duty to correct one's neighbor whose action is materially sinful. A private individual such as Dr. X in this case is obliged to give fraternal correction only when (1) the other person is in grave spiritual need, and (2) no one else can give it more fittingly, and (3) it is foreseen that the correction will be taken in good part, and (4) the correction can be given without grave inconvenience. All these conditions are in practice rarely verified. A physician is accounted a private individual in regard to the giving of spiritual advice. If, then, Dr. X could not impart the information without grave difficulty (because, for example, of the fear of causing resentment or anger with conse-

[15] Frank A. Pearson and Floyd A. Harper, *The World's Hunger*, p. 50. Ithaca: Cornell University Press, 1945.

[16] Robert M. Salter, "World Soil and Fertilizer Resources in Relation to Food Needs," *Science* 105:535, May 23, 1947. See also Jacob Rosin and Max Eastman, *The Road to Abundance* (New York: McGraw-Hill Book Company, 1953); Joseph C. Keeley, "Chlorella: Key to World Plenty," *Coronet* 35:32-34, February 1954; Grant Cannon, "Nitrogen Will Feed Us," *Atlantic Monthly* 192:50-53, September 1953; Norman Carlisle and Madelyn Carlisle, "Super-Animals for Super-Foods," *Coronet* 35:79-82, December 1953.

quent unfavorable criticism of him to other patients), he need not correct the patient's false conscience. If there is little hope that she would reform, he should say nothing.

Case 68
Recommending Artificial Birth Control

Dr. M has attended Mrs. C during her last two childbirths. "You must absolutely avoid having another baby," he warns her. "Another pregnancy will almost certainly mean your death. You had better persuade your husband to use artificial birth control in the future. Your children still need you, and for their sake at least you must not risk your life in this matter."

Solution. Dr. M is guilty of grave sin when he advises the practice of artificial birth control.

Explanation. If Dr. M is convinced that another pregnancy will cost Mrs. C her life, he is certainly justified in drawing her attention to this danger. He may not, however, licitly counsel as a means of avoiding the danger methods which are directly opposed to the law of nature. Artificial birth control is intrinsically evil. For the sake of her children who need her loving care Mrs. C should employ every licit means possible to conserve her health, but artificial birth control is not a licit means. Prior to her duty toward her children are Mrs. C's obligations toward God. She must do His will. His claims come first and His will requires that she avoid all violations of the natural law. With regard to Dr. M's prediction that the next pregnancy will bring death to Mrs. C, Dr. McGoldrick's statement (pages 196-97) is worthy of careful study.[17]

THE USE OF RHYTHM

R HYTHM is a practice by which the marital act is restricted, for the purpose of avoiding offspring, to the nonfertile periods of the wife. This practice is based on the theory that the period of a woman's ovulation can be determined with reasonable accuracy. This period of ovulation means the time when a mature ovum or egg cell is released from the ovary and passes into the female genital tract.[18] When the mature

[17] For a bibliography on artificial birth control see pp. 168-69.

[18] Facts concerning ovulation with which every physician is well acquainted are included for the benefit of the nonprofessional reader.

ovum appears there it can, for some hours at least, be fertilized by the male spermatozoon. The time during which the ovum can be impregnated is called the fertile period of the woman.

Competent medical authority teaches that the period of ovulation comes in cycles; that is, ovulation appears regularly at certain intervals. The space of time between the ovulations, however, differs in different women. The interval may consist of twenty-four days in one, of twenty-eight days in another, and of thirty or thirty-two days in a third. Determining the exact length of the interval between the end of one ovulation and the beginning of the next is essential to the successful practice of the rhythm theory. Because there is a biological connection between ovulation and the menstrual flow, knowledge of the time of the latter can aid in computing the time of the former.

Rhythm cannot be looked upon as a certain method of avoiding offspring. It provides at most only great probability of securing the desired results, but the extent of this probability varies with individual cases, and the outcome is sometimes definitely disappointing. The lack of certainty results from (1) the fact that it is difficult to be sure of the strict regularity of a particular woman's ovulation periods and (2) the fact that fertilization at times occurs during the periods which this theory regards as absolutely sterile.

The Morality of Rhythm

With regard to the use of rhythm two important questions arise. The first question has to do with the validity of the marriage when one or both parties contract marriage with the intention of using rhythm—that is, of restricting intercourse to the sterile periods. The second question has to do with the licitness of the use of rhythm in the married state. Because of their importance we shall analyze these two questions in detail.

1. *The Validity of the Marriage.* "It may be that at least one of the parties in contracting matrimony had the intention

to restrict the matrimonial *right,* and not only its *use,* to the periods of sterility; with the result that the other party would not have even the right to request intercourse at other times. In such a case there would be an essential defect in the matrimonial consent, involving the invalidity of the marriage itself, since the right that springs from the matrimonial contract is a permanent and uninterrupted right, belonging to each party in respect of the other."[19] In a valid matrimonial contract each party freely accords to the other the right to the use of his body in regard to those acts which are of a nature to produce offspring; namely, in regard to sexual intercourse. The contractual right thus given by the parties to each other must be permanent and uninterrupted. If at the time of the marriage either party intends to put time limits to that right—if, for example, he intends to accord that right only during the sterile periods of the wife—then he is not giving to the other party the true right of the matrimonial contract; and since this right pertains to the essence of matrimony, the marriage of the two parties is not a true or valid marriage.

2. *The Licitness of the Use of Rhythm in Marriage.* "But it may be that this limitation of intercourse to the periods of natural sterility does not relate to the right itself, but only to the use of the right. If this is so, the validity of the marriage is beyond question. But how far is such conduct of the parties morally permissible? The answer will depend on the motives on which their intention constantly to observe the sterile periods is based. Are these motives from a moral point of view sufficient and secure? The mere fact that the parties are not offending against the nature of the act, and that they are also prepared to accept and rear any offspring which may be born in spite of their precautions, would not alone suffice to guarantee the rightness of their intention and the unimpeachable morality of their motives.

[19] "Address of Pope Pius XII to the Italian Catholic Union of Midwives, 29 October 1951." *Clergy Review* 36:389, December 1951.

"The reason is that matrimony obliges to a state of life which, while carrying with it certain rights, also imposes the fulfillment of a positive work connected with that state of life. . . . Now upon the parties who make use of this right by the specific act of their state, nature and the Creator impose the function of providing for the conservation of the human race. . . . It follows from this that to enter upon the state of matrimony, to make constant use of the faculty proper to it and only in matrimony allowable, and on the other hand consistently and deliberately, and without a serious reason, to shirk the primary duty it imposes, would be to sin against the very meaning of married life.

"From the obligation of making this positive contribution it is possible to be exempt, for a long time and even for the whole duration of married life, if there are serious reasons, such as those often provided in the so-called 'indications' of the medical, eugenical, economic and social order. It therefore follows that the observance of the infertile periods may be *licit* from the moral point of view; and under the conditions mentioned it is so in fact. Nevertheless, in the absence—according to a reasonable and equitable judgment—of similar serious reasons, whether personal or circumstantial, the intention of married people to avoid habitually the fecundity of their union, while continuing to give full satisfaction to their sensual desires, can be based only on a false outlook on life or on motives that are foreign to true ethical standards."[20]

The use of rhythm can be sinful, also, if it unjustly deprives either the husband or the wife of the marital act when he or she earnestly and reasonably requests it outside the sterile periods. In this case the sin could be a grave one. If, moreover, either husband or wife cannot chastely observe the restraints involved in such periodic continence and one or the other is in proximate danger of sinning because of the limited periods

[20] *Ibid.*, pp. 389-90.

to which rhythm restricts sexual relations, the use of rhythm is illicit.

The morality, then, of an agreement between husband and wife to employ the rhythm theory in their marital relations may be briefly stated as follows. (1) If its use involves unjustly depriving one party of the marital act or placing either party in the proximate danger of serious sin, it would be gravely illicit. (2) If a couple already have several (that is, three or more) children, they have already substantially fulfilled their obligation to look to the propagation of the human race. Hence for them the use of rhythm would in itself be lawful. If, however, they do not have any reasonable cause for their desire to prevent the birth of more children, the practice of rhythm would usually involve venial sin because of the slightly sinful motive (for example, selfishness, avarice). (3) If a couple as yet have no children but intend to have several at some time in the future, the practice of rhythm for them would not be gravely sinful. Their motive in thus deferring the fulfillment of the obligation to propagate the race could be venially sinful. (4) If a childless couple were, without any excusing reason, to employ rhythm throughout the entire period of their married life, this would seem to be seriously sinful. This apparently is the common teaching of ethicians today, although there are some few who contend that the practice in the case here described would not in itself be gravely sinful.

Any of the following reasons would justify a married couple in employing rhythm for as long a period of time as the reason endures (even for the whole of married life): (1) Pregnancy will create for the mother either danger of death or danger of serious injury to her health. (2) All the children born to the mother will very probably be stillborn or will inherit a serious defect. (3) Very grave difficulty would be encountered by the parents in supporting more than the present family. Reasons which are less grave than these would justify the practice of rhythm for a short time. If one is in doubt about the sufficiency of his reason in this matter, he should consult a spiritual adviser.

Ordinarily speaking, when a couple practice rhythm their reason is to endeavor to avoid offspring. There is, however, another purpose which can be served by use of rhythm. Knowledge of the exact date of ovulation will often enable a married couple to determine the time when sexual relations are most likely to bring about a pregnancy. Rhythm's findings, then, may be of great help to married parties whose sexual unions have proved unfruitful and who desire to have children.[21]

BASAL BODY TEMPERATURE

WOMEN who are of childbearing age show during their menstrual cycle some variation of body temperature. The period of time which elapses between the beginning of one menstruation and the beginning of the next is in most women of about the same length month after month. Since these periods recur regularly and are of approximately the same duration, they form what is called the menstrual cycle. During this menstrual cycle the woman's temperature slightly rises and falls. The precise degree of temperature during the cycle is not of great importance. The chief consideration is the sequence of changes of temperature. The lowest temperature recording is to be especially noted, for, immediately after arriving at the lowest point, the temperature suddenly rises rap-

[21] For material on the use of rhythm see Gerald Kelly, S.J., "Rhythm in Marriage: Duty and Idealism," *America* 87:128-30, May 3, 1952; Gerald Kelly, S.J., *Medico-Moral Problems*, pt. 4, "Official Statement on Rhythm," pp. 29-34 (St. Louis: Catholic Hospital Association of the United States and Canada, 1952); E. J. Mahoney, "Papal Teaching on the Infertile Period," *Clergy Review* 37:235-37, April 1952; John McCarthy, "Some Problems Regarding the Use of the Sterile Periods," *Irish Ecclesiastical Record* 78:372-76, November 1952; Nicholas Orville Griese, *"Rhythm" in Marriage and Christian Morality* (Westminster: Newman Bookshop, 1944); Joseph B. Doyle, M.D., "Concurrent Calculation of Ovulation Rhythm," *Linacre Quarterly* 17:23-31, February 1950; Henry A. Fallon, *Rhythm-Cal*, third revised edition (Kansas City: R-C Publishing Company, 1945); Pius XII, "Apostolate of the Midwife," *Catholic Mind* 50:49-64, January 1952.

idly and it is thought that during this sudden rise ovulation occurs.[22] The morality of using basal body temperature in order to avoid having offspring is the same as the morality of using rhythm for the same purpose.

REFERENCES

Bickers, William, M.D. "Do We Want Birth Control?" *Catholic Digest* 6:90-93, September 1942.

Bonnar, Alphonsus, O.F.M. *Catholic Doctor,* chap. 6, "Birth Prevention and Birth Control," pp. 63-80. London: Burns Oates and Washbourne, 1951.

Chartier, M., and E. Tesson. "Fécondité et continence périodique." *Cahiers Laënnec* 14:1-44, decembre 1954.

Cooper, John M.; Henry Davis, S.J.; and John A. Ryan. "Birth Control: The Perverted Faculty Argument." *Ecclesiastical Review* 81:54-79, July 1929.

Cummins, Damian, O.S.B. "Birth Control Platform." *Ecclesiastical Review* 92:164-73, February 1935.

Davis, Henry, S.J. *Artificial Human Fecundation.* New York: Sheed and Ward, 1951.

Doyle, Joseph B., M.D. "The Cervical Spoon: An Aid to Spermigration and Semen Sampling." *Linacre Quarterly* 16:41-47, January-April 1949.

———— "Concurrent Calculation of Ovulation Rhythm." *Linacre Quarterly* 17:23-31, February 1950.

Ficarra, Bernard J., M.D. *Newer Ethical Problems in Medicine and Surgery,* chap. 9, "Artificial Insemination," pp. 97-107. Westminster: Newman Press, 1951.

Gardiner, Harold C., S.J. "Enemy of the West—Birth Control." *America* 77:513-15, August 9, 1947.

Glover, William Kevin, S.M. *Artificial Insemination among Human Beings.* Washington: Catholic University of America, 1948.

Goldstein, David. *Suicide Bent: Sangerizing Mankind.* St. Paul: Radio Replies Press, 1945.

---

[22] See Pendleton Tompkins, M.D., "The Use of Basal Temperature Graphs in Determining the Date of Ovulation," *Journal of the American Medical Association* 124:698-700, March 11, 1944; Mary Barton and B. P. Wiesner, "Waking Temperature in Relation to Female Fecundity," *Lancet* 2:663-68, November 24, 1945.

Guchteneere, Raoul de. *Judgment on Birth Control.* New York: The Macmillan Company, 1931.

Hartnett, Robert C., S.J. "Britain's Dwindling Birthrate Is the Empire's Direst Threat." *America* 67:596-97, September 5, 1942.

Hicks, Nathaniel W. "By 'Planned Parenthood' the People May Perish." *America* 68:709-11, April 3, 1943.

McFadden, Charles J., O.S.A. *Medical Ethics,* second edition, chap. 4, "Contraception," pp. 74-101. Philadelphia: F. A. Davis Company, 1949.

Schmiedeler, Edgar, O.S.B. "Putting Birth Control Over." *Catholic Mind* 41:34-44, April 1943.

Schwitalla, Alphonse M., S.J. "Contraception." *Catholic Encyclopedia,* vol. XVIII (Supplement II). New York: Gilmary Society, 1951.

Sheil, Bernard J. "Birth Control." *Catholic Mind* 45:526-35, September 1947.

Sutherland, Halliday, M.D. *Control of Life,* chap. 1, "How Nations Die," pp. 7-24; chap. 11, "Does Nature Control Birth-Rates?" pp. 136-52. London: Burns Oates and Washbourne, 1944.

——— *Laws of Life,* chap. 9, "The False Law of Malthus," pp. 143-59; chap. 11, "Neo-Malthusian Claims," pp. 177-96. New York: Sheed and Ward, 1936.

PREGNANCY CASES

AND STERILIZATIONS

I N THE present chapter we endeavor to discuss all the conditions that can give rise to ethical problems during pregnancy. Various associated questions are included, such as tests for pregnancy and measures used to prevent pregnancy. Among the cases discussed is one of a husband who wishes to have himself sterilized in order to prevent a pregnancy in his wife.

TESTS FOR PREGNANCY

THERE ARE TIMES when a woman who is scheduled for a major operation is, unknown to the surgeon and perhaps even to herself, pregnant. It is of course important that the surgeon have knowledge of a patient's pregnancy, for ignorance about this fact will often jeopardize the life of the young fetus. There are various ways of discovering whether or not a woman is pregnant. The Ascheim-Zondek test, in which the woman's urine is injected subcutaneously into mice, has a high degree of accuracy. The Friedman test is a modification of the Ascheim-Zondek test. In another test, known as the Xenopus test of Hogben, some of the patient's urine is injected into a male bullfrog. If the woman is pregnant, the frog will, within from two to four hours, discharge male sex cells. Is some such test ever obligatory in the case of a woman of childbearing age who is to undergo surgery?

Some reliable pregnancy test is obligatory if the surgical operation would probably endanger the life of the fetus and if the surgeon has a positive suspicion that the woman is with child.[1] "To have positive suspicion" means that one has good reason for believing that pregnancy exists. If the surgeon after investigation has no sound reason for suspecting pregnancy and if he judges from the absence of ordinary signs that no pregnancy exists, a test, if inconvenient to administer, is not obligatory. Even here, however, a test is advisable. Knowledge of the patient's pregnancy will not necessarily mean that surgery must be deferred, but only that the surgeon will proceed in a more than ordinarily cautious manner. As is evident from what is said on pages 231-35, there are cases in which, in spite of grave proximate danger to the fetus, surgery necessary to save the mother may licitly be performed.

DIRECT STERILIZATION

STERILIZATION in the case of a female can be brought about by the removal of the uterus, the removal or ligating of the Fallopian tubes, or the removal or irradiation of the ovaries. The general principle is that any one of these procedures is licit if a pathological condition of the organ renders it necessary for the preservation of the patient's life or health, but that it is illicit if the purpose of the operation or treatment is to prevent the inconveniences or dangers of childbearing.

Sterilization in Pathological Menstruation

There are cases in which it is licit to excise or X-ray the ovaries because of menstrual disturbances that seriously affect the patient's health.

---

[1] If the surgery affects some organ not connected with the genital tract (for example, the gall bladder, appendix, or kidney), no danger to the fetus would necessarily be connected with the operation.

Case 69
Sterilization of Ovaries To Ease Menorrhagia

The patient, a 30-year-old woman, has protracted and very copious menstrual periods which seriously affect her health. The physician wishes to relieve this pathological condition by excising or X-raying her ovaries. May he employ either of these procedures?

Solution. If the physician judges that the pathological menstruation is so grave that either of these procedures is medically indicated, the procedure is morally justified.

Explanation. To this case we may rightly apply the principle of the twofold effect. The physician's intention in removing or X-raying the ovaries is the arresting of an abnormal condition which is causing grave injury to the patient's health. His action in excising the ovaries or spraying these organs with X ray is immediately aimed at destroying their hormonal activity and not their production of ova. Hence the physician's action is not one of direct sterilization. It consists in suppressing a function which is gravely harmful here and now to the health of the patient. The evil effect of his action (the complete termination of ovulation) is not the cause of the good effect (the safeguarding of the patient's health). The woman's health is harmed, not by the ovulation, but by the hormonal activity of the ovaries. It is for the physician to decide whether there is due proportion between the foreseen good and evil effects of the procedure. The patient's condition would, it seems, be sufficiently grave if the bleeding is so pathological that it habitually causes severe pain or grave inconvenience during a notable part of the month. Perhaps most physicians today would use other remedies for this ailment. That is for them to decide. The ethician passes judgment on what is permissible if the physician prescribes certain measures as necessary.

Sterilization because of the Dangers of Pregnancy

There are numerous cases in which the physician judges that another pregnancy might be fatal or that it would at least result in grave danger to the mother and in serious impairment of her health. While there is reason for believing that physicians sometimes exaggerate the danger and give too little thought to what a courageous and well-intentioned woman can do, it is not the part of the ethician to challenge their judgment when there is question of the medical aspects of the case. The ethician confines himself to affirming that it is illicit to perform any sterilization for the sole purpose of making marital relations possible without the consequent danger of a pregnancy. If the patient accepts the physician's judgment and is unwilling to risk another pregnancy, she can do no more than abstain from marital relations or depend upon the use of rhythm (see pages 162-67). The six cases that follow are identical insofar as the application of principles is concerned. All are included for the purpose of covering the medical conditions that have been found to provide a reason, though an unsound one, for this type of sterilization.

Case 70

Sterilization because of a Heart Ailment

The patient, a 30-year-old married woman, has rheumatic heart disease of a severe degree. Pregnancy will almost certainly bring death to the mother and possibly to the fetus also. The physician proposes the irradiation of both the patient's ovaries in order to sterilize her and thus protect her against the dangers of childbirth. May he licitly employ this procedure?

Solution. The physician may not licitly irradiate the ovaries.

Explanation. The physician's purpose in irradiating the ovaries of the patient would be to prevent them from producing fertilizable ova. His direct intention, therefore, would be to sterilize the patient, and direct sterilization is never permissible. There is now no danger arising from the functioning of the ovaries; danger will be present only if the patient becomes pregnant. Hence the physician's action would not be remedial in reference to a present ailment with which the woman is afflicted; it would be contraceptive in reference to a merely threatened evil.

Case 71

Sterilization in a Case of Tuberculosis

The patient, a married woman, has severe pulmonary tuberculosis. She is being operated on for appendicitis. The surgeon, fearing that pregnancy will kill her, excises part of her Fallopian tubes. His intention is to save her life by preventing future pregnancies.

Solution. The surgeon's act is gravely illicit.

Explanation. The surgeon in this case is removing a healthy part of the body which is not a present threat to her life. His act is one of direct contraceptive sterilization. His intention is, it is true, to save her life, but he accomplishes this purpose by means of a gravely illicit mutilation.[2] It may also be noted that the surgeon excises part of the Fallopian tubes without the patient's consent. This would make his action doubly illicit. With present-day therapy very few feel that women with tuberculosis cannot bear children.

Case 72
Sterilization because of a Scarred and Weakened Uterus

The patient has had several caesarean sections and is now pregnant again. Her physician warns her that her uterus has been greatly weakened and badly scarred. Another pregnancy, he says, will gravely endanger her life, and he asks her permission to do a hysterectomy after delivering her next baby.

Solution. A hysterectomy may not licitly be performed in this case.[3]

Explanation. The scarred uterus of the patient, it is true, may in the future cause her grave danger, but this danger will occur only on condition that she becomes pregnant again. If she has no future pregnancy, this organ will cause her no difficulty. The surgeon is not justified in excising the uterus as a useless organ, now unfit to fulfill its proper function. The scarred condition of the uterine wall is in no wise detrimental to the health of the patient. Moreover, the uterus at present cannot be called useless, since it serves as a flooring for the support of the abdominal cavity. It will, moreover, function normally in the woman's orgasm during marital relations. Excising the uterus can bring somewhat pronounced reactions such as beset a woman at menopause. Besides, one may not resort to surgery, especially to that which involves some danger, merely to rid the body of an altogether harmless part that does not function effectively. If some part of the body were actually to be considered useless and if it were nevertheless in no way a source of inconvenience, pain, or hindrance of some sort, one would not risk the

[2] As an example of one writer who suggests that sterilization is indicated in some cases of heart, kidney, or lung weakness, as a birth-control measure, and for eugenic purposes in other cases see Clarence J. Gamble, M.D., "Human Sterilization," *American Journal of Nursing* 51:625-26, October 1951.

[3] There is another opinion about this case which is explained in *Theological Studies* 12:70, March 1951 and 15:68-71, March 1954. The author of MEDICAL ETHICS does not consider the opinion there expounded solidly probable, and therefore he would not permit its use in practice.

Direct Sterilization *it may be removed.*

complications which an operation might cause, nor would he be justified in doing so.

see case #83 pg 182

Despite any opinion to the contrary, it is difficult to see how the surgeon's intention in excising the uterus could be anything but contraceptive. His purpose in operating is to rid this woman of a part of the body which will prove dangerous if, and only if, conception occurs. Hence he intends to excise the uterus as a means of preventing a danger which would substantially arise from pregnancy alone. His intention, then, is evil, for he directly seeks sterilization, and direct sterilization is gravely illicit. But could not the surgeon "purify" his intention? Could he not intend merely the removal from the woman's body of a useless organ? The answer is that here there is no other reason for the operation except that of preventing a future pregnancy. The surgeon cannot claim that the purpose of the excision is to rid the body of what he considers to be an obstruction, for actually the uterus when not pregnant is not a source of inconvenience, of pain, or of any other physical disturbance. The operation does not tend to promote the health of the patient's body except insofar as it is contraceptive. The chief reason for condemning this operation is that it appears to be one of direct sterilization. One may ask the surgeon whether, if he were absolutely certain that the patient would never again become pregnant (because, for example, she is a widow who has a vow not to remarry), he would wish to excise the scarred uterus. In this case would the hoped-for physical benefit to her body compensate for such a mutilation?

A case different from the one described above may perhaps occur in which the uterus after the caesarean section cannot be adequately closed and consequently, if left in situ would probably produce a seriously pathological condition such as that of an intestinal obstruction. Because excision of the uterus in this case is necessary to prevent grave danger which may arise, not from a pregnancy, but from the pathological state of the organ itself, a hysterectomy appears clearly licit. A similar case is that in which the uterine wall has a rent which, because it will not heal, will prove gravely dangerous.

Case 73

Sterilization because of Vulvar Varices

The patient, a 25-year-old female, has vulvar varices. After performing the surgery required to relieve this pathological condition, the surgeon, using the vaginal route, employs electro-coagulation of the tubal cornua. Although the Fallopian tubes are in the state of normal

175

health, the surgeon wishes to obviate, by cauterization, any danger which a future pregnancy could cause the patient.

Solution. The surgeon acts in a gravely illicit manner when he thus blocks off the lumen of the tubes.

Explanation. A ligating of the patient's Fallopian tubes is in no wise required for remedying the present condition of a pathological organ of the patient. The purpose of this procedure is to prevent the woman from becoming pregnant. Hence the surgeon's act of cauterizing the tubes comprises contraceptive sterilization and is gravely illicit. The act is doubly illicit if it is done without the patient's knowledge and consent.

Case 74
Sterilization because of Danger of Uterine Rupture

Mrs. M is having her sixth caesarean. From the second caesarean on, at each succeeding operation, the old scar was removed. The area around the old scar is so thin that the surgeon cannot understand why rupture has not already occurred. The danger of rupture will become more imminent with each pregnancy. "Any further child-bearing," says the surgeon, "is absolutely impossible and would gravely jeopardize the mother's life." To save the mother so that she can care for her children, he ligates both Fallopian tubes.

Solution. The surgeon's act of ligating the tubes is illicit.

Explanation. The surgeon's action consists in binding the tubes so that fertilization cannot occur in the patient. His act is intentionally and directly contraceptive. This type of sterilization is of its nature evil and is never permitted. As in Cases 70 and 71, the surgeon is apparently assuming the patient's permission.

Case 75
Sterilization because of a Pathological Uterus

The patient is multipara, and during previous deliveries there have been lacerations of the cervix and perineum. The large and boggy uterus is retroverted and prolapsed well down in the pelvis. The physician prescribes amputating the cervix and doing anterior and posterior colporrhaphy and ventral suspension. After ventral suspension he will ligate and bury the Fallopian tubes, because a pregnancy would probably bring grave danger to the patient.

Solution. Ligating and burying the tubes would here be gravely illicit.

Explanation. Ligating the tubes in this case would constitute direct sterilization. The purpose of this procedure is contraceptive, and therefore the operation is rightly classified as contraceptive sterilization, which is always immoral.

Case 76
Illicit Double Vasectomy

Because he has already six young children and his wife is but 30 years of age, the patient has himself doubly vasectomized. "To have any more children," he contends, "would be gravely unfair to my wife and I want to protect her happiness."

Solution. The bilateral vasectomy was gravely illicit.

Explanation. Obviously the surgery referred to in this case is directly contraceptive and therefore, like all other forms of artificial birth control, it must be condemned. If, moreover, the patient is seeking thus to safeguard his wife's happiness, he is employing not only an evil means but an ineffective one to accomplish his objective. Dr. Vincent J. O'Conor, a professor of urology, makes the following observation about cases such as the present one: "Making a man 'safe sexually' has often resulted in marital infidelity, domestic discord, separation and divorce. These experiences are frequent in our records in contrast with those quoted by the authors in their 50 cases. . . . Most experienced urologists will agree that profound sexual neuroses and imaginative ills often follow vasectomy when it has been performed purely to prevent pregnancy."[4]

Temporary Sterilization

Physicians are sometimes requested to bring about temporary sterilization, the purpose usually being to make intercourse possible without the consequent danger of pregnancy. Direct temporary sterilization is always illicit.

One means by which, it is contended, fertility may be controlled is through the use of phosphorylated hesperidin. Temporary sterility, it is thought, can be produced by impregnating the female ova, the male sperm, and the surrounding fluids with a hesperidin derivative.[5] If we assume that the effect

[4] Vincent J. O'Conor, M.D., "Sexual Effects of Vasectomy." *Journal of the American Medical Association* 144:1502, December 23, 1950.

[5] See Benjamin F. Sieve, "A New Antifertility Factor," *Science* 116:373-85, October 10, 1952; John J. Lynch, S.J., "Fertility Control and the Moral Law," *Linacre Quarterly* 20:83-88, August 1953.

sought in the use of phosphorylated hesperidin is that of temporary sterilization, this manner of rendering sexual intercourse infertile is clearly illicit, for it consists in directly sterilizing the generative function. It makes little difference, from the viewpoint of the moralist, whether the means employed to effect the direct sterilization be surgery, X ray, or chemicals; the action is one of direct, illicit mutilation of the reproductive faculty and therefore it is morally unjustifiable.

Another method of bringing about temporary sterilization consists in severing the Fallopian tubes and burying the distal ends in the folds of the broad ligament. The later attempt to restore the passageway is not always successful. At present medical authorities do not promise success in a later attempt to restore the tubes so that the lumen will function normally as a passageway for the ova and spermatozoa.

Case 77

Temporary Sterilization

Mrs. L asks Dr. K to sterilize her for a period of 8 or 10 months. Dr. K plans to inject gonadotropic hormones into the patient in order to bring about temporary sterilization. The result will be that Mrs. L can have normal marital relations with her husband without fear of becoming pregnant.

Solution. Dr. K may not licitly sterilize the patient in this manner. Even though gonadotropic hormones are doubtfully effective, his intention is to do something that is illicit.

Explanation. Direct sterilization offends against the law of nature. The means by which the sterilization is effected are of little importance; it is the act itself, no matter how it is accomplished, which violates God's law. Hence all types of direct sterilization by surgery, X ray, drugs, and so forth, are illicit.

INDIRECT STERILIZATION

IN DIRECT sterilization the first and principal purpose of the physician is to render the patient sterile. There is no pathological condition present that renders an attack upon an organ necessary. The physician's intention is usually to safeguard the health of the patient, but a good intention does not justify the use of illicit means. Were such a principle accepted, men would be free to commit the most heinous crimes in order to accomplish some good purpose.

In indirect sterilization the first and only purpose of the physician is very definitely different. His first and only purpose is to correct a pathological condition presenting danger to his patient. The steps that must be taken to correct this condition will result in sterilization, but he intends this sterilization only indirectly, not directly. The licitness of thus acting is explained in the discussion of the twofold effect, pages 94-101.

In nine of the eleven cases about to be discussed the procedure is licit. In two cases there is an erroneous application of the principle of the twofold effect. In the cases here discussed the patient is not pregnant. Cases involving a pregnant uterus will be treated later in the chapter.

Case 78
Removal of a Pathological Uterus

The patient has had many vaginal deliveries and as a result lacerations, infections, and erosions have occurred in the cervix uteri. Moreover, there has been subinvolution of the uterus and the organ itself has become heavy, boggy, enlarged, and weakened, and is now causing the patient great physical debility, pain, and distress. May the physician excise the uterus for the present relief of the patient?

Solution. If the physician considers the removing of the uterus to be the only effective remedy for this condition, the organ may be excised.

Explanation. The uterus may not be excised unless its removal is required for the present health of the patient. The condition described above would be sufficiently grave to justify this operation if less radical treatment would not prove effective. Because this organ is helpful in preserving for the patient complete physiological equilibrium, the physician will be slow to sacrifice it.

Case 79
Preventive Oophorectomy

The patient, a woman of childbearing age, has carcinoma of the breast. A radical mastectomy has been performed. The surgeon, judging

X-ray therapy and the use of androgens ineffective in this case as a means of preventing metastases, wishes to perform a bilateral oophorectomy. Is the excision of the ovaries in this case licit?

Solution. An oophorectomy in these circumstances is licit.

Explanation. In order to conserve the general health of the body it is permitted to sacrifice one of its parts. The part which is excised need not in all cases be diseased or pathological. While the best medical practice might not call for an oophorectomy in the present case, the ethician must pronounce it licit if the physician insists that he considers it necessary. The operation cannot properly be classified as one of direct sterilization. The act of the surgeon is the removing of certain glands, the ovaries, because they are sending into the blood stream hormones which are thought to help to spread the cancer. The surgeon has no intention nor desire to prevent by his act future pregnancies. He is removing the organs insofar as they constitute a present danger for the patient. If the patient's health could be safeguarded by medication, it would not be good medical practice to operate. If medication would prove effective and would not involve grave inconvenience, the physician must use it in preference to oophorectomy, for in such circumstances no proportionate reason would exist which would justify the surgery.

Case 80
Irradiation of the Ovaries because of Carcinoma

The patient, aged 30, has carcinoma of the breast. After excising the breast the physician advises the irradiation of the apparently healthy ovaries in order to prevent metastases. May the physician licitly perform the irradiation?

Solution. The degree of irradiation is licit which is judged to be necessary to prevent metastases.

Explanation. To this irradiation we may apply the principle of the twofold effect. The physician's intention is to safeguard the life of the patient. The evil effect (rendering the woman sterile) does not cause the good effect (arresting the spread of the cancer), for whether the woman is able to conceive a child or not does not have any bearing on the cure which is sought. The physician's action is not evil in itself. His act consists in suppressing the endocrine function of the ovaries. These are perfectly healthy, but to render an operation licit it is not always required that the part to be excised be itself diseased. If, then, the ovaries are at present endangering the patient's life independently of any outside influence, they may licitly be sacrificed

180

for the good of the whole body. The operation is not a direct sterilization, for the action is aimed principally, not at rendering conception
impossible by killing the ova, but at suppressing the manufacture of
hormones which threaten the woman's life.

If, therefore, irradiation of the ovaries is medically advisable, this
may be licitly done, but the degree of irradiation must not be greater
than that which is required for preventing metastasis. If prolonged
X ray is necessary to ward off the danger, this procedure is justified,
even though permanent sterility will result. If, however, milder irradiation which would not destroy the patient's reproductive power
would suffice, the stronger irradiation would be illicit for lack of a
reason to justify the additional destruction produced. In the patient
who is pregnant and has carcinoma of the breast the harmful effects
of the ovaries are practically negligible while the pregnancy continues, and therefore irradiation or excision of the ovaries would not
be morally permissible nor medically advisable. After the termination
of the pregnancy the ovaries in such a patient may be either excised
or irradiated if this is medically necessary. See also Case 124.

Case 81
Hysterectomy because of Suspected Cancer

In order to detect the presence of cancer of the uterus the patient is
given the Papanicolaou test. The results of the test, together with
other clinical findings, fail to establish with certainty the presence of
carcinoma but indicate that the uterus is *probably* cancerous. The
physician wishes to do a hysterectomy if this is morally permissible.
The patient is not pregnant.

Solution. If the test indicates that there is solid probability that the womb
is cancerous, a hysterectomy may be licitly performed.

Explanation. If an organ is probably endangering the life of a person,
that organ may be licitly sacrificed in order to safeguard the rest of
the body. By the phrase "probably endangering" is meant that there
is some positive, weighty reason for believing that danger is present.
The mere unfounded fear that danger is at hand would of course
not justify the operation. If the Papanicolaou test in a large percentage of cases is trustworthy in revealing the presence of cancer, it
would give sufficient probability to make the hysterectomy licit.[6]

[6] In the event that the patient is pregnant with a nonviable fetus, the hysterectomy may not licitly be performed unless the danger to the woman is
certain and not merely probable.

Case 82
Hysterectomy because of Prolapsus Uteri

The patient has prolapsus uteri. The cervix of the uterus is protruding several inches. The cervix is eroded and infected. The physician believes that the cervix may become cancerous and that amputation of the cervix is therefore indicated. A complete hysterectomy, however, is preferable for the permanent cure of the patient.

Solution. If the complete hysterectomy is in this case necessary for a permanent cure, the operation is licit.

Explanation. If the excision of the uterus is necessary for the present health of the patient, it is justified on the principle of the twofold effect. If, however, there is no positive evidence of carcinoma such as would be provided by a positive Papanicolaou smear or a positive biopsy specimen, the excision would be illicit. Unfounded fears or mere suspicion would not justify so radical a remedy.

Case 83
Bilateral Salpingo-Oophorectomy because of Carcinoma

The patient is a female 46 years of age, and the surgeon performs a hysterectomy because of the presence of multiple leiomyomata of the uterine fundus. Both the ovaries and the tubes appear healthy but he wishes to excise them, for he is afraid that they may develop cancer. Bilateral salpingo-oophorectomy is, in all such cases, routine procedure.

Solution. The surgeon may in these circumstances excise both the Fallopian tubes and both the ovaries.

Explanation. The solution which here permits the excision of the healthy tubes and ovaries is based on the principle already explained (see pages 122-23) that mutilation of the body is licit when necessary for preserving the health of the whole body. When the uterus must be excised because of multiple leiomyomata, medical records indicate that cancer will develop in the tubes and ovaries in a high percentage of cases. Because of this great probability bilateral salpingo-oophorectomy constitutes a lawful means of safeguarding the life of the patient. The doctrine expounded in Case 52, page 126, and Case 79, pages 179-80, may be rightly applied to Case 83.

Case 84
Hysterectomy To Prevent Atrophy of Uterus

The surgeon finds it necessary to remove both ovaries and Fallopian tubes because they are in a diseased state. He then proceeds to excise the uterus also, for he asserts that, left in place, this organ will very probably atrophy.

Solution. The surgeon's action is licit.

Explanation. After the ovaries and the Fallopian tubes have been excised, the uterus obviously cannot function as a childbearing organ. If, then, after the removal of the tubes and ovaries it would probably atrophy and cause some physical disturbance, there would be sufficient reason for its removal. Some medical authorities assert that in the present case excising the uterus would be inadvisable, for the uterus, left in place, will not be useless. It will serve as a flooring for the abdominal cavity, and this good compensates for the disturbance which atrophy would produce. It is for the surgeon to decide what is the best medical procedure. If he favors the excising of the uterus in the present case, its removal is morally justifiable.

Case 85
Excision of a Second Uterus

The patient has a double uterus. In order to prevent a double simultaneous pregnancy and to reduce the danger of premature labor, dystocia, and third-trimester bleeding, the surgeon, with the patient's consent, excises one uterus. A year after he has removed the organ, the woman suffers very severe hemorrhage from a large fibroid in the remaining uterus and the surgeon states that he must remove the second uterus in order to save the patient's life. May he do so?

Solution. The surgeon may remove the second uterus.

Explanation. Safeguarding the patient's life here and now depends upon excising the second uterus. This bleeding organ is a present source of grave danger to the patient, and hence it may licitly be removed. As to the lawfulness of removing one uterus to prevent a double simultaneous pregnancy which would jeopardize the patient's life, the surgeon is not suppressing the generative function nor preventing future fertilization. He is merely eliminating a part of the body which is unnecessary and which would hinder the proper functioning of the other uterus, for the space it occupies will serve during pregnancy for the healthy growth of the fetus. Hence the surgeon is aiding the generation of children and remedying a defect of nature.

Case 86
Ligation of Fallopian Tubes

In order to rectify a prolapsus uteri the surgeon does a Watkins interposition operation. Since in this procedure the fundus of the uterus .

is flexed forward and sutured to the bladder, a pregnancy cannot remain long and develop in the uterus. The surgeon in these circumstances ligates the Fallopian tubes to prevent the dangers which pregnancy will involve for the mother.

Solution. The surgeon may not licitly ligate the tubes.

Explanation. The ligating of the Fallopian tubes would have as its primary purpose the prevention of conception by making it impossible for semen to reach any of the patient's ova. Such contraceptive procedure is against the natural law and is gravely illicit. It would be an erroneous application of the principle of the twofold effect to argue that the Fallopian tubes may be ligated because they are a menace to the patient. If they are a menace, it is not because they are pathological but only because the patient may voluntarily become pregnant. It may also be observed, however, that a surgeon would probably be sharply criticized on strictly medical grounds for performing a Watkins interposition operation on a woman who is still menstruating.

Case 87
Needless and Illicit Oophorectomy

The surgeon has excised one ovary because of a dermoid cyst. In order to prevent the development of a dermoid cyst in the other ovary and to obviate the necessity of operating on the patient a second time, the surgeon excises the other ovary. The second ovary is unquestionably in the state of normal health. Does the surgeon act licitly?

Solution. The surgeon's excision of the healthy ovary is illicit.

Explanation. The assumption in the present case is that the second ovary is in sound health and that its presence in the body of the woman does not jeopardize her life in any way. Excising such an organ would be gravely illicit, for it would suppress the ovarian function needlessly. Such an excision is not necessary to prevent the spread of a disease in her body.

Case 88
Licitness of Olshausen and Gilliam Operations

In order to correct the retrodisplacement of the uterus in a patient of childbearing age, Dr. X wishes to do an Olshausen or Gilliam operation. The patient believes that the operation would be contrary to the Catholic code of ethics.

Solution. This operation is licit.

184

Explanation. The Olshausen operation and the Gilliam operation are intended to relieve distress caused by the uterus and to facilitate childbearing. Hence there is no moral objection to this procedure.[7] The patient misunderstands the purpose of the operation, and her fears should be set at rest.

THE USE OF DRUGS DURING PREGNANCY

I N ALL the cases that have been discussed up to this point the patient is not actually pregnant. The various procedures occurring in the cases do not affect a present pregnancy but will or might affect or prevent a future one. We now turn to cases in which the patient is pregnant at the time. We will first speak briefly of the use of drugs.

Drugs may be used either for the purpose of curing a disease or for the purpose of relieving pain. Quinine is the principal drug that is of interest when there is question of curing a disease. Although the use of quinine does not by any means result in an abortion in all cases and at all stages of pregnancy, it does sometimes produce this effect, and women of loose morals often keep themselves supplied with it because its use is traditional in their group and because it is easy to obtain. Ergot is used in cases of hemorrhage. Morphine, Demerol, and other drugs are used to relieve pain. Even moderate doses of analgesics can harm the fetus just before delivery, when its delicate respiratory centers will no longer receive their oxygen through placental circulation, and heavy doses may harm the fetus at earlier stages of pregnancy.

The general principle governing the use of drugs during pregnancy is that any drug may be used if it is necessary to save the life of the patient, injury to the fetus being merely permitted as an unsought secondary effect. Because of the advances in medical science, cases in which a very dangerous drug must be used occur rarely if at all, although they might occur in areas where the newer drugs are not available. In

[7] See Nicholson J. Eastman, M.D., *Williams Obstetrics,* tenth edition, pp. 890-91. New York: Appleton-Century-Crofts, 1950.

cases in which drugs are used for the relief of pain rather than for the cure of disease the dosage can be so controlled that the edge is taken off the patient's pain without injury to the fetus. It is the responsibility of the physician to weigh in all cases the several factors involved, among them the seriousness of the disease or the acuteness of the pain, the stage to which pregnancy has advanced, and the possibility of employing other means to which no danger is attached. The application of these principles is illustrated in the following cases.

Case 89
The Use of Quinine for Malaria during Pregnancy

The patient, pregnant with a nonviable fetus, is afflicted with malaria. In order to counteract the malaria organism the physician prescribes the use of quinine.

Solution. If there is available no other effective treatment which would be less likely to harm the fetus, quinine may be used.

Explanation. The use of quinine during the pregnancy creates some but very little danger for the fetus. There is a just proportion between the greatly beneficial effects of the medicine on the mother and the very slight risk which its use involves for the child. Needless to remark, a drug which would produce the good effect of curing the mother without the evil effect of endangering the fetus in any way must if possible be given preference. A number of drugs for the treatment of malaria that are even more effective than quinine and that have little or no effect upon uterine contractility are now available. Among them are Atabrine, Aralen, and Pamaquine.

Case 90
The Use of Quinine for a Cold during Pregnancy

The patient, 2 months pregnant, has a severe cold. The physician has found that in her case the use of quinine proves an effective remedy. He is convinced that the dosage which he prescribes for her will not injure the fetus.

Solution. If there is no danger of harming the fetus, the patient may be given quinine as a cure.

Explanation. Large doses of quinine do, at times, bring about in a pregnant woman the emptying of the uterus. There is, moreover, the danger that generous doses of quinine would have an injurious effect on the fetus. The use of quinine would be illicit if either of these evil effects would probably follow, for there would then be no proportion between the probable evil effect (abortion or narcotizing the fetus) and the good effect (curing the patient's cold).

Case 91
The Use of Ergot for Hemorrhage during Pregnancy

The patient is 3 months pregnant and is now hemorrhaging severely. The physician wishes to employ ergot to stop the bleeding, but he knows that the use of this drug may bring on an abortion.

Solution. If the mother's life is gravely endangered by the bleeding and if there is no other less drastic way of stopping the hemorrhage, the physician may licitly employ ergot for this purpose. His intention in the use of ergot must not be to induce an abortion.

Explanation. Ergot is fairly effective in arresting hemorrhage, but it also stimulates uterine contractions which may produce abortion. The skilled physician, even if he regards abortion as licit, does not employ ergot for expelling the fetus; for although the drug does at first increase uterine contractions, this effect soon disappears and afterwards the expulsive power of the uterus is lessened. If the physician judges that the use of ergot is urgently indicated to save the woman from a fatal hemorrhage, he may, according to the principle of the twofold effect, licitly employ this drug. This solution assumes that there is no other drug available whose use would be equally effective as that of ergot and which would not entail the dangers that are present in employing ergot. It is asserted that diethylstilbestrol in such cases as the present one would produce the good effects that follow the use of ergot but without ergot's dangers.[8] If in a particular case satisfactory results are to be looked for from the use of diethylstilbestrol and if it is at the time obtainable, the use of ergot in that case would not be morally justifiable.

Case 92
The Use of Morphine To Relieve Pain during Pregnancy

The patient, who is pregnant with a nonviable fetus, is suffering acutely from a renal stone. In order to relieve the mother's pain the physician prescribes large doses of morphine. Is he justified in so acting?

[8] See O. Watkins Smith, M.D., "Diethylstilbestrol in the Prevention and Treatment of Complications in Pregnancy." *American Journal of Obstetrics and Gynecology* 56:821-34, November 1948.

Solution. Morphine may be licitly administered in this case provided there are no indications that premature labor is beginning.

Explanation. Morphine produces narcosis in the fetus just as it produces narcosis in the mother. If the fetus remains in the womb, the narcosis passes away as the effects of the drug wear off. If delivery occurs before the effects of the drug have worn off, the life of the infant, especially if he is premature, will be in danger. It is therefore illicit to use heavy sedation shortly before delivery, since there is no just proportion between the good effect of reducing or eliminating the mother's pain and the evil effect of causing grave danger to the infant's life. This remains true even though the infant is so premature as to be altogether nonviable. Impending death does not justify such a shortening of life.

DIRECT ABORTION

ABORTION, as the word is employed in this book,[9] means the intentional expulsion of a nonviable, living fetus from the mother's uterus. In order to constitute abortion the act must be directly intended; that is, the abortion must be attempted either as the end to be accomplished or as a means to achieve some desired purpose. A nonviable fetus is one that is so immature that it is unable to survive outside the uterus of the mother. It may be said in general that in ordinary circumstances a fetus is considered viable at the end of the twenty-eighth week of gestation. If the child is to be born in a modern hospital, where it will receive skilled care and where it can be placed in an incubator, the fetus is judged to be viable at the end of its twenty-sixth week in the womb. It is for the physician who is handling the case to decide whether the fetus, in a particular instance, should be considered viable.

At times the fetus, because of shock or of some pathological condition, is born before it is viable. This is not an abortion in the strict sense. In medical terminology it is called spontaneous abortion, but laymen refer to it as miscarriage. Since sponta-

---

[9] In this book abortion, unless otherwise noted, is used in the sense of "direct abortion." In medical books and in some theological treatises abortion is not employed in this meaning.

neous abortions are entirely unintentional and beyond man's control, they do not constitute a moral act. The present discussion will be limited to therapeutic and criminal abortion. An abortion which is deemed necessary to safeguard the health of the mother is called therapeutic. An abortion is termed criminal when it is not considered necessary for the conservation of the mother's health. The motive for inducing a criminal abortion is not a medical one; it is rather to preserve the mother's reputation if she is an unmarried woman, or to save her the inconvenience involved in carrying the child to term, or for some other such reason.

The medical profession justly looks with contempt upon those physicians who for the sake of gain, or even for a better reason, procure criminal abortions. The attitude of the profession toward therapeutic abortions, however, is quite different. Here the purpose is, not to protect a woman against the inconvenient social or economic effects of her own free act, but to save her life. It is easy to understand how a truly upright man could err in such a matter by failing to think of the fundamental moral principles that are applicable and of the logical consequences of the principles that he accepts in place of the correct ones. The vast majority of those physicians who perform or prescribe therapeutic abortions have no intention of doing something morally wrong. On the contrary, they would consider it morally wrong not to take the action that they think should be taken. If we condemn their action, it does not follow that we look upon them as evil-minded. A physician can sincerely desire to do what is right and still be in error as to what is or is not right in a given situation.

The fact that therapeutic abortions, not too many years ago, were looked upon as medically indicated and as morally justifiable in very many situations is well known to the profession. Dr. Charles O. McCormick stated the ethical principle upon which defenders of therapeutic abortion depend when he said: "The artificial termination of pregnancy during the early weeks of gestation . . . is ethically justified *only to save life, health, and reason of the mother.*"[10] In order to remove a condition which might jeopardize a woman's life abortion was prescribed in some cases of severe vomiting of pregnancy, in some instances of preeclampsia, renal disease, heart disease, and pulmonary tuberculosis, and occasionally when the patient was suffering from severe diabetes, leukemia, pernicious anemia, chorea, or epilepsy.[11] Dr. Richard W. Te Linde stated the attitude existing some ten years ago when he wrote: "As to the general principles, medical and moral, which guide us in determining whether or not a woman should be aborted, there is a great difference of opinion in the medical profession. . . . The difference in opinion is well illustrated by answers obtained by J. C. Ayres to a questionnaire that he sent out to 62 obstetricians living in the southern part of the United States. These replies have been tabulated, and here is the summary of the findings:

	Yes	*No*
For social reasons to prevent disgrace	10	51
For economic reasons, poverty	6	56
For health reasons (life not involved)	22	37
To save mother's life	61	1
In case of rape	36	20
For dominant hereditary taint in both parents	21	34

"In a recent study at the New York Lying-In Hospital by Kuder and Finn their listed indications are more in keeping with the view of obstetricians generally. They grouped 44 indications under 9 main headings."[12]

In a 1950 number of the *Journal of the American Medical Association* the editor quotes the textbook on obstetrics by

[10] Charles O. McCormick, M.D., *A Textbook on Pathology of Labor, the Puerperium and the Newborn*, second edition, p. 208. St. Louis: C. V. Mosby Company, 1947.

[11] See Henricus J. Stander, M.D., *Williams Obstetrics*, eighth edition, pp. 1113-16. New York: D. Appleton-Century Company, 1941.

[12] Richard W. Te Linde, M.D., *Operative Gynecology*, first edition, p. 475. Philadelphia: J. B. Lippincott Company, 1946.

De Lee and Greenhill that describes eight different conditions in which therapeutic abortion is considered to be indicated.[13]

There is at the present time a marked trend toward reducing the number of situations in which therapeutic abortions are said to be indicated. This is due in part to the fact that therapeutic abortions have so often produced disastrous effects on the mother; in part, no doubt, to a sincere and praiseworthy desire to save both lives whenever possible; and in part to the development of newer drugs and therapies.

The medical profession is well aware that the Catholic Church is most firmly opposed to all direct abortions. Such abortions were condemned by Innocent XI as early as the seventeenth century, and the position taken by the Church has never changed. We will present as briefly and as clearly as we can the ethical and moral principles that support this position.

As soon as the male and female cells unite vitally after intercourse—or, in other words, as soon as conception takes place—we have present a human being. True, a long period of development lies ahead, not only during prenatal life, but during infancy, childhood, and adolescence, until finally the individual reaches full maturity; but during all this period the body receives no organ or part that it did not have in an undeveloped state from the beginning. In its prenatal state and in its postnatal state the body receives nothing from the outside except the nourishment that makes growth possible. Now, if the Creator decreed that new human beings should come into existence through the mating of men and women and if He made the body so complete that the ovum need do no more than develop without any addition from without, it is not un-

[13] *Journal of the American Medical Association* 142:608, February 25, 1950. Because he believes that the infant would probably be defective, Dr. Greenhill in his *1952 Year Book of Obstetrics and Gynecology* advocates (p. 277) emptying the uterus of a mother who contracts rubella in the first trimester of her pregnancy. See Gerald Kelly, S.J., *Medico-Moral Problems*, pt. 5, pp. 16-19 (St. Louis: Catholic Hospital Association of the United States and Canada, 1954).

reasonable to assume that He infuses into the ovum at the instant when it is to become a living being the soul without which it would be a mere animal and not a man.

If there are any who contend that the soul is not indeed present from the moment of conception, the burden of proof would seem to rest upon them. If the soul is not present from the moment of conception, precisely when does it begin to exist? Is it at the beginning of the twenty-eighth week, when the fetus becomes capable of living outside the womb? Is it at the time of delivery, when the newborn infant draws its first breath? If we postpone the appearance of the soul to some such time as this, we might almost as logically postpone it to the time when the infant ceases to live as an animal lives and becomes able to reason—a theory which would free us from the guilt of murder if we did away, not only with unwanted fetuses, but with unwanted infants as well.

It is true that there are some authorities within the Catholic Church, even today, who hold that the soul is not present from the first moment of conception.[14] Their opinion, however, does not tend in any way to change an abortion from an illicit into a licit act, nor do they intend that it should. The reasons for this are as follows.

First, even if a fetus at the moment when an abortion is committed does not possess a human soul, it was intended by God to become in course of time a human being in the full sense of the word and to receive a human soul. If a human life is not destroyed, the beginnings at least of a human life are destroyed. To kill a human fetus, even if that fetus did not as yet possess a soul, would therefore be a quite different thing from killing a mere animal. The term "potential murder" has been used to describe the act by those who feel that "murder" would not be so clear and precise a word as might be used.

14 On this subject see Hyacinthus-M. Hering, O.P., "De tempore animationis foetus humani," *Angelicum,* January-March 1951, pp. 18-29; Benedictus H. Merkelbach, O.P., *Quaestiones de embryologia et de ministratione baptismatis,* Q. IV, pp. 65-69 (Liége: La Pensée Catholique, 1928).

Second, those who maintain that the soul is not present from the first moment of conception do not and cannot claim that their opinion is certain. They offer their opinion as something for which they think that some arguments can be adduced. But the opinion opposed to theirs, to the effect that the soul is present from the first moment of conception, is more commonly favored by moralists. Now, if it is probable, though not certain, that the object which one is attacking is a human being, the attacker is guilty of murder in his heart whether or not the object is a human being. A deer hunter, for example, sees toward dusk a moving object that might be a deer or that might be a man. If he tells himself that he will shoot first and find out later what it was that he shot, he is guilty of intending to murder even though he finds that what he shot was actually a deer. It is not necessary, then, that a physician should be able to say with absolute certainty that a soul is present if he is to be guilty of murder when he commits an abortion. It is sufficient that he should know and realize that a soul is *probably* present. If he inflicts a deathblow upon something that he knows may be a man, not caring whether it is a man or not, he incurs the guilt of murder.

Finally, the opinion of those who believe it is possible that the soul is not present in the fertilized ovum or in the embryo stage is a merely personal opinion which enjoys no official approval of the Church and which applies to the early stages of gestation only. Concerning the later stages there is no difference of opinion. Even the civil law in the United States of America recognizes the unborn child's right to life. See, for example, the case *Kine* versus *Zuckerman* (Pa. 1924). In the state of California the civil law recognized (1931) the right of inheritance of the fetus immediately after its conception.

It is precisely at such points as these that the Catholic turns to his Church for an authoritative, if not a fuller, statement of what the natural law requires. If God's promise to preserve His Church from error in matters falling within her proper field is to be fulfilled, the Church should know to whom her sacraments can be administered and when the fundamental natural rights of man are being invaded. Now, the law of the Church (Canon 747) prescribes that all living aborted fetuses, regardless of their age, should be baptized, not conditionally but unconditionally; and the Church does not baptize the dead nor any living being that is not human. Again, Pius XI, when speaking of abortions, says: "However much we may pity the mother whose health and even life is gravely imperiled in the performance of the duty allotted to her by nature, nevertheless what could ever be a sufficient reason for excusing in any way the direct murder of the innocent? This is precisely what we are dealing with here. Whether inflicted upon the mother or upon the child, it is against the precept of God and the law of nature: 'Thou shalt not kill' (Exodus 20:13). The life of each is equally sacred, and no one has the power, not even the public authority, to destroy it. It is of no use to appeal to the right of taking away life for here it is a question of the innocent, whereas that right has regard only to the guilty; nor is there here question of defense by bloodshed against an unjust aggressor (for who would call an innocent child an unjust aggressor?)"[15]

Even the desire to protect one's good name, which is a very precious thing, cannot be recognized as a reason for committing an abortion. If an unmarried woman were to become pregnant and were to permit the pregnancy to go to term, this would, in some cases at least, result in the loss of her reputation. The physician, however, is not free to induce an abortion in order to prevent the grave evil of the loss of her good name. Evil may never be done that good may come of it. The act of directly inducing abortion is intrinsically evil, and therefore morally wrong. The purpose for which the surgeon wishes to perform the abortion is indeed praiseworthy, for his intention

[15] Pius XI, *Christian Marriage*. In *Five Great Encyclicals*, p. 95. New York: Paulist Press, 1939.

is to preserve the woman's reputation in the community. The manner in which he would accomplish this noble end, however, is evil, for actually it is murder.

But, it may be asked, is not the life of a mother of a family of far greater value than that of the unborn baby? The first answer to that question is: Even though the mother's life were a thousand times more precious than that of the fetus, it would still be gravely wrong directly to kill the innocent child enclosed within the womb in order to safeguard the mother's life, for this would constitute murder. But in the second place, we reply that one human life is just as valuable basically as any other. Hence the life of the unborn fetus may not be directly terminated, even in order to provide for the best interests of the mother of a large number of small children.

What is to be said of the case where it is necessary to save *either* the mother *or* the child? The attending obstetrician cannot save both, he says. If he attempts to save the baby, the mother will certainly die. And perhaps the preservation of the mother's life is very important, for it may be that she has several young children who would suffer gravely were they to be deprived of her care. In such a dilemma may not the physician sacrifice the life of the baby, who is not at all needed (and is perhaps even unwanted) in order to safeguard the woman who is so necessary for the well-being of her family? The answer is that evil may never be done in order that good may come of it. The physician is not permitted to murder the fetus in order to preserve the mother's life. "But," one may object, "let us suppose that, if an abortion is not performed, both the mother and the child will die. In this case is not the physician who commits an abortion really choosing the lesser of two evils? The two evils are the loss of the child and the loss of both the child and the mother. Obviously the loss of the child alone is a lesser evil than the loss of both mother and child."

The one who raises this objection misstates the case. He does not accurately describe the evils involved. There are two evils in question, it is true, but they are evils of two different kinds. One of them is merely a physical evil; the other is a moral evil.[16] The true choice lies between the following: (1) directly killing an innocent human being and (2) permitting (not causing) the death of both mother and child. The first, a moral evil, is immeasurably worse than the second, a merely physical evil. Hence, even considering the physician's action as a choice between two evils, it must be condemned. It is never permissible to commit sin, a moral evil, in order to prevent any other evil, physical or moral. It is preferable by far that a million mothers and fetuses perish than that a physician stain his soul with murder. In a case which the physician considers absolutely desperate, when he feels sure that the mother will die unless he performs an abortion, he can but leave the patient in the hands of her Creator. This is not the only drastic situation which he encounters where he is helpless to apply an effective remedy. His patients will die of other incurable ailments too. He can do nothing for them but commit them to God.

As a matter of fact, is the physician placed at times in the dilemma described in the preceding paragraph? Let Dr. Joseph L. McGoldrick reply to that question. "The mother-or-child dilemma," says Dr. McGoldrick, "is a relic of the early days of obstetrics. If it is talked about today by any medical men, it is only by those whose training and experience evidently do not qualify them to perform modern obstetrics. In one of the largest hospitals in New York City, where the average number of deliveries is over 3000 a year, no such dilemma has been encountered in my experience during the last twenty years. I have had the same experience in the private hospitals I attend. Cases of pregnancy with heart, lung or kidney complications, which were formerly regarded as necessitating therapeutic

---

[16] A physical evil is something that is opposed to the perfection of a being's physical nature; blindness, for example, sickness, and death are physical evils. A moral evil, on the other hand, is a violation of the eternal law.

abortion . . . are now carried through to term or at least to viability, and in most cases result in an improved physical condition of the mother."[17] The facts given by Dr. McGoldrick would seem to indicate that therapeutic abortion is never a necessary means of saving the mother.

Dr. Roy J. Heffernan, nationally known authority in this field, has the following to say about the matter:

"For thirty-five years it has been my privilege to observe the tremendous progress made during that period in all branches of the healing art, particularly in my specialty, obstetrics and gynecology. One of the most gratifying advances has been the change in the attitude of the profession with regard to the deliberate interruption of pregnancy . . .

"When I was in training and for several years afterwards, therapeutic abortions were frequently performed in most of the leading non-Catholic obstetrical clinics. Tuberculosis, diabetes, hyperemesis gravidarum, chronic nephritis, hypertension, severe anemia, chorea, thyroid dysfunction, disturbances of the nervous system and psychiatric disorders—in fact, in almost any complication of early pregnancy which did not promptly respond to conservative therapy, evacuation of the uterus would be considered. . . .

"Strangely enough, during this time those of us who held intrauterine life inviolate were not piling up tremendous maternal mortality lists. Our task was not easy. Many patients with serious complications required long, painstaking, expert care. . . . With proper care, these women *did not die.* There are scores of well-trained Catholic obstetricians, like myself,

[17] Joseph L. McGoldrick, M.D., "Mr. Blanshard in Medicine," *Homiletic and Pastoral Review* 48:361, February 1948. This opinion is confirmed by leading obstetricians of Spain such as Drs. Nubiola, Oreja, Ruiz Contreras, and Gomez Ibar. See Jacobus Puiula, S.J., *De medicina pastorali,* pp. 107-08 (Rome: Marietti, 1948). See also Roy J. Heffernan, M.D., and William A. Lynch, M.D., "Is Therapeutic Abortion Scientifically Justified?" *Linacre Quarterly* 19:11-27, February 1952; Frederick L. Good, M.D., and Otis F. Kelly, M.D., *Marriage, Morals and Medical Ethics,* p. 149 (New York: P. J. Kenedy and Sons, 1951).

and not a few non-Catholic obstetricians, who have success-fully attended thousands of women during pregnancy with all the complications one sees in private and hospital practice. Many of us have never had a death from hyperemesis gravidarum, from tuberculosis, diabetes, eclampsia or many of the other severe complications of pregnancy.

"It has been most pleasing in recent years, to watch how Science is at last catching up, so to speak, with Ethics. Following bitter experiences, the advocates of therapeutic abortion have, in the past twenty years particularly, consistently narrowed down what they felt were proper indications for this procedure. When therapeutic abortion in the presence of pneumonia increased the mortality by 50 per cent, when therapeutic abortion in cardiac disease reached the state that obstetricians and cardiologists alike were publishing the statement that cardiac decompensation plus interruption of pregnancy equaled death and when succeeding reports of successful management of the complications of pregnancy *without* therapeutic abortion were published in the literature, so much professional embarrassment was engendered that therapeutic abortion lost much of its popularity. In the past ten years the indications for interruption of pregnancy for organic disease have fallen off sharply and during that time so-called psychiatric disorders became more popular substitutes. This popularity bids fair to be short lived as psychiatrists are beginning to point out in the literature that the anxiety state, guilt complex and conversion neuroses, which have followed therapeutic abortion, have made the patient's psychiatric condition worse.

"Modern medical literature is not only revealing this narrowing of indications for therapeutic abortions, but it is also disclosing a definite positive trend toward our viewpoint.

"Speaking of 'Tuberculosis and Childbearing' Dr. Edwin Jameson of Saranac Lake, New York, (*Proceedings of 3rd. American Congress Obstetrics and Gynecology,* 1947) said: 'The occurrence of pregnancy in a woman with active Pulmonary Tuberculosis is to be avoided if at all possible as it complicates the picture medically, economically and socially, although there is ample evidence at the present time to lead us to believe that if the tuberculous woman receives adequate treatment for her pulmonary disease, as well as proper antepartum, intrapartum and postpartum obstetrical care, the pregnancy need give rise to no particular worry from a medical viewpoint.'

"In 'Heart Disease Complicating Pregnancy' Gorenberg (*American Journal of Obstetrics and Gynecology*, May 1943) wrote: 'Absolute bed rest for certain classes of cardiac patients is stressed. By this means alone the incidence of decompensation in pregnant women with heart disease has been reduced from 22.3 per cent to 2.5 per cent, four cases out of a total of 157 and 3 of the failures (of compensation) may have been preventable. The mortality rate has dropped from 3.5 per cent to 0.64 per cent. If only part of the difference between the failure incidence in private and clinic cases, 35.4 per cent to 2.5 per cent, and if only part of the difference in mortality rates between these two groups of cases, 9.1 per cent to 0.64 per cent, is due to financial difficulties encountered by application of this therapy in private cases, some plan must be instituted by maternity hospitals and the associated communities to overcome such difficulties. However, the private doctor plays a most important part, too, and his responsibility in this condition must be stressed. . . .

" 'Considering a previous report of 345 cases together with this series of 223 cases, in which no therapeutic abortion was performed, it is probable that practically every pregnancy encountered in a patient with heart disease can be brought to a successful spontaneous termination, if adequate prenatal care is instituted and if absolute bed rest is enforced . . .'

"The effect of pregnancy on mental disease is discussed by Arbuse and Schechtman (*American Practitioner,* October 1950) who writes: 'There does not seem to be any one condition

199

which absolutely indicates interruption of a pregnancy. . . . The mental state is seldom justification for the induction of abortion. . . . Abortion, per se, is unquestionably a shock and may conceivably be even more detrimental than continuation of the pregnancy. . . . If it could be shown that conception may lead to permanent psychosis in certain defined cases, then the termination of pregnancy would clearly be in the best interests of the patient and the operation would conform to the desired standards. The contrary appears to be the rule, for psychoses initiated by pregnancy rarely persist, but tend to recover after a comparatively short period and in some cases may clear up spontaneously before full term is reached. Women who show permanent impairment of mentality following childbirth belong to the class of the potential psychotic for whom pregnancy is merely a subsidiary factor in the pathogenesis of the psychosis. Upon the mentality of such women a therapeutic abortion cannot be curative and it may exert a deleterious effect that is more harmful than the continuation of pregnancy.'

"And for those who recommend interruption of pregnancy for 'eugenic' reasons, they say: 'There is no psychiatric disorder that is hereditary to the degree that the occurrence of mental illness in the offspring of the patient can be predicated with reasonable certainty.'

"These few examples quoted from men who are preeminent in their field and obviously not prejudicially Catholic are but recent striking examples of many such similar articles occurring in modern medical literature. Dr. Samuel Cosgrove, the director of the Margaret Hague Maternity Hospital, the second-largest institution in this country of its kind, has on several occasions spoken rather strongly about therapeutic abortions. In a paper delivered in 1944 (*American Journal of Obstetrics and Gynecology* 48:299, September 1944) he developed the thesis that the medical profession must vehemently work to maintain the ethical principle that the foetus is a human individual and that its destruction is murder, and in 1946 (*New England Journal of Medicine,* December 1946), he summarized the entire situation as follows, 'Finally, it is believed that there is a continuing and increasing trend toward what Dr. Willard Cooke, of the University of Texas, calls "rationalism" in obstetrics.' This is considered a better term than 'conservatism' or 'radicalism,' which are hard to define and often interchangeable. Perhaps the wish is father to the thought that this trend is wholly desirable. Rationalism includes such objectives as Bingham's fine phrase 'Keep the normal obstetric case normal,' and the principle that medical and surgical complications of pregnancy should be appropriately medically and surgically treated, without interference with pregnancy. It does not embrace, on the one hand, blind confidence that pregnancy is and will remain physiologic, or on the other, a baseless fear that pregnancy may not be successfully managed in the presence of almost any complication. Intelligent improvement in obstetric practice will be principally predicated on thoughtful individualization of cases on the basis of such rationalism.

"If doctors are to be worthy of their calling, if they are to hold to the traditional standards of the profession—above all to do no harm and to work always for the best interest of the patient, they must first accept the obvious fact that patients are human beings and not scientific studies. A three month foetus must be safeguarded as zealously as a three year old child. Human dignity must be respected and human ills in all their vagaries, complex and simple, difficult and easy, must be accepted and managed on a plane in keeping with the highest traditions of our calling."[18]

---

[18] Quoted from a letter received by the author from Dr. Heffernan. Dr. Heffernan is connected with Tufts College of Medicine and Carney Hospital, Boston. See also Roy J. Heffernan, M.D., and William A. Lynch, M.D., "Is Therapeutic Abortion Scientifically Justified?" *Linacre Quarterly* 19:11-27, February 1952; "What Is the Status of Therapeutic Abortion in Modern Obstetrics?" *American Journal of Obstetrics and Gynecology* 66:335-45, August 1953.

Others have had the same experience in this matter. Dr. Keith P. Russell thus describes conditions in the Los Angeles County Hospital: "Whereas the average incidence of therapeutic abortion in the Los Angeles County Hospital 20 years ago was 1 in every 106 deliveries, during the past five years it has been 1 in 2,864 deliveries and in the past year, 1 in 8,383 deliveries. . . . No abortions have been performed for hyperemesis gravidarum since 1937. None has been performed for pyelitis since 1939. . . . No abortions have been performed for fetal indications in the past 20 years. . . . No abortions have been performed for mental or nervous system diseases since 1942. . . . Despite a greatly lowered incidence of therapeutic abortion, the maternal mortality rate in the hospital has not risen; rather, it has shown a progressive decline."[19]

Even from the medical point of view abortion is a remedy that is not infrequently far worse than the disease. Abortion can, and frequently does, cause very serious infection and hemorrhage. Dr. Thomas Parran, former Surgeon General, U.S.A. Public Health Service, asserts that one fourth of all maternal deaths are caused by aborted pregnancies.[20] It is undoubtedly true that abortion has killed some mothers who might have lived many years after the normal delivery of the child. Dr. Frederick Taussig states that "spontaneous abortions have complications in one-quarter of the cases, as compared with more than half in the induced. . . . Under late complications we have conditions such as menstrual disturbances, sterility, tendency to repeated abortions, and various neurasthenias." He also mentions that Zomakion, in an analysis of 24 of 81 curetted abortions, noticed the occurrence of "relative and absolute sterility." Dr. Taussig refers to the fact that I. C. Rubin

[19] Keith P. Russell, M.D., "Changing Indications for Therapeutic Abortion." *Journal of the American Medical Association* 151:108-11, January 10, 1953.

[20] Jane Ward, "What Everyone Should Know about Abortion," *American Mercury* 53:194-200, August 1941. In the *Linacre Quarterly* 21:137, November 1954, Dr. Jose Martinez, Mexican delegate to the Sixth International Congress of Catholic Doctors, emphasizes the point made by Dr. Thomas Parran.

found in the 219 induced abortions and the 239 spontaneous ones which he studied that the induced abortions "were far more frequently followed by sterility."[21]

Perhaps few physicians who have practiced their profession for many years, unless they restrict their practice to certain fields, have not been asked to perform an abortion. The temptation to accede to such a request may be severe for one who is involved in financial difficulties, for the compensation accorded such illicit practice may be very generous. No conscientious physician, however, will perpetrate so evil a deed as abortion, no matter how great his need of money may be. When a woman approaches a physician in this matter, he should be interested not only in keeping his own hands clean of murder, but in trying to protect if possible the baby whose life is in danger. To this end he could have a heart-to-heart talk with the young mother. He might stress the dangers that would arise for her were an abortion performed. He might emphasize the horror of the crime of murder and the grave sin with which her soul would be stained were she to carry out her plan. He might describe the helpless condition of the baby that is nestling under its mother's heart, dependent upon her for protection and love, totally unaware that she may mete out to it hatred and destruction.

One wise physician who was asked by a mother criminally to terminate her pregnancy prematurely told her to bring down to his office her three-year-old son, Jimmy, to whom she was greatly attached. When the two arrived, the physician placed the little boy on the operating table, and, putting a hammer into the woman's hand, he ordered: "Hit Jimmy three strong blows just above the temple." "Why," said the amazed mother, "I could never do such a terrible thing as that. That would be murder." "That's right," rejoined the physician, "and that is exactly what you want me to do to the baby within your

[21] See Frederick J. Taussig, M.D., *Abortion: Spontaneous and Induced,* pp. 272, 274. St. Louis: C. V. Mosby Company, 1936.

womb. If it would be murder to kill Jimmy here, it would also be murder to kill your unborn baby."

When there is question of a young unmarried woman who is now with child, the physician is in a position to help her make arrangements so that the fact of her pregnancy will remain secret. The physician will usually know of some out-of-town home or hospital to which the unmarried mother may retire until after the birth of the baby. He can acquaint the woman with this possibility, advise her concerning the time when she should go away, and suggest reasons for leaving that she can give to her family, employer, and friends. In such cases it would ordinarily be preferable for the young mother herself not to undertake the rearing of the baby but to provide, through the hospital authorities, for a good home for him.

We may conclude the discussion of direct abortion by quoting from Canon E. J. Mahoney, a most competent moralist who has written for many years on this and associated problems and who fully understands the difficulties with which members of the profession are confronted. He says:

"The attitude of the priest or of the professional theologian towards members of the medical profession, whether doctors or nurses, contrary to what they may imagine to be the case, is one of very deep sympathy which expresses itself as helpfully as possible by endeavouring to discover a *modus vivendi,* whilst preserving intact the moral teaching of the Church, in cases where their professional reputation or even their employment in hospitals is at stake. In the last resort, some material loss may have to be faced rather than offend against the law of God in so grave a matter. The issue between causing and not causing direct abortion is, at all events, a matter which has wider interests than purely medical ones. We find it hard to believe, though we are open to persuasion, that the professional reputation of a doctor would gravely suffer, in the long run, if he pleaded these wider interests, religious or legal or social or moral or whatever they may be, in justification of refusal directly to cause an abortion."[22]

Cases Illustrating Direct Abortion

In some of the following cases the physician's action would always constitute a direct abortion; in others it would or would not be a direct abortion according to the conditions described as existing.

Case 93
Aborting the Fetus because of Oligohydramnios

The patient is 18 weeks pregnant. Oligohydramnios is discovered at this time. The physician wishes to empty the uterus at once because of the danger to the mother and the serious fetal deformities that may result if the pregnancy is permitted to go to term. May he do this?

Solution. The physician's action of emptying the uterus at once would be gravely illicit.

Explanation. As long as an immature fetus remains within the uterus with the placenta attached to the uterine wall, there is some hope that it will survive to viability. Extracting a nonviable fetus from the uterus would be to inflict on it a fatal blow, for this act would remove the fetus from the only place where it can live.

Case 94
Aborting the Fetus because of Rape

A girl 15 years of age has been criminally attacked and the physician discovers later that she is pregnant. The father of the girl asks him to do an abortion, for, he says, "This fetus is the fruit of an act of injustice. I have the right to protect my daughter against the loss of her reputation and against all the inconvenience involved in illegitimate motherhood."

Solution. Even in the case of a raped girl direct abortion is illicit.

Explanation. The fetus within this girl's womb is a human being who has done no wrong. It is true that an evil action, that of the rapist, has produced this innocent child and brought about his presence in this place, but that does not alter the fact that the child himself has done

[22] E. J. Mahoney, *Questions and Answers,* vol. II, *Precepts,* p. 54. London: Burns Oates and Washbourne, 1949.

nothing evil. We may not punish one man for the crime of another. Hence no injury may be inflicted on this innocent fetus because of the crime of his rapist father. The girl's father in this case may defend her reputation, but in so doing he may use only legitimate means. Murder is in all circumstances a gravely illicit manner of remedying an undesirable situation.

Case 95
Aborting the Fetus because of an Infected Kidney

The patient is 5 months pregnant. An infected and hydronephrotic kidney resulting from pressure from the enlarged uterus on the corresponding ureter is causing uremic poisoning which may soon kill the mother unless the pressure is removed. The physician proposes that he compress the uterus to relieve the pressure.

Solution. The physician's action would not be licit.

Explanation. Since there is no procedure known to medical science by means of which a uterus can be permanently compressed so as to relieve pressure, the physician's proposal that he compress the uterus can mean only this, that he will reduce its size by removing the nonviable fetus. It is true that in cases of chronic glomerulonephritis or hydronephrosis some medical manuals teach that the "pregnancy should be terminated as soon as serious symptoms appear, without attaching too much importance to the life of the child."[23] The action of the physician, however, in compressing the uterus to relieve the kidney, in order to be effective, would be directed at producing the emptying of the uterus, and this obviously would constitute direct abortion. The act of compressing would have for its purpose reducing the womb to a size where it would no longer press against the kidney. In order to accomplish this desired objective, the uterus would have to expel the fetus. Hence the act of the physician, like all direct abortions, would be gravely illicit.

Case 96
Aborting the Fetus because of Eclampsia

The patient, although only in her second trimester of pregnancy, is suffering from eclampsia which is so severe that her life is in jeopardy. In order to relieve the mother of her danger the physician wishes to empty the uterus of the nonviable fetus.

[23] See Henricus J. Stander, M.D., *Williams Obstetrics*, eighth edition, p. 654. New York: D. Appleton-Century Company, 1941.

Solution. This action would be gravely illicit.

Explanation. Obviously in this case the physician directly intends to produce an abortion. What he desires to do is to save the mother's life; but no matter how noble his purpose may be in trying to produce this effect, his action is of its very nature gravely evil and is never permitted. The physician must, moreover, admit in all honesty that he cannot be certain that the mother will die unless a direct abortion is performed, nor can he be sure that an induced abortion will not cause her death.

Case 97
Aborting the Fetus because of Hemorrhage

The patient, 4 months pregnant, is hemorrhaging from a premature partial detachment of the placenta. The fetus will very probably abort within a short time. The hemorrhage presents a grave danger to the mother, and to control it hastening the expulsion of the fetus is necessary. May the physician administer a drug which will directly produce this effect?

Solution. If the drug is administered directly to expel the fetus from the uterus, the procedure would be gravely illicit.

Explanation. Because of the present partial separation of the placenta from the uterine wall, the fetus will very probably soon become completely detached. This probability, however, does not justify the physician in directly bringing about an abortion, even to save the life of the mother, for his act would constitute the direct killing of a nonviable fetus. The reader will note the difference between Case 97 and Case 130 (pages 239-40), for in the latter case there is question of *complete* abruptio placentae.

Case 98
Aborting the Fetus because of Hyperemesis Gravidarum

The patient, who is pregnant with a nonviable fetus, goes into pernicious or uncontrollable vomiting. The attending physician says that a therapeutic abortion is absolutely necessary in order to save the woman's life. May the abortion be performed?

Solution. Therapeutic abortion, even in this case, would be gravely illicit.

Explanation. The operation would be illicit because it would be a direct and fatal attack upon the living fetus. This case is intentionally included with a full realization of the fact that well-informed physicians no longer consider therapeutic abortion indicated when the patient is suffering from hyperemesis gravidarum. Effective therapies have recently been introduced, among them the use of dramamine and thiamine. There was a time, however, when a therapeutic abortion was recommended in such cases.[24] It should be significant to physicians that the refusal to commit a direct abortion under any circumstances leads to increased efforts to develop better therapies, with the resultant saving of many lives, not only of unborn children, but also of mothers to whom the shock of an abortion is often fatal. As early as 1928 one physician was able to write that it is of the greatest interest to observe that at a certain hospital, out of 10,000 deliveries in six years, there were 25 cases of *hyperemesis gravidarum*, in most of which—and five were almost on the verge of dissolution—the textbooks would have advised the emptying of the uterus. In point of fact, all the cases recovered and went to full term, being delivered of healthy living children.[25]

Case 99
Aborting the Fetus because of Carcinoma of the Breast

An operable carcinoma of the breast is discovered in a woman 3 months pregnant. The physician wishes to do a radical mastectomy, and a total hysterectomy and bilateral salpingo-oophorectomy in order to remove the stimulating effect of the estrogen secreted by the placenta and the ovaries on the possible residual cancer cells left after the mastectomy. He also feels that it is desirable to eliminate the possible stimulating effect of the postabortal uterus.

Solution. It is permissible to do the radical mastectomy and to follow through with deep X-ray therapy to the breast. It is not morally justifiable to remove the uterus.

Explanation. The death of the fetus is not secondary to the purpose of taking out the uterus, but is the direct purpose of the operation, which is to eliminate the placental secretion of the hormones. The placenta is an integral part of fetal life, since it contains fetal blood vessels. When the fetus reaches a real viability a caesarean section may be done, followed by the surgical removal of the ovaries. The uterus need not be removed, since its stimulating effect is questionable. It must also be remembered estrogen is also probably secreted by the adrenals.

[24] See Henricus J. Stander, M.D., *Williams Obstetrics*, eighth edition, p. 637. New York: D. Appleton-Century Company, 1941.
[25] See a communication of Louis Cassidy in "Deontology. Questions Regarding Craniotomy and Abortus Provocatus," *Catholic Medical Guardian* 6:56, April 1928.

In four of the following five cases a nonviable fetus might be either alive or dead. The solution given is consistently the same: that the fetus may licitly be removed only if it is certainly dead. In such a case, of course, no abortion is committed, for abortion as that term has been defined is the direct expulsion of a living and nonviable fetus. In the fifth and last case the physician refrains from performing an abortion that might (though illicitly) have been performed.

Case 100
Procedure after an Attempted Abortion

The physician is called during the night to a home where he finds a
    woman hemorrhaging very dangerously. Examination reveals the fact
    that she has attempted to procure an abortion. The fetus is still in
    utero, but the physician is certain that the placenta is detached from
    the wall of the uterus. May he complete the abortion in order to save
    the patient's life?

Solution. If the placenta is completely detached, the physician may now
    completely empty the uterus. He should then at once baptize the
    fetus if it is not certainly dead.

Explanation. When the physician examines the patient he finds that she
    has already pulled the placenta loose from the inner wall of the
    uterus, by doing which she has already dealt a fatal blow to the
    fetus. In extracting the fetus, the physician does nothing to injure
    it. It would die within some minutes whether it remained inside the
    uterus or were brought forth. Its ultimate death is due, not to the
    physician's act, but to the mother's.

In order to understand Case 100 and some of the cases to be explained on the following pages, it is well to remember that one is never permitted *directly* to kill an innocent person nor *directly* to shorten his life. As has been explained above (see page 96), "directly to kill another" means that the death of that person is either the end or purpose which one sets out to accomplish or that it is a means for arriving at the accomplishment of the end in view. Directly to kill an innocent person constitutes the crime of murder. Moreover, directly to hasten another's death is a violation of the law of nature. Such an action would be evil, even though one were directly to hasten another's death by only an hour or even by only a few minutes. The reason for this assertion is that God has supreme and exclusive ownership over the lives of all human beings. He and He alone has supreme dominion over every moment of their lives from their conception up to the time of their last breath. It is He, therefore, and He alone who has the right directly to terminate or to abbreviate human life. It is for this reason that mercy killing (see page 267) is intrinsically evil. When a person is mortally wounded or incurably sick, and has only a few days or hours to live, no one is justified in administering to him a *coup de grace* either for the sake of ending his agony or for any other reason. Such an action would have as its purpose the termination of life; the hastening of death, therefore, would be directly intended.

Quite different, however, from the *direct* hastening of death is the act of *indirectly* shortening life. A physician, for example, because his services are in constant demand, works strenuously over a long period of time in caring for the plague-stricken. He may feel certain that his heroic devotion to the sick will shorten his life notably; his actions nevertheless are not therefore evil. Obviously the physician does not desire nor intend the shortening of his life; he merely permits it for a weighty reason. In some of the cases[26] discussed in this chapter there may be question of some hastening of the death of the fetus. This hastening of death is not, however, sought or intended. The death of the fetus would be prevented if this were at all possible, and the hastening of death involves no desired advantage. The hastening of death in these and similar cases is merely permitted. In other words, we say that life is shortened, not directly, but indirectly only. For a proportionately grave reason this is justified according to the teaching explained in the application of the principle of the twofold effect (see pages 98-101).

[26] See for example Cases 105, 107, 110, 111, 113, and 114.

Case 101
Procedure in a Case of Suspected Carcinoma

The patient, a woman of 35, is in very critical condition. The physician discovers in the uterus something which may prove to be a carcinoma, though he is not certain that it is not a fetus. In order to save the woman's life he wishes to perform a dilatation and curettage or a hysterectomy. May he licitly do so?

Solution. The physician should wait until he can ascertain whether the growth is a tumor or a fetus. If the ordinary positive or probable signs of pregnancy are absent, if the pregnancy tests are negative, and if there is some definite evidence of malignancy, he may licitly perform a curettage or a hysterectomy.

Explanation. In the case as described the physician uses all available means of determining whether or not a fetus is present and refrains from acting until he knows that all signs and tests of pregnancy are negative. He is therefore justified in telling himself that a fetus is not present and that he is not performing an abortion.

Case 102
Procedure in a Case of Hydatidiform Mole

The patient is diagnosed as having in utero a hydatidiform mole. The physician does not know whether or not a living fetus is present, but he wishes to empty the uterus at once because in a certain percentage of cases the chorion becomes a malignant tumor (chorionepithelioma).[27] May he empty the uterus if he believes that this is necessary to save the patient's life?

Solution. If the physician doubts whether or not a living fetus is now in utero, he may not adopt this procedure.

Explanation. The hydatidiform mole is a diseased condition of the chorionic villi produced by a pathological proliferation with degeneration. In this case the degenerated chorion resembles a bunch of grapes. "Hydatidiform degeneration usually begins about the fifth week of pregnancy, but may begin earlier or later. If it begins early, the fetus is absent, but if it starts later, only part of the placenta may be involved and a well-formed fetus may be present. It can develop in one of twins. Cases are on record where a living child has been

---

[27] At one time hydatidiform moles were thought to develop into chorionepitheliomas in 10 per cent or more of the cases. Recent figures as given by Crossen reduce the incidence to less than 2 per cent. See Robert J. Crossen, M.D., *Diseases of Women,* tenth edition, p. 579 (St. Louis: C. V. Mosby Company, 1953).

born with hydatidiform mole present, but such happenings are rare."[28] What means the physician can employ to ascertain whether or not a living fetus is within the uterus is a medical problem. It is true that, if a fetus is present, it is usually dead, or at least that it would rarely be able to survive to viability. If, however, the uterus even *probably* contains a living fetus, that fetus may not be directly attacked by a death-dealing blow. The evacuation of the uterus would constitute such a fatal blow, for it would remove the nonviable fetus from the only place where it could possibly live. Even if the physician knows that the fetus cannot live much longer, he may not licitly remove it from the uterus, for so to act would be a direct and unjust attack on the life of an innocent human being.[29]

Case 103
Curettage after an Attempted Abortion

The patient, 7 weeks pregnant, is suffering a severe uterine hemorrhage. She summons her physician and asks him to terminate her pregnancy. The physician dilates the cervix, thinking that this dilatation may stimulate the uterus to expel the fetus. After this dilatation the patient continues to hemorrhage and still feels that she may be pregnant. She then consults a second physician, presenting him with all the facts. May the second physician curette the uterus?

Solution. The second physician may do a curettage only on condition that it is certain that the fetus is now dead or that it has already been expelled. The presence of a living fetus can ordinarily be established, but the results of laboratory and clinical examinations are sometimes equivocal. If there is genuine probability that the fetus is still attached to the uterine wall and that it is at least probably alive, curettage is not permissible, and every means possible must be used to save the fetus.

Explanation. If the fetus is not certainly dead, the second physician by using curettage would intend to abort it even if it is alive. If the fetus is certainly dead, the physician not only may but should expel it. The purpose of the curettage would be to stop the hemorrhage and to prevent the danger of infection. In such a case the fact that the patient has maliciously effected an abortion should not deter the

[28] John F. Cunningham, M.D., *Textbook of Obstetrics*, p. 240. New York: Grune and Stratton, 1951.

[29] For the procedure followed by one conscientious physician in such cases see Frederick L. Good, M.D., and Otis F. Kelly, M.D., *Marriage, Morals and Medical Ethics*, pp. 106-09 (New York: P. J. Kenedy and Sons, 1951).

physician from coming to her aid. Healing and protecting from death
the sinning woman is a commendable action.

Case **104**

Refraining from an Abortion in a Case of a Hemorrhage

The patient, who is the mother of several children, is 3 months pregnant.
She has a severe hemorrhage about every 10 days, and with each
hemorrhage she becomes weaker. All efforts to stop the hemorrhaging have been made. The physician judges that the only effective means left is removing the fetus, but he does not disturb the
fetus because it is not viable. When the fetus is 6 months old the
mother dies. Was the physician justified in thus treating the case,
even though he felt certain that the mother could not live long
enough for the fetus to become viable?

Solution. The physician acted licitly.

Explanation. The physician could not have acted other than he did, for
directly to empty the uterus of the nonviable fetus would have been
to commit the crime of abortion. Even in the event that the physician
were certain that both mother and child would die unless a direct
abortion were performed, that procedure would nevertheless still be
forbidden. In the case as described nothing is said of an attempt by
the physician to save the mother's life by blood transfusions. He was
at fault if he failed to use all available means.

INDIRECT ABORTION

IN DIRECT abortion a living and nonviable fetus is removed
from the uterus. The reason for the removal is that the
pregnancy, added to some pathological condition from which
the mother is suffering, increases her difficulties or even lessens
her chances of survival. No condition exists, however, which
makes the removal of the uterus itself necessary as a means of
saving the mother's life.

The abortion is termed indirect when the pregnant uterus
itself is excised because its condition is such that its removal
is medically necessary. If the uterus contains a living and
nonviable fetus, the fetus will of course inevitably die. There
is no direct attack upon the fetus, however, and its death is
merely permitted as a secondary effect of an act which needs

to be performed and which, as we shall see immediately, it is permissible to perform.

It is licit to excise a diseased uterus which is gravely dangerous, even though the operation will indirectly kill the fetus which is enclosed in the womb. The reason is that we may rightly apply the four conditions of the principle of the twofold effect. (See pages 98-101.) The first condition is fulfilled, for the operating surgeon's intention is to save the life of the mother. He, of course, foresees the death of the fetus, but he does not desire this evil effect. The second condition is fulfilled, for the surgeon's act consists in ridding the woman of a diseased part of her body which is jeopardizing her life. Hence that which he sets out to accomplish is licit. If the fetus were not present, the surgical operation of removing a diseased and dangerous part of the woman's body, the cancerous uterus, would obviously be an act which of its nature is not evil. The presence of the living fetus in the diseased womb does not alter the nature of the act which the surgeon performs. The operation is directly remedial regarding the mother's body and is in itself unconnected with the pregnancy. The third condition is fulfilled, for the evil effect (the death of the fetus) does not cause the good effect (saving the life of the mother). Whether the fetus were harmed by the operation or not would make no difference in regard to producing the good effect. The fourth condition is fulfilled, for safeguarding the mother's health is a proportionately grave reason for permitting the death of the fetus.

The physician who performs an operation of this kind should have a nurse procure beforehand a basin of lukewarm water in which the fetus may be baptized immediately after the uterus is removed from the mother. When the diseased womb has been extracted from the woman's body, it should be cut open at once and the fetus should be baptized. If the fetus is very small, baptism by immersion would be preferable. If the fetus is enclosed in the sacs or membranes, the latter must of course be removed, so that in the baptism the water will touch the head of the infant.[30]

In all such operations, where the surgery has important bearing on two lives and not merely one, the surgeon must be sure that the reason for operating is a proportionately grave one. If, for example, the fetus is near viability and an immediate hysterectomy would only *probably,* and *not certainly,* diminish the danger of death to the mother, the operation would be illicit. In this case the pregnant uterus may not be excised; for since the surgery would bring certain death to the fetus, the latter's certain right to life must take precedence over the mother's right to a doubtful benefit. Again, if excising the uterus would only *probably* indirectly cause the death of the fetus, surgery would be licit if needed to remove *probable* danger to the mother's life. If, moreover, the operation would *rarely* result in death for the fetus, it would be licitly performed when necessary, not to save the mother's life, but to cure her of a grave disease. A remote hope of saving the mother justifies surgery which is necessary to prevent death of *both* the mother and the child, for the surgeon is doing all in his power to save both. It is taken for granted that there are no other effective means which would not endanger the fetus.

The cases that follow illustrate the application of these principles. Case 105 is a typical case involving cancer of the uterus. Cases 106, 107, 108, and 109 give the rules to be applied under the four possible conditions that can exist; if the cancer is operable, if the cancer is inoperable, if the fetus is viable, and if the fetus is nonviable.

Case 105
Hysterectomy because of Carcinoma of the Uterus
The patient during the second month of her pregnancy is found to have a carcinoma of the uterine cervix. The lesion has not as yet spread

[30] For a fuller discussion of baptism see pp. 357-69. In the cases discussed in this section it is always assumed that a living fetus will be baptized, and the fact that it should be baptized is not mentioned.

beyond the confines of the underlying uterine wall, but the physician judges that it will do so within one or two months.

Solution. The physician is free to use either radium and X-ray therapy or a radical hysterectomy. If radium and X ray are used, the physician is not free to use a dilatation and curettage first in order to clean out the pregnant uterus.

Explanation. The uterus is now a grave danger to the mother; hence it may be excised. Immediate action will shorten the life of the fetus (which can in no case be saved), but this indirect and merely permitted effect is outweighed by the good result. If radium and X ray are used, the fetus will die and be aborted, but the purpose of the therapy is not to kill the fetus but to arrest the carcinoma. To provide for baptism, hysterectomy is preferable. The immediate purpose of a dilatation and curettage, however, would be to remove and hence to kill the fetus, and this direct attack upon the living fetus would not be licit.

Case 106
Operable Carcinoma and a Viable Fetus

The patient, who is pregnant with a viable fetus, has an operable carcinoma of the uterine cervix. How should the physician proceed?

Solution. At the time that he judges best the physician should perform a caesarean section to deliver the child. He should then use surgery or irradiation to remove or arrest the carcinoma.

Explanation. Since the fetus is viable, there is present a just and proportionate reason for hastening the birth of the child in order to save the life of the mother. The physician is free to perform a caesarean section when the fetus reaches absolute viability at 28 weeks. If it is safe to permit the fetus to come somewhat closer to term, the physician will decide how long to wait before delivering the child.

Case 107
Operable Carcinoma and a Nonviable Fetus

A pregnant patient has an operable carcinoma of the uterus and the fetus is not viable. What should the physician do?

Solution. If the pregnancy is in the first trimester, the physician may proceed as if it did not exist, as explained in Case 105. If the fetus is so close to viability that it might be saved, the physician will use doses of radium which will hold the carcinoma in check without harming the fetus and then deliver the fetus by caesarean section when viability is reached. If at any stage in the case it becomes evident to the

216

physician that the attempt to save the fetus will certainly or very probably result in the mother's death, he is free to use surgery or radiation that is so heavy that the fetus cannot survive.

Explanation. The mother has a moral obligation of giving the fetus a chance to reach viability, but not if this would appreciably increase the danger to her own life. If surgery would be as effective as irradiation that would prove fatal to the child, surgery must be preferred so as to provide, insofar as possible, for the baptism of the fetus.

Case 108
Inoperable Carcinoma and a Viable Fetus

The patient, who is pregnant with a viable fetus, has an inoperable carcinoma. What should the physician do?

Solution. The delivery of the child should be delayed until the fetus is as close to term as possible.

Explanation. The mother's condition will not be appreciably worsened by the delay, and the fetus' chance of more perfect development and continued life will be improved.

Case 109
Inoperable Carcinoma and a Nonviable Fetus

The patient, who is pregnant with a nonviable fetus, has an inoperable carcinoma of the uterus. What should the physician do?

Solution. The physician should wait until the fetus is viable and then deliver the child by caesarean section.

Explanation. Since the carcinoma is inoperable and nothing can be done to save the mother, the physician's chief concern will be to provide for the best interests of the fetus. Even though the fetus is so far removed from viability that any attempt to save it seems hopeless, irradiation which is so heavy that it would prove fatal to the fetus may not be used. Measures that could be defended under the principle of the twofold effect as a means of saving the mother's life cannot be defended when saving her life has ceased to be possible. Heavy irradiation fatal to the fetus would, moreover, eliminate, without a justifying reason, all hope of baptizing the infant.

Case 110
Carcinoma of the Uterus and the Use of X Rays

The patient, 3 months pregnant, has carcinoma of the uterus. The physician believes that he can cure the patient if he X-rays the uterus at once, but he realizes too that this procedure will very probably cause the death of the nonviable fetus. May he nevertheless irradiate the uterus?

Solution. If this drastic procedure alone will cure the mother, the physician may X-ray the uterus. If, however, a hysterectomy would be equally effective, this is to be preferred, for then one could probably administer baptism to the infant as soon as the uterus is excised.

Explanation. The principle of the twofold effect would justify the use of X rays even though death might result for the fetus. The death of the fetus would be indirectly produced, and there is a proportionately grave reason for permitting this evil effect to occur. The child's spiritual welfare, however, must be safeguarded if this is possible. If in the present case a hysterectomy would afford the opportunity of baptizing the fetus, this operation must be given the preference.

Case 111
Excision of a Gangrenous Fibroid Tumor

The pregnant patient has a gangrenous subserous pedunculated leiomyoma. Its immediate removal is necessary to save the woman's life, but the operation may mean the death of a nonviable fetus. May the physician excise the myoma?

Solution. This operation may be licitly performed.

Explanation. The physician's act of removing the fibroid tumor is directly aimed at saving the mother's life, although indirectly it will bring about the death of the fetus. The evil effect is fully compensated for by the good effect. If, however, it is possible without causing grave risk to the patient to delay the surgery until the fetus is viable, this must be done.

Case 112
Hysterectomy because of Discovery of a Myoma

The patient is 3 months pregnant. Her abdomen has been opened for an appendectomy. The physician discovers a myoma in the uterus. He wishes to do a hysterectomy after the appendectomy.

Solution. The physician may do neither a hysterectomy nor a myomectomy if the surgery can safely be delayed until the child is viable. Moreover, if surgery is necessary, a hysterectomy is illicit if a myomectomy would suffice to safeguard the patient's health.

Explanation. In order to justify the indirect killing of the fetus by a hysterectomy or running the risk of bringing about an abortion through myomectomy, the surgeon must have a proportionately grave reason. If an immediate hysterectomy is required to save the

218

mother's life, he may operate at once. If, however, without causing danger of death to the mother, he can delay operating until the fetus is viable, he must wait, for in that case there would not be present a sufficient reason for permitting the death of the fetus. Moreover, if a myomectomy would suffice to relieve the present danger to the mother, there would be no reason to justify the added evil involved in a hysterectomy. A hysterectomy would mean certain death for the fetus; in a myomectomy there would be hope of saving the life of the fetus. In order to justify excising a pregnant uterus the surgeon must be certain of two points: (1) that the myoma cannot be effectively cut from the uterus without destroying that organ and (2) that the fetus cannot be carried to viability. It may be added that if the physician wishes to excise the uterus merely to avoid a delivery made difficult by a myomatous organ, the operation could not be justified.

Case 113
Excision of a Ruptured Uterus

The patient has a ruptured uterus and the fetus is nonviable. May the physician remove the uterus, now hemorrhaging dangerously?

Solution. The ruptured uterus may be licitly excised if this is necessary to stop a hemorrhage which is a grave threat to the mother's life.

Explanation. The excision of the uterus is justified on the principle that a part of the body may be sacrificed in order to preserve the rest. Unless the hemorrhaging uterus is removed, the mother will die. To prevent death the source of the danger may be excised. The principle of the twofold effect justifies the operation in the case where a nonviable fetus is enclosed within the ruptured uterus.

Case 114
Excision of a Scarred Uterus

The patient is pregnant. During the course of an emergency appendectomy the surgeon discovers that her uterus is so severely scarred that even now it is in grave danger of rupturing and it will certainly rupture if the pregnancy is allowed to continue for any great length of time. The fetus cannot possibly live to viability. May the surgeon at once excise the uterus?

Solution. If the fetus is sufficiently large to permit its being baptized, it is lawful to excise the scarred uterus at once. If delay would not notably augment the danger to the mother's life and if it would give greater hope of validly baptizing the fetus, the surgeon must wait. If any delay is dangerous, he may operate at once.

Explanation. The reasoning that justifies this operation is the same as that which permits the excision of the Fallopian tube in certain cases of ectopic tubal pregnancy. (See pages 221-26.) The uterus is now in a dangerously pathological condition. Its removal is necessary to safeguard the mother's life. Hence the surgeon may licitly excise this part of her body in order to conserve the rest. The fetus, enclosed in the womb, will die when the uterus is excised, it is true; but while its death is certainly foreseen, it is neither directly intended nor directly procured.

If the fetus is not yet large enough to establish sound probability that it can be validly baptized, charity demands that the surgeon wait if possible until there is greater hope of administering valid baptism. If, however, a delay in excising the uterus would considerably increase the danger to the mother's life, the surgeon may operate at once, for the certain good which an immediate operation would effect for the mother would outweigh the probable benefit which delay would bring to the child.

Case 115
A Craniotomy When Fetus Is Known To Be Dead

The patient, 8 months pregnant, is hemorrhaging severely. It is evident that the fetus is dead, but its head is so large that extraction is difficult. The physician does a craniotomy.

Solution. The physician's action is licit.

Explanation. The physician's action does not injure the fetus, for the latter is already dead before the craniotomy is performed. The mutilation of the head of a dead fetus is licit for a sufficient reason. In the present instance there is obviously a justifying reason.

INDIRECT ABORTION IN ECTOPIC PREGNANCIES

A N ECTOPIC pregnancy is one which is implanted in the body of the mother somewhere else than in the uterus. The fertilized ovum will normally lodge in the uterus. If it does not do so, it is called an ectopic (that is, "out-of-place") pregnancy. Such extrauterine pregnancies are classified according to their location. If the fertilized ovum settles in the Fallopian tube, it is called a *tubal* pregnancy. If it clings to an ovary, it is an *ovarian* pregnancy. If it develops in some other part of the abdominal cavity, it bears the name of *abdominal* pregnancy. By far the most common type of ectopic pregnancy is the tubal.

Tubal Ectopic Pregnancy

In the tubal ectopic pregnancy the fertilized ovum lodges in some part of the Fallopian tube. The reason that it does not continue its descent into the uterus may be the pathological condition of the tube itself or of the ovum. Once the fertilized ovum takes up its nesting place in the tube, it begins to bore into the wall of the tube, seeking as it does life-giving nourishment. This "boring-in" action on the part of the tiny embryo perforates the inner layers of the tube and the tube soon becomes weakened by internal hemorrhaging. There is present a pathological condition of the tube, caused by the erosive action of the trophoblast which is destroying the muscle wall and penetrating blood vessels. The growing fetus causes the tube to swell, and this swelling dangerously stretches the tube's outer wall. Left in this condition, the tube will ordinarily rupture; and unless surgery is performed very soon after the rupturing, the mother may die.

When the Fallopian tube is in this condition, would it be licit to slit it open and remove the fetus? Obviously this action would be gravely evil, for it would constitute a direct, unjust attack on the life of an innocent fetus. It would, in short, be murder. In such a procedure the operating surgeon would set out to destroy the fetus as a means of curing the mother, and thus he would directly intend its death. The same conclusion would follow if the physician used drugs, X ray, or any other method directly to terminate the life of the fetus.

Would it, however, be likewise illicit to excise a Fallopian tube which contains a living fetus? If the tube itself is healthy, there would of course be no justifying reason for the excision. But in the case of an ectopic pregnancy the Fallopian tube is in a definitely pathological condition. Its inner portion is riddled, greatly weakened, and full of internal hemorrhaging.

Once the tube has ruptured externally, the physician may and should immediately tie off the arteries which supply blood to the tube and then remove the tube by surgery. This operation is obviously justified, for in it are fully verified the four conditions required for the application of the principle of the two-fold effect. The excision of this ruptured and gravely dangerous part of the mother's body is similar, in respect to the moral law, to the removal of a pregnant uterus whose cancerous condition is at present gravely threatening the mother's life. (See pages 213-15.)

But let us suppose that the tube in the case of an ectopic pregnancy has not yet ruptured. Must the surgeon, before the excision, wait until an external rupture occurs? The answer is that, if the tube is at present in a gravely dangerous condition and if its excision cannot be delayed without a notable increase of danger to the mother, this Fallopian tube may be removed at once. This conclusion is based on two principles: (1) Mutilation is licit if it is required to conserve the health of the whole body. (2) An act which has two effects, one good, the other bad, may be licitly performed, given certain conditions. The latter principle is correctly applied to the present case. The first condition is fulfilled, for the surgeon's intention is good. He has as his purpose in operating the saving of the mother's life. He foresees, it is true, that the fetus will die when the tube where it is resting is removed from the woman's body, but he does not desire its death. This is a merely permitted evil effect. The second condition is fulfilled, for the surgeon's action is not intrinsically evil. That which he sets out to accomplish is cutting away a pathological or diseased part of the woman's body. The third condition is fulfilled, for the action's evil effect (the death of the fetus) does not cause the good effect (the preserving of the mother's health). Whether the fetus died or not would hardly affect the mother's health. It is the ridding the body of a seriously corrupted part which directly promotes the mother's well-being. It is not the fetus which at present constitutes the threat to the mother's life; it is the diseased organ. The fourth condition is fulfilled, for there is due proportion between the evil effect and the good effect. The death that will result for the fetus is compensated for by the life that will be saved for the mother.

In the analysis of the application of the fourth condition to our present case, it is well to bear in mind the following facts. Tubal pregnancies practically never go to term. In about ninety-nine cases out of a hundred the fetus is aborted (and usually this will occur before the twelfth week), or the tube ruptures externally; and in either case the fetus will perish. Hence when one considers excising a dangerously weakened but externally unruptured tube in ectopic pregnancy, the choice lies between the following two modes of procedure: (1) permitting the tube to remain in the woman's body until it ruptures externally. This will bring death to the fetus and will imperil the life of the mother; or (2) excising the tube at once. This latter operation will bring to the mother safety but to the fetus death. In the first procedure the fetus is, practically speaking, just as certain to die as in the second procedure. As far as the fetus is concerned, the difference between the first procedure and the second procedure is that in the first procedure its life probably would be lengthened by a few weeks. Hence in evaluating the fourth condition the physician must have sufficient cause for permitting the life of the fetus to be shortened because of the excision of the tube.

Is it, then, licit in every case of ectopic pregnancy to excise the diseased Fallopian tube? The answer is that the operation is licit if the tube is at present gravely dangerous to the mother, or if putting off the operation would involve grave danger. The physician is the one who must decide when the tube may be considered to be gravely dangerous. He must judge each individual case on its own merits. The general rule which should be followed is this: *If delay in excising the diseased Fallopian tube would gravely jeopardize the mother's life, the physician may operate at once.* The ultimate decision in a particular case is in the hands of the physician. It may be that in most cases where an ectopic pregnancy is found, the removal of the tube at once is required to avert existing and grave danger from the mother. But this is not true in all cases. In some few cases at least there is no grave danger to the mother when the ectopic is first discovered. In these few cases the immediate removal of the tube is not licit. The diseased tube may not be excised until it is a source of grave danger to the mother. To excise the tube before this time would indirectly shorten the life of the ectopic fetus without a sufficient reason, and this would be illicit. Hence in all cases in which grave danger is not actually present the physician must adopt the expectant treatment.

There are cases in which the surgeon discovers an ectopic pregnancy during the course of a surgical operation; for example, an appendectomy. May he immediately excise the tube if to wait would necessitate performing another grave operation? In this event, because the expectant treatment would involve so great an added danger to the mother, the surgeon may at once remove the pathological tube. The same solution is to be given when the patient would have to be kept under constant observation in a hospital and she refuses to be hospitalized because she cannot afford the expense.

There are circumstances when the physician will sincerely doubt about the gravity of the danger in a particular ectopic pregnancy. In that event he may and should give the mother the benefit of the doubt. The reason is that an immediate operation will probably have the good effect of saving the mother's life, and will probably have the bad effect of indirectly shortening to some extent the fetus' life. The good effect will thus greatly outweigh the evil effect. Hence the physician preferably will excise the diseased tube at once.

Misconceptions concerning the principles involved can arise because of the fact that the diseased condition of the tube is due to the fetus. Is it not true, one may argue, that the tube's weakened and hemorrhaging condition was brought about by the fetus? Is not the excision of the tube intended to rid the mother of the fetus, the cause of her danger? We reply to this objection by admitting that the fetus did cause the present riddled condition of the tube; but, we add, the tube itself is now seriously diseased and would remain diseased quite independently of the fetus. It is the tube itself, not the fetus, which constitutes the present grave danger to the mother; and so, given certain conditions, it may be excised.

Some who are not acquainted with the facts believe that the Catholic Church has changed her attitude in regard to the licitness of doing surgery on ectopic pregnancies. Up to the present day the Church has made only a few official pronouncements on this question, and these pronouncements refer to the direct attack of the surgeon on the fetus or to the direct removal of a nonviable fetus from the mother's womb.[31] Such procedures even today are condemned by all Catholic moralists. On these questions the Church has not changed her view. Catholic ethicians, however, have changed their view with regard to the licitness of excising the unruptured Fallopian tube in an ectopic pregnancy, but this change of opinion stemmed from new medical findings on this matter. Fifty years ago there was little medical knowledge available with reference to the pathology of an ectopic pregnancy. When medical authorities provided the information that the diseased condition of the Fallopian tube, even before its external rupture, in many

[31] See T. Lincoln Bouscaren, S.J., *Ethics of Ectopic Operations*, pp. 21-22, 48-64 (Milwaukee: Bruce Publishing Company, 1944). See also Henry Davis, S.J., *Moral and Pastoral Theology*, vol. II, chap. 6, "The Ectopic Embryo," pp. 171-86 (London: Sheed and Ward, 1949); Gerald Kelly, S.J., "Morality of Ectopic Operations," *Linacre Quarterly* 15:2-8, April 1948; John McCarthy, "Direct and Indirect Abortion—Ectopic Pregnancy," *Irish Ecclesiastical Record* 55:59-66, January 1940; James O'Brien, "Ectopic Gestation: Moral Aspects," *Ecclesiastical Review* 105:95-103, August 1941; Elmer A. Schlueter, M.D., "Ectopic Gestation: Medical Aspects," *Ecclesiastical Review* 105:81-94, August 1941.

cases of ectopic pregnancy constituted a grave and present danger to the mother's life, the moralists declared that the excision of the tube was licit even though the death of the fetus could not be prevented. The moralists made no change in regard to principles or in the application of principles. They merely applied the principles to new facts and arrived at a new conclusion. It is for physicians accurately to present the facts to the moralist. He depends on them for medical information. Given the medical information necessary, he will then apply the ethical principles to the case and pronounce upon the licitness or illicitness of certain procedures.

Ovarian and Abdominal Pregnancies

If an ectopic pregnancy is clinging to an ovary or to the woman's viscera, may the surgeon remove it? The solution to this case is similar to that given in the case of a tubal pregnancy. If the organ to which the fetus is clinging has become so diseased or weakened that it is now a grave source of danger to the woman, the organ may be licitly excised. The organ may have become diseased independently of the fetus or it may have become riddled and weakened because of the "boring-in" action of the fetus. The initial source of the danger does not matter. If at present the condition of the organ is actually pathological and if it is a grave threat to the mother's life, that part of her body may licitly be removed in order to preserve the rest of the body. The same norms about delaying the operation when delay is possible apply in this case as in that of a tubal pregnancy.

It will be noted that, in all the solutions which have been given, the fetus itself is never directly attacked. A pathological organ which is threatening the mother's life is removed, just as it would be removed if it contained no fetus; and the death of the fetus is permitted as a secondary effect of the operation. It is conceivable that there might be a rare case in which the fetus has taken up its lodging next to a vital organ which cannot be removed, such as the liver. If the fetus continues its riddling process, the organ will soon be destroyed and the mother will die. Should such a case ever occur in medical practice, the only thing that could be done to save the mother would be to remove the fetus; and the only argument that could be alleged to justify the removal would be that the fetus, now actually attacking a vital organ of the mother, is an unjust aggressor. The claim that the fetus can ever be, under any circumstances, an unjust aggressor cannot be accepted as correct. The fetus is a living human being. It has been placed by nature where it now resides. It had no voice in the decision. It cannot be called an unjust aggressor, for it is engaged in a purely natural process. Surely we may not call nature unjust. To do so would be to call into question the justice of God, the Author of nature, and this is unthinkable. Hence we must conclude that the fetus may, in no conceivable set of circumstances, be directly killed, for this would be murder. This judgment is confirmed by the words of Pius XI: "What could ever be a sufficient reason for excusing in any way the direct murder of the innocent? . . . Who would call an innocent child an unjust aggressor?"[32]

Case 116
Illicit Excision of a Fetus from a Fallopian Tube

The patient's abdomen is open for an appendectomy. The surgeon discovers a pregnancy in the Fallopian tube. The fetus is probably dead, and therefore the surgeon slits open the tube and extracts the fetus. "If it was not already dead when I took it out," says the surgeon, "it surely would not have had long to live anyway. Hence my procedure was fully justified." What is to be said of the morality of the surgeon's action?

Solution. The surgeon acted in a gravely illicit manner.

Explanation. The surgeon here directly attacked a fetus which was only probably dead. If the fetus was only probably dead, it was possibly alive. Hence the surgeon ran the risk of directly killing an innocent

[32] Pius XI, *Christian Marriage.* In *Five Great Encyclicals*, p. 95. New York: Paulist Press, 1939.

person. This is never licit. If the fetus were certainly dead, the surgeon could of course remove it from the Fallopian tube. He could also remove the tube with the fetus, as in Case 117, if he found the tube so pathological that it was an immediate and grave threat to the mother; but apparently he did not find it so. The principle expressed by him, to the effect that it is licit to kill one who will soon die anyway, is ethically unsound, and its acceptance would lead to the gravest possible abuses.

Case 117
Licit Excision of Fallopian Tube Containing Fetus

It is discovered during the course of an operation that the patient's Fallopian tube contains a 6-week-old fetus. The patient's general condition is not good, and the surgeon has strong reason for fearing that she could not survive another laparotomy if it were performed within a month. In other cases where the tube's condition is similar to that of this patient's, the surgeon would postpone excising it. May he remove the tube at once?

Solution. The surgeon may licitly remove the tube at once.

Explanation. The condition of the tube, it is assumed, is gravely pathological. Removing it now is necessary to safeguard the patient's life. Delay in making the excision, because it would require another operation, would notably increase the danger to the patient. Because of these circumstances the surgeon would be justified in at once removing the Fallopian tube. When an immediate operation on the tube provides notably greater probability of saving the patient's life, it is licitly performed. This "greater probability" can arise from the fact that the patient could not be operated on again for some weeks, either because of her delicate condition or because surgical facilities would not be available.

Case 118
Excision of an Abdominal Pregnancy

The fetus is now mature, but the placenta is hopelessly attached to the mother's bowels. If the surgeon were to remove the fetus, the probability is that the operation would kill the mother. If he were to let the fetus die before removing it, the operation would be far less dangerous to the mother. What is the surgeon to do?

Solution. The surgeon must weigh well the probable results of operating at once: (1) the probable danger to the mother and (2) the probability of saving the child. If the probability of saving the child is equal to, or greater than, the probability of causing the mother's death, the surgeon will preferably operate. The mother has an obligation of submitting to this operation, even at such danger to her own life, if it is certain that the child can thus be brought forth alive and be baptized.[33]

Explanation. The reason for the fact that the mother is obliged to submit to the surgery when it is certain that this will permit the child to be baptized is that she must prefer the child's spiritual life to her own physical life. The child within her abdominal cavity, if left there very much longer, will die, and will die without baptism. Hence the child is in very grave spiritual necessity. To relieve this necessity she must be ready to sacrifice any temporal good, even life itself. If, however, it is uncertain that the child can be brought forth alive, the mother would not be obliged to undergo this dangerous operation. She would not be under the obligation of encountering the grave danger involved in the operation in order to effect for the child a benefit which merely probably (not certainly) would result.

Case 119
Excision of Tube with Fetus Approaching Viability

The patient has a tubal pregnancy of 5 months, and the Fallopian tube is not yet externally ruptured.[34] The surgeon judges, however, that, unless the tube is removed at once, the patient will surely die. May he proceed with the excision of the tube?

Solution. The surgeon may licitly do so.

Explanation. In very extraordinary cases in which the ectopic tubal pregnancy is close to viability, the excision of the tube is justified, as a general rule, only when the present danger to the mother is so great that any delay in excising the tube would certainly cost her her life. In such a case mere probability that the delay would endanger the

---

[33] If the surgeon knows that the mother does not believe in the necessity of baptism, he may prudently refrain from attempting to explain it, since his efforts would in all probability merely distress the mother and produce no good effect.

[34] Such cases as this, though very rare, do occur. T. Lincoln Bouscaren, in his very thorough survey of the literature on the subject, describes cases in which the ectopic fetus reached full development and viability, but says that an early ectopic has only a very slight chance of developing to viability. See T. Lincoln Bouscaren, S.J., *Ethics of Ectopic Operations,* pp. 102-05 (Milwaukee: Bruce Publishing Company, 1944).

mother's life would not be sufficient, for there is here well-founded hope that, without the operation, the fetus can be brought to viability. In Case 117 the hope of bringing the fetus to maturity was so slight as to be negligible.

Case 120
Excision of a Fallopian Tube in a Double Pregnancy

The patient is carrying a 2-month-old intrauterine fetus and it is now discovered that she has a second pregnancy, also 2 months old, in a Fallopian tube. May the physician perform a salpingectomy in order to safeguard the uterine pregnancy?

Solution. If the Fallopian tube is at present a grave threat to the mother's life, it may be excised. If it is not in such a condition, it must not be tampered with.

Explanation. The fact that the tubal pregnancy occurs simultaneously with a uterine pregnancy does not make the tubal fetus in any sense an unjust aggressor. This second fetus is located in the place where nature has placed it and is guilty of no attack. The tube may be excised if it is so pathological as to be a grave threat to the mother, but not in order to safeguard the uterine pregnancy.

Case 121
A Myomectomy during Pregnancy

A laparotomy is performed on the patient so that the surgeon may operate on what he has diagnosed as a myomatous uterus. After the abdomen is opened the uterus is split and a live fetus is discovered. The surgeon is at a loss to know what his obligations now are.

Solution. The surgeon must at once carefully suture the uterus and abdomen and permit the pregnancy to go to term.

Explanation. Before preparing to operate on a myomatous uterus the surgeon should ascertain whether or not the patient is pregnant. If it is found that she is pregnant and the fetus is not yet viable, the operation should be deferred unless it is immediately necessary to save the mother's life. Mistakes do occur in the operating room. In the present case the surgeon should do whatever he can to rectify his mistake. Hence he must make every effort possible to help the fetus arrive at viability.

We may close this discussion of the morality of direct and of indirect abortion with a quotation from Canon E. J. Mahoney. What he says of the difficulties experienced by the lay mind scarcely applies to the highly trained members of the medical profession of today.

"The lay mind, untrained in Catholic ethical theory, cannot usually perceive why the instances we have discussed [on the lawfulness of excising a cancerous womb containing an unviable fetus and of removing an ectopic fetus] do not also justify *direct* therapeutic abortion; their reasoning is from particular case to particular case, instead of from a general principle to a particular deduction. The justification of indirect abortion, with its accompanying distinctions, is often condemned as a contemptible exercise in hair-splitting, which can have no place where a human life is hanging in the balance. But every law, human as well as divine, needs applying to concrete cases— *qui bene distinguit bene intelligit* [one truly understands if he can distinguish well]; the judgments, for example, given by an appeal court, on which a human life may depend, often turn on the finest of legal distinctions which to a lay person are hair-splitting. Catholics who cannot understand the reason why (direct) therapeutic abortion is condemned must accept it solely because the Church teaches it, and this they are certainly bound to do."[35]

EXPOSING THE FETUS TO DANGER

IN CASES of direct abortion and in cases of indirect abortion the fetus is killed. We will now discuss cases in which death is not inevitable for the fetus but in which some danger is present.

Case 122
Cholecystectomy during Pregnancy
The patient is 5 months pregnant and is suffering an acute attack of cholecystitis. The physician judges that immediate surgery is re-

[35] E. J. Mahoney, *Questions and Answers*, vol. II, *Precepts*, p. 54. London: Burns Oates and Washbourne, 1949.

quired because of the imminent danger of gangrene, but he realizes that the cholecystectomy may cause the fetus to abort.

Solution. If the operation is urgently demanded for saving the mother's life, the physician may proceed without scruple. In less urgent cases he must wait until the fetus is viable. In any event he must do the operation with great care so as not to disturb the pregnancy any more than is strictly necessary.

Explanation. The principle of the twofold effect may rightly be applied to this case. If the mother's life is now in jeopardy and can be saved only by surgery, the physician may operate at once. There is due proportion in this case between the evil and the good effect of his action. The danger to which the fetus will be exposed by the operation is compensated for by the cure of the mother.

Case 123
An Appendectomy during Pregnancy

The patient, who is pregnant with a nonviable fetus, has an acute attack of appendicitis. If she is not operated on, she may die; and if the appendectomy is performed, premature labor may follow. What is the physician to do?

Solution. If the physician judges that an appendectomy is necessary to safeguard the mother's life, he may perform this operation.

Explanation. The physician should of course employ all his skill and care to prevent if possible a premature birth; but if premature labor follows the appendectomy, the physician is not to be held accountable for this evil effect, which he does not desire nor directly produce. In this operation we find verified the four conditions of the principle of the twofold effect. The surgeon's intention is upright, for his purpose in performing the operation is to remove from the mother's body a diseased and dangerous organ. His action (the appendectomy) is not evil in itself. The good effect (the mother's cure) is not produced by means of the evil effect (the premature labor). There is due proportion between the good and the evil effects. The same solution would hold true if, in similar circumstances, some other organ were dangerously diseased and immediate excision were indicated.

Case 124
Removal of an Ovarian Tumor

The patient, 4 months pregnant, has an ovarian tumor. The physician is convinced that the tumor must be excised at once if the mother's life is to be saved, but an operation of this kind may cause an abortion.

Solution. The physician may remove the ovarian tumor.

Explanation. The action of the physician is not evil in itself, for it is aimed at relieving the mother's body of a part which is jeopardizing the whole. His intention is praiseworthy, for his purpose in performing the surgery is to safeguard the mother's life. The good effect of his action, the cure of the mother, is not caused by the evil effect, the danger of abortion. There is due proportion between the two effects, for on the one hand the mother's life will be saved, and on the other the fetus may be lost.

Case 125
Electric Shock Therapy in Pernicious Vomiting of Pregnancy

The patient, 3 months pregnant, is suffering pernicious vomiting of pregnancy. Intravenous therapy, psychotherapy, and hypnosis have proved ineffectual in reversing the condition. The physician now wishes to use electric shock therapy. May he licitly do so?

Solution. Electric shock therapy may licitly be used in this case.

Explanation. The purpose of the physician is to control a condition that might prove fatal to the mother. If death or injury results for the fetus, this evil effect would be caused indirectly only. The harm that may overtake the fetus is not desired either as a means or as an end in the effort to effect the mother's cure. As a matter of fact, electric shock therapy does not appear to create any special danger for the fetus. If, however, danger is present because of existing conditions, the treatment may still be licitly used provided no other means of saving the mother's life with which danger to the fetus is unassociated can be found. Whatever is here said concerning the licitness of using shock therapy in cases of pernicious vomiting is equally applicable to the use of shock therapy because of psychoses during pregnancy that threaten the mother's life.

Case 126
Irradiation of Ovaries because of Carcinoma

The patient has cancer of the breast. After he has removed the breast the physician wishes to irradiate the ovaries. The patient is pregnant and the irradiation of the ovaries will probably cause the abortion of the nonviable fetus.

Solution. If irradiation is probably necessary in order to arrest the spread of the cancer and if it cannot, without danger to the patient's life, be delayed until the fetus is viable, the physician may spray the ovaries with X ray.

Explanation. One may rightly apply to this case the principle of the two-fold effect. The physician's purpose is good, for he intends merely to safeguard the mother's life; he has no wish to harm the fetus. The act of irradiating the ovaries in this case is not intrinsically evil. The good effect sought (the health of the mother's body) is not to be caused by means of the evil effect (the danger of abortion). There is due proportion between the good and evil effects; that is, between the saving of the mother's life and the probable abortion or destruction of the fetus.

The solution would be the same if the child would probably be killed in utero by the X ray, provided the following condition is verified: If the ovaries are not irradiated at present, the fetus will probably die before viability. This condition would be fulfilled if the fetus would not survive the mother, and if the mother without irradiation of the ovaries would probably die before the viability of the child. The reason for requiring the fulfillment of this condition is that the child's spiritual welfare, insured through baptism, would take precedence over the mother's physical good; namely, her life. Hence if the choice were between *probably* causing the fetus to die without baptism and *probably* saving the mother's life, there would not be a sufficient reason for running the risk of depriving the child of the beatific vision, which would be gained for him by baptism.

Case 127

Removal of a Ureteral Calculus during Pregnancy

The patient is pregnant with a 4-month-old fetus. The physician discovers a ureteral calculus which is causing grave pain and danger. To operate for the removal of the calculus may bring on an abortion. May the physician licitly operate?

Solution. If there is grave danger to the woman's life unless the calculus is removed, the physician may operate despite the danger of abortion. He must use the operative procedure which is best calculated to leave the gestation uninterrupted. During the first four months the danger of an abortion as a result of surgery is not ordinarily great. The danger would increase at a later stage, and the surgeon would in addition be confronted with great mechanical difficulties. The enlarged uterus would interfere with a proper exposure of the ureters, and bleeding would be free and possibly hard to control because of the dilation of the blood vessels. Even at this stage the surgeon may operate if he is convinced that an operation is necessary to save the life of the mother.

234

Explanation. The principle of the twofold effect may be licitly applied
in this case. The surgeon's act in dislodging the stone is good and
his intention is honest. The evil of exposing the fetus to the danger of abortion is not the cause of the good effect of relieving the
mother's danger. There is due proportion between the good effect
and the evil effect.

Case 128
Hastening Delivery in a Spontaneous Abortion

The patient, 4 months pregnant, has already begun to abort and the
contractions of labor are completely beyond control. They will continue until the fetus is ejected from the uterus and nothing can be
done to arrest them. The physician is eager to baptize the fetus
before it dies; and consequently, in order to expel it from the womb
more quickly, he uses hand pressure on the mother's abdomen. Is he
justified in so acting?

Solution. The physician here acts licitly.

Explanation. In this case, where the uterine contractions of labor are
completely beyond control, the fate of the fetus is already sealed.
The deathblow—namely, the uncontrollable contractions of labor—
has already befallen the fetus. Hence the action of the physician in
hastening the expulsion is not the cause of the death of the fetus.
Before he begins to act the cause of the abortion has been placed,
the abortion itself has already begun, and it is now merely a matter
of time before the effect of that causative action will be produced
completely. The fetus is doomed to die as soon as it is expelled, or
perhaps during its passage from the uterus to the vagina if the labor
is protracted. In exerting pressure to expel the fetus sooner than it
would otherwise be expelled the physician is merely helping to bring
it from a place where it cannot be baptized to a place where it can
be baptized. He is not inflicting on it a deathblow. The deathblow
has already been inflicted, for the convulsions of labor are beyond
all control. The physician's action merely hastens the birth process,
not the child's death.

Chorea Gravidarum or Sydenham's Chorea

One of the very rare complications which may be present
in pregnancy is that of chorea gravidarum or Sydenham's
chorea. The physician may employ typhoid-paratyphoid vac-

cine in the treatment of the patient, in spite of its probable fatal effect on the fetus, if there is available no other effective way of treating the mother which would not involve the same danger to the fetus. There is no direct attack upon the fetus; its death, if it does occur, will be but the indirect effect of the medication. (See "The Principle of the Twofold Effect," pages 98-101.) For an interesting case report on this subject see Harold M. Groden, M.D., "Chorea Gravidarum," *Linacre Quarterly* 17:17-20, May 1950. Direct termination of the pregnancy while the fetus is nonviable is not only morally wrong but is considered by at least some competent physicians to be medically inadvisable.

HYDRAMNIOS

HYDRAMNIOS is an abnormality of pregnancy in which an excessive quantity of amniotic fluid accumulates within the amniotic sac. In some cases this pathological condition may present serious danger for the mother unless the pressure on some vital organ which the abnormal swelling of the fluid-filled amniotic sac is causing is soon relieved. If the fetus is viable, there is generally no moral problem, for the birth may be hastened by rupturing the membranes. This premature delivery of a viable infant is justified if there is a proportionately grave reason for permitting the ensuing danger to the child's life, and removing from the mother a grave threat to her life would be a proportionate reason that would compensate for exposing the child's health to serious danger.

If the fetus is not yet viable, the surgeon may not of course directly empty the uterus. Even though he judges that this action is necessary to safeguard the mother's health, it is not permitted, for the action is intrinsically evil. Is it likewise forbidden to puncture the amniotic sac in order to drain off the excessive fluid and thus relieve the dangerous pressure on the organs of the mother? In reply to this question we must distinguish between two kinds of puncture of the membrane:

(1) that which will gravely rupture the fetal sac and (2) that which causes no such rupture.

If the puncturing will produce a grave rupture of the fetal membrane, the fluid will be released and abortion will as a rule soon follow. Deprived of the amniotic fluid, the nonviable fetus will generally die, for at its present stage of development its survival depends to a very great extent on the amniotic fluid. When the surgeon punctures the amniotic membrane, he is directly administering a blow to the child which most probably will prove fatal, and therefore his action is gravely evil.

[handwritten margin note: This fluid recurs rapidly in this case is producti... so removal ... may be don safely —]

If the puncturing were so small and so skillfully done that it would not rupture the amniotic sac, it would be permitted. It has been contended that a skilled surgeon can perforate the amniotic membrane in so delicate a manner that, without danger of a complete rupture, he can thus drain off the desired quantity of excessive fluid. Morally speaking, there is no objection to this practice. Before attempting this procedure, however, the surgeon must be certain that he will not tear the membrane so severely that all the fluid would be lost. The question as to whether the procedure is medically necessary is discussed in Case 129. *[handwritten: Today patients with ruptured membranes are frequently carried for weeks without delivery of infection —.]*

Case 129

Draining the Amniotic Fluid

The pregnant uterus of the patient is retroflexed and imprisoned in the pelvic cavity. The attending physician wishes to perforate the sac in order to drain off the amniotic fluid and thus to bring the uterus back to its normal size. The release of the amniotic fluid will mean the aborting of the fetus. If the fetus is nonviable, is this operation licit?

Solution. If the fetus is nonviable, the perforation of the sac with the consequent loss of the amniotic fluid is illicit.

Explanation. This is a problem much discussed many years ago which today offers little difficulty, for means other than the draining off of the amniotic fluid are available. Manual replacement and surgery are some of the measures which make unnecessary the rupturing of the membranes enclosing the fetus. If, however, no remedy other than draining off the amniotic fluid is at hand, this may not be done if the fetus is nonviable, for this act would be a direct attack on the fetus. The amniotic fluid is a very important element for the well-being of the fetus. To drain it off completely would be to cause a very grave injury to the infant; for though in such an event some fetuses do go on to term, it ordinarily happens that the complete loss of the amniotic fluid is soon followed by the aborting of the fetus. Puncturing the sacs and thus causing the loss of the fluid would immediately and directly cause grave injury to the fetus and only mediately procure the good effect on the mother.[36]

If, however, the puncture of the sacs were small so that some of the fluid could be drained off without producing an abortion, this procedure would, for a grave reason, be permitted. The difficulty in this case would be to control the size of the outlet; for once the sacs are pierced, even slightly, the rupture tends to get out of hand and very probably would release all the amniotic fluid, bringing about an abortion.

PLACENTA PRAEVIA

IF THE placenta or a part of it covers the inner mouth of the uterus, it is called placenta praevia. When the cervix dilates and the upper uterus contracts, the placenta is often detached, wholly or partially, from the uterine wall, and hemorrhage results. Some maintain that the pregnancy should be terminated as soon as the diagnosis is made,[37] but this opinion cannot be accepted without restrictions. We must distin-

[36] For the opinion of other moralists on this problem see Henry Davis, S.J., *Moral and Pastoral Theology*, vol. II, pp. 189-90 (London: Sheed and Ward, 1949); Patrick A. Finney, C.M., *Moral Problems in Hospital Practice*, p. 72 (St. Louis: B. Herder Book Company, 1942); P. G. Payen, *Déontologie médicale d'après le droit naturel*, nn. 407-08, pp. 513-16 (Zi-Ka-Wei près Chang-Hai: Imprimerie de la Mission Catholique, 1935).

[37] De Lee and Greenhill say: "With two exceptions every pregnancy complicated by placenta praevia should be terminated as soon as the diagnosis is made" (Joseph B. De Lee, M.D., and J. P. Greenhill, M.D., *Principles and Practice of Obstetrics*, tenth edition, p. 425. Philadelphia: W. B. Saunders Company, 1951). The two exceptions are: (1) when bleeding is slight and (2) when the child is nearly viable. We should remember however that directly to terminate the pregnancy of a nonviable fetus is intrinsically evil, insofar as it consists in directly administering to the child a fatal blow.

guish between the case where the fetus is viable and where it is not. If the fetus is viable, it may be delivered whenever there is a proportionately grave reason for this hastening of birth. If leaving the viable fetus in the uterus would be dangerous for the mother, it may be delivered at once. If, however, the fetus is not yet viable, it may not be delivered while still alive, even in order to save the mother's life. To withdraw the nonviable fetus from the uterus would be to take it from the only site where it can possibly survive, and this, directly performed, would constitute murder. If the fetus is nonviable and hemorrhage threatens the mother's life, the physician can try to control the hemorrhage by means of tamponing. There is danger that tamponing may bring about an abortion; but if the fetus is aborted, its ejection from the womb would be produced indirectly, not directly, by the tamponing, and the reason for tamponing is sufficiently grave to permit the risk of an indirect abortion. Here the act of tamponing is directed at the curtailment of the hemorrhage, not at producing an abortion. Because the principle of the twofold effect is rightly applied to this case of tamponing as a means of arresting the hemorrhage, the physician may licitly employ this method. It must be noted, however, the dangerous procedure of tamponing would not be licit if resting in bed would suffice to avert the danger from the patient.

Case 130
Hastening Birth after Complete Abruptio Placentae

The patient is 4 months pregnant. The physician discovers that the placenta has been torn loose from the uterine wall and that the woman is having a severe hemorrhage. May he at once remove the fetus from the womb?

Solution. When the abruptio placentae is complete, the physician may and should remove the child at once, and this holds true even in cases in which the child is not yet viable. After removal he should see that it is baptized immediately.

Explanation. Once the complete abruptio placentae has occurred, the fetus will die within ten minutes or less whether it be removed from or left in the uterus. In delivering this nonviable fetus the physician is not committing an abortion. A fatal blow has already been administered to the child, and this blow was inflicted by natural causes. The physician in extracting the fetus is not making its lot worse. He may be benefiting the child spiritually; for if the fetus is still alive when he baptizes it, he will be the means of gaining for it the beatific vision. If, however, the abruptio placentae is but partial, to empty the uterus would be a direct attack on a living fetus. The latter circumstance is quite different from the preceding one, for here no fatal blow has already been dealt the fetus by natural causes. Actually it happens at times that, even though partial abruptio placentae has occurred, the fetus goes to term and is born alive, though perhaps with some physical defect. In the event, then, that the abruptio is not complete, the fetus may not licitly be brought forth from the uterus, neither in order to save the mother nor in order to baptize the child.

There are cases where the abruptio placentae is such that the placenta cannot be said to be wholly detached, but the part of it which clings to the wall of the uterus is insignificant and no longer serves as a source of life for the fetus. The abruptio is such that the nonviable fetus cannot possibly be saved. At present it is bleeding to death. In such circumstances the complete deathblow has already been struck and the fetus may and should be delivered at once in order to administer baptism.

REFERENCES

Bonzelet, Honoratius, O.F.M. "The Morality of Indirect Sterilization." *Ecclesiastical Review* 109:125-27, August 1943.

Dunne, George H., S.J. "The Blanshard Charges." *Commonweal* 47:536-42, March 12, 1948.

——— "Paul Blanshard and the Catholic Church: The Church and Medicine." *America* 81:438-40, July 16, 1949.

Kelly, Gerald, S.J. *Medico-Moral Problems*, pt. 2, "Moral Aspects of Sterility Tests and Artificial Insemination," pp. 14-21. St. Louis: Catholic Hospital Association of the United States and Canada, 1950.

——— "Moral Aspects of Sterility Tests and Artificial Insemination." *Linacre Quarterly* 16:30-40, January 1949.

——— "Suppression of Ovarian Function To Prevent Metastasis." *Linacre Quarterly* 15:27-30, July 1948.

Kremer, Peter, O.S.Cam. "Some Ethical Considerations in X-Ray Treatment of Irradiation of Ovaries in Cancer of the Breast." *Ecclesiastical Review* 108:271-73, April 1943.

Mahoney, E. J. "The Morality of Sterilization." *Catholic Mind* 34:205-16, May 22, 1936.

McCarthy, John. "A Report on Abortion." *Irish Ecclesiastical Record* 55:337-53, April 1940.

Moore, Thomas Verner, O.S.B., M.D. "Morality of a Sterilizing Operation." *Ecclesiastical Review* 106:444-46, June 1942.

Schmitt, Alexander Hunter, M.D., F.A.C.S. "Comparative Safety in Five or More Repeated Cesarian Sections." *Linacre Quarterly* 13:16-18, October 1945.

Schwitalla, Alphonse M., S.J., "Recent Studies of Therapeutic Abortion." *Linacre Quarterly* 13:25-34, January-April 1945.

IN THIS chapter we discuss problems with moral issues that occur during delivery. The problems are connected with the use of drugs during labor; hastening delivery; caesarean sections under various conditions; complications arising during delivery, especially those in which craniotomy or embryotomy might be employed; the delivery of twins; and the delivery of hydrocephalics.

THE USE OF DRUGS DURING CHILDBIRTH

THE USE OF NARCOTICS during parturition to relieve the pain of the mother or to facilitate the obstetrician's handling of a difficult case is justified, provided there is due proportion between the estimated good and evil effects. The use of drugs to alleviate pain would be illicit if it were to endanger the life of either the mother or the child, for in that event the evil effect (exposing someone to the danger of death) would not be duly compensated for by the good effect (the alleviation of suffering), no matter how great the mother's pain might be. Because, however, the foreseeable ill effects on mother and child, if they result at all, would be slight, the skillful use of caudal analgesia, rectal ether, and similar medication during parturition is morally permissible. It is taken for granted that the physician will employ what he judges to be the least dangerous anesthetic and the safest dosage.

242

Even when there is present a grave reason for resorting to an anesthetic in parturition, some physicians are opposed to its use. It is impossible, they say, to know whether or not the unborn fetus is perfectly normal. It may have a heart ailment or it may be suffering from some other malady. If an anesthetic were employed, its use might cause the fetus just enough harm to make its survival impossible. Because of these borderline cases they try to avoid, insofar as they reasonably can, the use of drugs during parturitions.[1]

The physician should remember that some religious-minded women, realizing that pain and suffering generously accepted from a supernatural motive can enrich one spiritually, prefer to forgo during childbirth the use of any drug which would lessen their pain.

The punishment imposed by God on Eve and on all women who were to live after her cannot be used as an argument against the use of drugs during childbirth. When God said to Eve, "In pain shall you bring forth children" (Genesis 3:16), He meant: "Up to the present moment, Eve, you have enjoyed the preternatural gift of immunity to all pain and suffering. From now on you will be deprived of this privilege." In giving birth to children the mother ordinarily experiences some inconvenience or pain, though these are not necessarily grave. This pain and inconvenience are natural effects of childbirth from which Eve, before the fall, was exempt. Once original sin came into the world, parturition involved some degree of suffering. The words of Genesis are not a command. They are

---

[1] J. D. Ratcliffe comments as follows on the danger connected with the use of drugs: "Drugs given within one to four hours before birth depress the respiratory center in the baby's brain—dulling its urge to breathe. . . . The too liberal use of analgesia and anesthesia *may* endanger the life or health of the baby" (J. D. Ratcliffe, "Surviving the First Day," *Today's Health* 30:24-26, September 1952). The danger may be expected to decrease as drugs are improved. Drs. Cappe and Pallin describe analgesic methods that "provide relief from the pains of labor without respiratory depression in the newborn" (Bernard E. Cappe, M.D., and Irving M. Pallin, M.D., "Recent Advances in Obstetric Analgesia," *Journal of the American Medical Association* 154:377-79, January 30, 1954).

merely a statement of the effects produced by man's fallen nature. There is, therefore, according to Catholic teaching, no prohibition of a scriptural source against alleviating the pains of a woman during childbirth.

DELIVERING PREMATURELY

PREMATURE delivery means hastening the birth of a viable fetus. To remove the fetus from the womb at any time before it has reached term exposes it to greater or less danger, the degree depending upon the stage of the fetus' development. Since the fetus in cases of premature delivery is viable, taking it from the uterus does not inflict on it a fatal blow. Because, however, of the harmful effects which hastening birth has upon the fetus,[2] the physician is not permitted artificially to remove the viable child from the uterus prematurely unless a proportionately grave reason is present to justify exposing the child to the dangers involved in this procedure. The premature induction of delivery is licit in the following and in similar cases.

1. Unless birth is hastened, the infant will die in utero without baptism.

2. The child could not be born at term normally because of the mother's narrow pelvis.

3. Delay in the matter would bring graver danger to the mother than that which premature delivery would involve for the child.

4. Delay would bring grave danger to the child. If the mother is in imminent danger of death, the birth of the viable child may and should be hastened, provided this would not appreciably shorten the patient's life. In this manner the phy-

---

[2] In certain cases, when the patient is near term, the induction of labor is safe, but it is recognized that this practice is open to abuse. See "Induction of Labor," *Journal of the American Medical Association* 147:1719, December 22, 1951. See also Gerald Kelly, S.J., *Medico-Moral Problems*, pt. 4, "Induction of Labor," pp. 24-28 (St. Louis: Catholic Hospital Association of the United States and Canada, 1952).

sician can save the child, which otherwise would very probably die with the mother.

If the infant is only *probably* viable and hastening birth is necessary to save the mother's life, the procedure is licit, provided there is also genuine hope of saving the child's life. The obstetrician's act of hastening the birth in this case is not necessarily fatal to the child; it merely exposes it to grave danger. Actually, his purpose in hastening delivery is to save the life, not only of the mother, but also of the child, for the latter would die with the mother if delivery was not prematurely induced. The physician is therefore doing what is best for both parties.

Case 131
Hastening Delivery because of Toxemia

The patient, 27 weeks pregnant, is suffering severely from headache resulting ·from a toxemia of pregnancy. In order to end her pain the physician induces the delivery of the fetus.

Solution. Hastening birth in this case is justified only when the following three conditions are present: (1) if the newborn child can at once be placed in an incubator, (2) if the patient's suffering is very grave, and (3) if no less drastic means, such as the use of antihypertensive agents and other medical treatment, can relieve her pain. The physician can decide without difficulty whether the child can be placed at once in an incubator and whether less drastic means are available. To decide whether the pain is sufficiently severe is quite another matter. Here the physician must form an honest judgment on the basis of his past experience and of what he observes in the patient.

Explanation. When all three conditions mentioned above are verified, we may licitly apply the principles of the twofold effect. If, however, any one of the three conditions is not fulfilled, hastening the birth would be morally reprehensible.

Case 132
Hastening Delivery in an Abdominal Pregnancy

The patient, a woman 30 years of age, has a secondary abdominal pregnancy. The physician decides to open the abdomen and deliver this viable fetus at 28 weeks gestation. May he licitly do so?

Solution. This viable fetus may licitly be delivered at once.

Explanation. If the mother is doing well, the physician will let the pregnancy continue to eight and one-half months, for thus the fetus is better provided for and the danger in removing it is less for the mother. If, however, grave complications arise, the physician may wish to operate at once. If the fetus is viable, he may licitly do so.

CAESAREAN SECTIONS

CAESAREAN sections may be performed under various conditions, at various stages of gestation, and for reasons that are more or less valid. The following cases illustrate the principles that should be observed.

Case 133
A Caesarean Section To Avoid the Pains of Childbirth

The patient, who is near term, wishes to have the physician perform a caesarean section. Her reason for requesting this operation is that she may avoid the pains involved in natural childbirth. Would the physician be justified in acceding to her request?

Solution. There is no reason here which would justify the physician in performing a caesarean section.

Explanation. The caesarean section involves major surgery and brings with it risk of infection, of surgical shock, and of pulmonary complications. Birth by caesarean section is more dangerous to the mother than is natural vaginal birth. A woman is not permitted to run the added risks involved in a caesarean section unless she has a proportionately grave reason for doing so. Merely to avoid the pains that are ordinarily attendant upon natural parturition would not constitute such a reason.[3]

Case 134
A Caesarean Section in a Case of Tuberculosis

The patient, 27 years of age, is pregnant with an 8-month-old fetus. She is at the point of death from tuberculosis. The only means of extracting the child alive is by caesarean section, but this operation would cause the death of the mother on the operating table. May the attending physician perform a caesarean section in order to save the child?

[3] See Paul Titus, M.D., *The Management of Obstetric Difficulties,* third edition, p. 700 (St. Louis: C. V. Mosby Company, 1945); John F. Cunningham, M.D., *Textbook of Obstetrics,* p. 434 (New York: Grune and Stratton, 1951).

Solution. In these circumstances a caesarean section would not be permissible. As soon as the mother dies from the tuberculosis, the child must be extracted at once and baptized.

Explanation. The Fifth Commandment and the natural law forbid directly taking the life of an innocent person. It is never permitted to kill one man in order to save another. A caesarean section in the present case would be a direct and death-dealing attack on an innocent person. A caesarean section when performed on a strong and healthy patient would, it is true, entail no proximate danger of death; but we must evaluate the nature of an operation by its ordinary effects on patients of a particular class—for example, on normally healthy men, or on children, or on young women, or on those weakened by age. We judge the nature of an operation by this norm: Does it as a rule bring some danger, or extreme danger, to this category of patient? If the operation—for example, a caesarean section—would, *as a rule,* cause death to a woman who is in the last stages of tuberculosis or whose heart is extremely weak, then it must be considered a direct, fatal attack on the patient. If the operation is thus classified, it could never be licitly performed.

In the present case a caesarean section would be of the nature of a lethal attack; and although it would produce the good effect of liberating the imprisoned fetus, it would be an evil means to a good end. This means would be evil, for it would be a direct deathblow administered to the mother. The operation performed on this patient, weakened as she is by the ravages of disease, would simply kill her.

But, it may be urged, unless this operation is performed, both mother and child will die. This conclusion is not certain, for it may be that the child can be extracted alive immediately after the mother's death. Even if it were certain that both would die, the physician would be forbidden to perform the caesarean section, for he may never do evil that good may come of it. If the mother is certain to die and if performing the operation would merely deprive her of a few days of life, she may not surrender her right to this short period of life in order to save the child. She possesses no power over her own life or any part of it, for God alone has supreme ownership over all human life.

Case 135

A Caesarean Section in a Case of Pneumonia

The patient, who is 7 months pregnant, is dying of pneumonia. She asks the physician whether she is obliged to have a caesarean section so

247

that the child's life may be better safeguarded and that he may be baptized.

Solution. If the caesarean section would offer no hope of survival for the mother, the operation would not be permitted. If the caesarean section would not appreciably shorten the mother's life, it would be licit; it would not, however, be obligatory unless (1) the child could not be baptized in utero or (2) it would not survive the mother long enough to be baptized. When it is foreseen that the mother, told of the obligation to have the operation, would still refuse to permit it, the physician should say nothing about her duty in the matter.

Explanation. The reason that silence is recommended in the latter case is that informing the patient would do more harm than good. Here it is prudently foreseen that mentioning to the mother her duty would not help the child; it would, moreover, change the mother's good faith into bad. Before being told of her obligation, she believed that she was doing nothing wrong. If, however, after being told of her duty in the matter, she were to refuse to permit the operation, she would be guilty of grave sin. Hence informing the mother in such circumstances would result in her grave spiritual harm, and the child's interests would in no wise be better provided for.

Case 136
A Caesarean Section When Patient Is in Coma

The patient, who is nearly at term, is in the state of coma. The physician wishes to do a caesarean section at once in order to save the child. The operation would, however, be very dangerous for the mother in her present condition. What is he to do?

Solution. If there is no immediate and grave danger to the child, a caesarean section would be illicit.

Explanation. If the child is at present in no grave danger, a caesarean section would not be permitted, for this operation would unnecessarily jeopardize the mother. If, moreover, the child were in grave danger but an operation would prove fatal to the patient, the section would not be licit, for it would be equivalent to killing the mother. If the child were in grave danger and an operation would merely expose the mother to danger of death, it would be lawful.

Case 137
A Caesarean Section after Death

The patient is pregnant and the fetus is near term. The mother is at the point of death. The physician wishes to do a caesarean section as soon as she dies, but the near relatives of the patient strenuously object to this procedure, which they term an autopsy. What is the physician to do?

Solution. As soon as the mother dies the physician should as a rule, extract the fetus, and provide for its baptism.[4]

Explanation. The fetus, imprisoned within the body of the dead mother, is in extreme necessity, and the physician has the obligation to come to its rescue. The husband and other near relatives of the deceased woman have no right to object to the act of liberating the child. They have no legal grounds for objecting, for the civil law recognizes the infant in the mother's womb as an individual who is endowed with all the rights of a born child. Moreover, the natural law imposes on the relatives especially the duty of coming to the aid of their own flesh and blood who is now in extreme spiritual need. This obligation is present from the moment that the mother is certainly dead until the time when the child is certainly dead. Although the child often dies at the same time as the mother, in some cases the imprisoned child lives for an hour or more after the mother's death. Fetuses have been known to survive the mother's death by as much as one hour and forty-five minutes.[5]

COMPLICATIONS DURING DELIVERY

THE numerous complications that can arise during delivery interest us only insofar as recourse is sometimes had to procedures the licitness of which must be decided. These procedures are discussed in the present section.

Symphysiectomy, Pubiotomy, and Cephalotripsy

In cases of complicated childbirth the operations of symphysiectomy or symphaiotomy (dividing the cartilage which binds together the two bones of the pelvis) and pubiotomy (cutting the pubic bone) are licit procedures when medically advisable. Actually, however, they are rarely done today because of the undesirable consequences which they produce.

[4] See *Codex juris canonici,* Canon 746. Roma: Typis Polyglottis Vaticanis, 1936.

[5] See Austin O'Malley, M.D., *The Ethics of Medical Homicide and Mutilation,* pp. 88-89. New York: Devin-Adair Company, 1919.

249

Cephalotripsy is an operation in which, by means of forceps, the head of the child is compressed in order to facilitate delivery in childbirth. It should be carefully noted that the skull of the unborn child is not crushed. The physician's action is not of such a nature as to kill the fetus. Because of the abnormal size of the head or because of the narrowness of the pelvic opening, the fetus cannot pass into the vagina. If the child's condition is observed early enough, the delivery will usually be by caesarean section. If a caesarean section is not feasible, the physician may employ cephalotripsy; for if without this extreme measure the child will die in utero and if no better means are available to effect delivery, cephalotripsy is licit. If no action is taken, the child would under the circumstances be doomed to certain death. Cephalotripsy does, it is true, involve grave danger for the infant, but it provides some hope of saving it. The physician may licitly run the risk provided he has a proportionately grave reason for exposing the child to this danger.

Embryotomy and Craniotomy

By embryotomy is understood any mutilating operation on the fetus. In craniotomy the skull is perforated, the contents are removed, and the skull is then compressed. Both these procedures are always gravely illicit if the fetus is still living or probably living, for they constitute a direct and fatal attack upon the fetus. The only possible exception would be an embryotomy in which only an arm or a leg were removed. Such a case would rarely if ever occur in obstetrical practice, but an obstetrician might think of using the procedure as a last resort in a desperate case if he were convinced of the fact that an embryotomy necessarily resulting in death was illicit. The removal of a single member would be licit if no other means of delivering the fetus alive could be found.

The following cases illustrate in general the application of these principles.

250

Case 138
Embryotomy in a Case of Transverse Presentation

The child is still alive and the case is one of neglected transverse presentation. Version is impossible and the physician considers a caesarean section contraindicated because it would jeopardize the mother too much. His solution to this difficulty is embryotomy.

Solution. As long as the fetus is certainly or even only probably living, embryotomy would be gravely illicit.

Explanation. Embryotomy would be a direct and fatal attack on a living innocent human being; namely, the fetus. Hence, though embryotomy in the present case is recommended by some medical writers,[6] it would constitute murder. The solution given for the present case applies to all others in which embryotomy might be used.

Case 139
Embryotomy because of a Distended Abdomen

The mother is in the second stage of labor. Delivery of the head has occurred without difficulty. Delivery of the abdomen and the remaining portions cannot be effected because of a distended abdomen resulting from polycystic disease of the liver and kidneys. Under the circumstances may evisceration be employed?

Solution. It is gravely illicit to dismember the body of the living fetus.

Explanation. Every direct and deadly attack on an innocent person is forbidden by the natural law. Directly to inflict fatal punctures or cuttings on the fetus would therefore be gravely illicit.

Case 140
Cleidotomy

The head of the child has emerged but the completion of the delivery is obstructed by the abnormal size of the shoulders. The obstetrician has found that in such cases cleidotomy is indicated, but he is not sure that it is morally unobjectionable.

Solution. When cleidotomy is medically indicated for the delivery of a living child, it is ethically unobjectionable.

Explanation. Cleidotomy (the dividing of the clavicles to cause the shoulder girdle to collapse) is an operation which is not of its nature

---

[6] See Charles O. McCormick, M.D., *A Textbook on Pathology of Labor, the Puerperium and the Newborn,* second edition, p. 109 (St. Louis: C. V. Mosby Company, 1947); Henricus J. Stander, M.D., *Williams Obstetrics,* eighth edition, pp. 1040-41 (New York: D. Appleton-Century Company, 1941).

fatal to the infant. In medical writings, it is true, this procedure is advised in order to facilitate the extraction of a fetus that is already dead. But cleidotomy need not inflict on the child either death or an irreparable mutilation. It can be indicated as a necessary means of effecting the delivery of a living fetus. The purpose of the obstetrician is not to kill the fetus, but rather to bring about a safe delivery, even though in doing so he must inflict an injury on the fetus. The injury done, however, is but of a temporary nature. Similarly, if brachiotomy is required for the delivery of the child, this procedure also is licit. It is obviously preferable that the infant suffer the loss of an arm rather than that it die.

Case 141
Procedure When Attempts To Deliver Might Be Fatal

The progress of the child during delivery has been arrested in such a way that the physician fears that it may be killed by his attempts to extract it. If, however, it is left in its present site, it is certain to die before long.

Solution. The physician may and should try to deliver this child as best he can.

Explanation. The choice here is between certain death for the child and the probable saving of the child. The physician's act in attempting to extract the fetus is good. If actually the fetus is killed in the process of attempting a safe delivery, its death certainly is not intended. There is due proportion between the good effect sought and the evil effect which may result. Needless to say, it is the good of the child himself which is directly sought in the recommended procedure.

Case 142
Delivery of a Two-headed Infant

The physician, engaged in delivering a baby, finds after a head has been brought forth that the infant has two heads. He wishes to amputate the second head to make the delivery of the child possible.

Solution. Amputating the second head would be gravely illicit.

Explanation. There are probably present in this case two infants, for there are two heads. Hence the excising of one head would probably be a direct, fatal attack on the life of one of the infants, and this would be gravely evil. If, however, the infant dies before delivery of both heads, the second head may be severed from the body.

In a case such as that described here the obstetrician may licitly proceed with the attempt to deliver the child, trying as best he can to force the second head through the birth passage. If during this procedure the child dies, this evil effect of the physician's action is not desired nor is it imputable to him. During such a dangerous parturition the physician should remember to administer baptism to both heads if both can be reached.

THE DELIVERY OF TWINS

THE delivery of twins can very naturally give rise to complications requiring procedures the morality of which needs to be decided. The following cases illustrate the governing principles.

Case 143
Severing Umbilical Cord That Is Strangling Second Twin

The obstetrician is attending a woman who is to have twins. While delivering the first child he discovers that the umbilical cord of the second twin is wound tightly around the neck of the first. In order to liberate the latter he severs the cord which is strangling it. Does he act licitly?

Solution. The obstetrician is permitted to cut the cord of the second twin in this very rare case, since this procedure, properly performed, would not unduly endanger the life of the second child.

Explanation. Actually it would be difficult for the physician to decide to which twin the cord belonged. In most cases the indicated procedure would perhaps be to sever and clamp off the cord and deliver one twin as quickly as possible. The delivery of the second twin could be accomplished within the theoretical limit of eight minutes which obstetricians accept as the time within which the second twin must be delivered if it is to live. Clamping the cord would eliminate the danger of hemorrhage, and the shortness of time required for the two deliveries would make possible the avoiding of the danger of asphyxia.

Case 144
Craniotomy in a Case of Collision

The obstetrician encounters the complication of collision while delivering twins. The head of the first child and that of the second child are locked at the inlet. In order to deliver the first child the obstetrician performs a craniotomy on the second fetus. Was the action of the obstetrician morally wrong?

Solution. If the second fetus was alive at the time of the craniotomy, the obstetrician's act was gravely illicit.

Explanation. In perforating the head of the second living fetus the obstetrician directly administered a fatal blow to an innocent human being. His action, then, was murder. His ultimate purpose in performing this action was, it is true, praiseworthy, for he wished to make the delivery of the first fetus possible. Evil, however, may never be done that good may come of it. This destructive perforation of the skull of a living innocent human being is a direct, unjust attack upon his life, and is clearly a very gravely sinful crime.

Case 145
Decapitation in a Case of Interlocked Twins

The mother has interlocking twins during labor. One twin presents the breech, the other the head, but the former's chin is tightly placed under the latter's chin. In order to bring about the safe delivery at least of one of them the physician wishes to decapitate the one whose head is most easily reached.

Solution. Decapitation of a living fetus would, even in this case, be gravely illicit.

Explanation. Decapitation here would be a direct, fatal attack on the living fetus and therefore could never be justified. An accepted mode of delivery would be displacement of the head of the second child and the delivery of the head of the first child by the Piper forceps, followed by the delivery of the second child. If this was not possible under the circumstances, both children might be removed by caesarean section. If, however, the choice is to decapitate one child to save the other or to permit both twins to die, the physician must choose the latter. Thus he will not be guilty of performing a murderous action and the death of the twins must be ascribed, not to him, but to an accident of nature.

Case 146
Curettage with a Second Twin Probably in Utero

The patient has just suffered a miscarriage which has brought profuse bleeding of the uterus. The physician wishes to perform a curettage and tampon the uterus. He hesitates to do this, however, for the uterus may still contain a twin fetus. May he licitly proceed with the curettage?

Solution. The physician must first do all he can to ascertain whether or not a twin fetus is present in utero. If he finds that another fetus is present, he must try to save it if this is possible. If, however, he cannot ascertain whether or not a twin is within the uterus and if curettage must be performed at once to save the mother's life, he may licitly curette the uterus.

Explanation. In performing the curettage the physician's purpose is to remedy the dangerous condition of the bleeding uterus. The curettage is directly aimed at scraping from the inner surface of the uterus any piece of the decidua or placenta which may be still clinging to the uterine wall. Until such remnants of the afterbirth are removed, the woman's life will be endangered by hemorrhage. That which the physician sets out to accomplish is to clear away these dangerous and useless remnants; hence his action is not in itself evil. His intention, moreover, is praiseworthy, for he is endeavoring to save the mother's life. It is true that, if there happens to be a twin fetus remaining in the uterus, the action of curetting will destroy it; this destruction, however, is not directly intended. Destroying a twin, if it is actually present, is not here directly desired, although it is foreseen as a probability, however slight this may be.[7] There is, moreover, a proportionately grave reason (the saving of the mother's life) for incurring this risk. The problematical existence of the fetus is outweighed by the mother's clear right to life. In this case, therefore, the principle of the twofold effect finds proper application.

HYDROCEPHALIC FETUSES

WHEN the unborn infant is hydrocephalic, his cerebral ventricles are enlarged by excessive fluid and the distended head may be several times the normal size. In many cases the hydrocephalus is unnoticed until the second-stage labor pains have begun. The obstetrician may then consider it too late to perform a caesarean section, although some are of the opinion that it is possible even at this stage. Even if such an infant is born alive, it will usually die within a few days. If the extraordinary occurs and it does survive, it will be a hopeless idiot. For the mother a hydrocephalic fetus is a serious matter, for it can rupture the uterus and bring her a fatal hemorrhage. To know what he may licitly do in the case where

---

[7] The probability is said to be approximately one in ninety that a twin is present.

a mother is carrying a viable hydrocephalic infant is often a matter of great moment for the obstetrician.

Directly to administer to the child a fatal blow is of course forbidden, because such an act would be murder. Even though the physician's intention were most praiseworthy—namely, to save the mother's life—his action would be intrinsically evil, and evil may never be done in order that good may come of it. The surgeon may licitly cut out a section of the brain in order to drain off some of the excessive fluid and thus permit the unhindered delivery of the child if this procedure is not in itself a fatal blow and if it is the best that can be done to save the child. Such an operation would not be a direct attack on the life of the fetus; it would consist rather in sacrificing a part of the child's body in order to endeavor to save the rest. The procedure does, it is true, involve very grave danger for the child, but it is the child's only hope of surviving. If the child is left in the uterus, it will die and will probably cause the mother's death also.

In a hydrocephalus head presentation the physician may licitly employ intraventricular tap and drainage per vaginam with a spinal needle. This procedure is recommended by some authorities, who contend that it is safer and simpler than the treatments usually recommended.[8] If this treatment is possible and if it offers less risk to the child than cutting out a section of the brain, it must of course be preferred to the latter more drastic operation.

After the hydrocephalic infant is fully born, it must be given all the supportive treatments in the way of nourishment,

[8] See Cornelius T. O'Connor, M.D., and Arthur J. Gorman, M.D., "The Treatment of Hydrocephalus in Cephalic Presentation," *American Journal of Obstetrics and Gynecology* 43:521-24, March 1942; Nicholson J. Eastman, M.D., *Williams Obstetrics,* tenth edition, pp. 1126-27 (New York: Appleton-Century-Crofts, 1950). Dr. Eastman remarks: "In a case of hydrocephalus . . . a spinal puncture needle may be inserted through the most accessible suture space and sufficient fluid withdrawn to allow descent of the head through the pelvis. In the few cases in which I have done this, delivery has been prompt and there have been no discernible effects of a harmful nature on the infant."

medication, and so forth, which are obligatory in the case of normal infants. The fact that the child is a monstrosity does not deprive it of its right to life.

Case 147
Craniotomy in the Case of a Hydrocephalic Fetus

The patient, a woman at term, is admitted to the delivery room. The examination discloses that she is carrying a hydrocephalic infant. Fetal heart tones are present. A trocar is inserted into the cranium to drain off some of the fluid. The infant is baptized in utero. After an hour dilation is complete and no fetal heart tones are present. A craniotomy is performed and the dead fetus is extracted.

Solution. The absence of fetal heart tones is not a certain sign of death. The craniotomy here performed was gravely illicit, for the physician was not certain that the fetus was already dead.

Explanation. If a physician does a craniotomy on the fetus when the latter is probably still alive, he runs the risk of directly administering a fatal blow to a living and innocent human being, and this is never permitted. Before the physician may licitly do a craniotomy, he must be morally certain that the infant is already dead.

Case 148
Permitting a Hydrocephalic To Die in Utero

The physician, delivering the child in a breech presentation, does not discover that it is hydrocephalic until the head is arrested at the pelvic inlet. Because of the patient's weakened condition the physician feels that the danger from a caesarean section is even greater than the danger from a uterine rupture and that a section is therefore contraindicated. How should he proceed?

Solution. If there is no way of delivering the child without bringing death to the mother, the physician must merely await the death of the child. Once the child is dead, the physician may remove it by any convenient method.

Explanation. Since the hydrocephalic child as a rule would not live long even if it were delivered alive, why may not the physician in the present case perform a destructive perforation of the head with a trocar, quickly extract the fetus, and thus bring greater security to the mother? The reason is that this would be a direct, fatal attack on a living and innocent person which must be looked upon as murder. But why is it necessary that the physician wait until the hydro-

257

cephalic child dies in utero, since its death is inevitable and delay in extracting it from the uterus may cause the mother's death? Why should it not be permissible to kill it in order to safeguard the mother's life? The answer is that evil may not be done in order that good may come of it. Unjust killing is never licit. The mother may undergo a caesarean section in order to save the child if the section would not certainly be fatal to herself; but in judging that a section is contraindicated the physician judges that it would be equivalent to the direct killing of the mother. The direct killing of the mother is never justifiable, no matter how grave may be the reason because of which it is done.

REFERENCE

Kelly, Gerald, S.J. *Medico-Moral Problems,* pt. 3, "Delivery of Hydrocephalic Infant," pp. 17-21. St. Louis: Catholic Hospital Association of the United States and Canada, 1951.

UNCLASSIFIED PROBLEMS

S IX medico-moral problems of a heterogeneous kind are grouped together in this chapter because they do not merit chapters of their own. Included are the experimental use of drugs and germs, the use of hypnotism, euthanasia, experiments with unnatural forms of fertilization, the use of douches after rape, and hygiene during menstruation.

THE EXPERIMENTAL USE OF DRUGS AND GERMS

THE PHYSICIAN has a general obligation to use the remedies that he considers best for his patient. This obligation was discussed in Chapter Two, pages 20-21. We shall here discuss the use of new drugs of uncertain value and self-inoculation for experimental purposes.[1] Although the use of hormones is definitely not in the experimental stage, a few words are said on the subject in order that it may not be omitted.

The Use of New Drugs of Uncertain Value

Let us suppose that the patient has a very troublesome disease, that there is no immediate danger that he will die from the ailment, and that there is no known remedy which will certainly bring about a cure. An example might be severe peripheral neuritis in old age. May the physician in these cir-

---

[1] For an authoritative statement of the physician's obligations in the field of experimentation see *Acta Apostolicae Sedis* 44:779-89, October 16, 1952.

259

cumstances administer a newly discovered drug which may cure the patient but which may cause his death? The answer will depend upon the degree of the hope of success offered by the new drug. If there is but slight assurance that the patient will survive the medication, the use of the drug would be illicit, for it would be tantamount to murder. If, however, there is well-founded hope that the patient will be cured, if all possible precautions have been taken, and if the patient, knowing the risk which the drug would involve, freely consents to its use, the physician may licitly administer such medication. In this case the principle of the twofold effect is rightly applied. The physician's intention is to restore his patient to the state of good health. The action which he performs is that of administering the drug as a cure for the disease in question. The evil effect is the danger incurred. The good effect is the cure of the patient. The cure is not to be caused by means of the danger. Even though no danger were actually present, the cure could be effected. But the important problem here is whether there is a sufficient reason for exposing oneself to the risk. A sufficient reason is considered present if the affliction is serious enough to warrant the risk. In this very difficult case, where nothing else avails, although one may use the drug prescribed, he is not obliged to do so.

Let us alter the case that has just been described. Let us suppose that there are other remedies for the patient's disease. The new drug in question will very probably effect a cure within a short time; the other remedies require several years of medication. The new drug involves some, though not great, danger of death; the other remedies are harmless. In this case the patient could licitly make use of the new drug. He is running some risk from the use of the new drug, but it is not too grave a one and he has a justifying reason for incurring the risk; that is, the hope of avoiding the tedium and the inconvenience which other remedies would involve. In this case the risk to which the patient is exposed ought to be less than in the preceding case, since other remedies would effect a cure, though more slowly.

Case 149
Use of a Doubtful Drug with a Dying Child

The 2-year-old daughter of Mrs. S is dying of leukemia. Physicians have advised the mother that there is no known remedy for the disease and that death will occur within a year. Through the Associated Press, in an appeal entitled "Mother Offers Daughter as a Guinea Pig," Mrs. S asks anyone who may think that he has a remedy for leukemia to send it to her, so that she may use it with her child. Was her proposed action licit?

Solution. The action of Mrs. S was licit provided she did not intend to use any remedy unless she had sound reason for thinking that it would not prove gravely harmful.

Explanation. Since Mrs. S wished only to save her child's life, she would certainly not think of using any remedy which she had reason to believe would hasten death rather than prolong life. Her action, medically considered, was unwise, for any effective remedy for leukemia would be known to the profession, and any remedy sent to her would almost certainly be the product of a quack.

Case 150
Use of a New and Doubtful Drug by Felons

The governor promises a pardon to any convict in the state penitentiary who will use a new and doubtful drug for experimental purposes. Could convicts licitly volunteer to use the drug?

Solution. The use of the drug would be licit provided that it would not be the direct cause of grave injury and that the risk of indirect grave injury be avoided insofar as possible.

Explanation. In this case it is taken for granted that the experimentation would probably produce harmful effects in the patient and that the danger would be grave. Unless this circumstance were present, there would be no need to promise pardons to convicts in order to induce them to become experimental subjects. The reason for the experimentation—namely, a notable advancement of science—is a grave one. If the experimenting physician intended to produce in the human experimental subjects serious bodily injury, his action could not of course be justified. If, however, the physician did not directly intend grave bodily injury, but merely foresaw it as a probable effect of the experimentation, he could proceed for a proportionately grave reason. The risk of indirectly causing grave injury must be reduced insofar as possible by means of clinical study and animal experimentation. The experiments would not of course be licit unless the men freely consented; but in the present case there is no difficulty about this point, since the convicts are volunteers.

Self-Inoculation for Experimental Purposes

Physicians will recall the case of Dr. Jesse W. Lazear and the yellow-fever germ.[2] At the time of this incident there was available a remedy for yellow fever, but it was not known how the germ of this disease was communicated. In order to discover the manner in which the disease was contracted, Dr. Lazear and several others permitted themselves to be subjected to the risk of infection. Dr. Lazear contracted the disease and died because of some error on the part of the physician who attended him. Dr. Lazear acted licitly, for he had sufficient reason for exposing himself to the risk of infection. The good to be accomplished was great and the danger of death was not serious. His death was accidental; the others who contracted the disease during the experiment recovered.

There is, however, another case which is different from that of Dr. Lazear. Medical research workers had established the fact that yellow fever was caused by some one of ten agents, and the problem was to determine which of the ten agents was actually the cause. At the time there was no known cure for yellow fever, which was generally considered a fatal disease. In these circumstances, in order to discover the carrier of the yellow-fever germ, the physicians called for ten volunteers. Each of the ten volunteers would be inoculated with one of the ten agents. Nine of the agents would prove harmless; the tenth would bring death.

The physicians were not justified in inoculating the volunteers as they did, for they knew that their injections would

---

[2] See *Encyclopedia Americana*, article "Yellow Fever."

kill one of the volunteers. They did not know precisely which man would be the victim, but they were conscious of the fact that to one of the ten they were going to administer a fatal blow, the deadly germ. Thus one inoculation would of its very nature be lethal. No matter how noble the purpose of these physicians, no matter how many and how far-reaching the benefits which would result from their act for the human race, they were not justified in performing an intrinsically evil act. Objectively, therefore, the action of the physicians in this case was evil. Subjectively, however, they were no doubt free of guilt, for in all probability they erroneously looked upon their act as perfectly licit.[3]

The Use of Hormones

Modern medicine has discovered many beneficial uses for the sex hormones. In the male the female hormone is administered in treating cancer of the prostate gland. In the female the male hormone is used in the treatment of cancer of the breast. The male hormone is used to rid male patients of gonadal deficiencies. In the female lutein is used for those who are threatening to abort or who are habitual aborters. There is nothing morally wrong in all such uses of hormones if the good effects fully compensate for any evil effects that may follow. The possible evil effect is abnormal sexual excitation, but this will rarely occur if the dosage is properly controlled.

THE USE OF HYPNOTISM

HYPNOTISM consists of a "state of mental absorption in which all distracting thoughts are for the moment warded off, and only such thoughts as are suggested by the hypnotist reach the consciousness of the patient. The essence of hypnotism is the concentration of mind on one idea or only

---

[3] See John C. Ford, S.J., "Notes on Moral Theology. The Catholic Doctor," *Theological Studies* 5:511-13, December 1944; Joseph P. Donovan, C.M., "Test Tube Killing," *Homiletic and Pastoral Review* 45:59-60, October 1944.

a few ideas dictated by the hypnotist."[4] If the hypnotist is not skilled in this practice, the patient may suffer various evil effects. Among the deleterious effects that may be produced are (1) an abnormal proneness to become drowsy and to fall asleep; (2) a detachment, more or less pronounced, from reality, even though the patient is to all appearances in a state of wakefulness; (3) an occasional loss of memory and of mental equilibrium resulting in increased irritability; (4) incoherence of speech. The hypnotist has the subject in his power and can strongly influence his mind. He is able, moreover, to force him to reveal secret knowledge, to fill his memory with unwholesome suggestions, and even to perpetrate immoral actions with him.

There is of course nothing wrong in itself with the practice of hypnotism, and therefore under certain conditions its use would be licit. Since hypnotism, however, violently deprives the subject of the full use of reason and free will, a justifying cause is required for allowing it to be practiced. Hypnotism may be licitly used provided three conditions are verified: (1) there is present a grave reason, (2) the consent of the subject is obtained, and (3) due precautions are observed. We shall explain in detail the meaning of these three conditions.

A Grave Reason. A proportionate cause is required in order that one licitly be hypnotized, for we are not permitted to give up, without a compensatory reason, our dominion over the faculties of the understanding and the will. A justifying reason would be, for example, the need to cure or to curtail an evil habit such as drunkenness, pyromania, masturbation, or kleptomania. If deemed medically advisable, hypnotism may be licitly employed in place of an anesthetic for surgical cases. If there is at hand another remedy which would be equally effective but would not involve the dangers that often accompany hypnotism, it must of course be preferred.

[4] James J. Walsh, M.D., *Psychotherapy*, p. 152. New York: D. Appleton and Company, 1929.

264

The Consent of the Subject. The consent of the patient must be procured, for no one has the right to deprive another, against his wishes, of the full use of his faculties. Hence forcibly to impose an hypnotic state on another, even for a short period, would be to violate his rights. It is not necessary, however, always to obtain the explicit consent of the patient. If the patient is in such circumstances that his explicit consent cannot prudently be sought and if one is convinced that he would not object to hypnotic treatment, this would be considered sufficient consent on the part of the patient. With regard to the insane and to children who have not reached the age of reason, the physician should not use hypnotism without first procuring the consent of the parents or of the one who is charged with their care.

Due Precautions. The first precaution which must be observed is that the hypnotist be one who is medically qualified to exercise this art. An unskillful hypnotist may injure the patient's mental faculties. A competent physician can as a rule prevent the evil effects which sometimes result from the use of hypnosis. The second requirement is that there be present an authorized witness of unimpeachable character who will serve as a protection both to the physician and to the patient. The witness (for example, a parent or the marriage partner of the patient) could afterward defend the physician against any false accusations of improper conduct.[5]

Case 151
Use of Hypnotism in Insomnia
The patient is of a nervous type and is suffering from insomnia. The physician wishes to try hypnosis to effect a cure, but he is doubtful whether it is licit to use hypnosis as a remedy for insomnia.
Solution. The use of hypnotism in this case is licit.

[5] For material on hypnotism and its morality see James J. Walsh, M.D., *Psychotherapy*, pp. 151-62 (New York: D. Appleton and Company, 1929); *Catholic Encyclopedia*, article "Hypnotism"; William T. Heron, *Clinical Applications of Suggestion and Hypnosis*, chap. 8, pp. 90-93 (Springfield: Charles C. Thomas, 1950).

Explanation. There is a sufficiently grave reason here to justify the use of hypnotism, even though it does violently deprive the subject of the use of his senses for a prolonged period of time.

EUTHANASIA

EUTHANASIA ("happy death") or mercy killing is administering, ordinarily at the victim's own request, an easy, painless death to one who is suffering from an incurable and perhaps agonizing ailment. There are today not a few who sincerely favor mercy killing, pointing with approval to cases such as the following. A girl twenty years of age poisoned her mother, whom she could not bear to see suffering acute pain from an incurable disease. A young mother shot a daughter who was born blind. It is said in defense of mercy killing that modern civilization has developed a sensitiveness to the sufferings of others; that the law which looks upon euthanasia as murder was framed in an age when indifference to human suffering was normal and is now out of date. Public sympathy tends to defend euthanasia, and many modern juries have refused to convict the mercy killer.

In December 1947 two thousand New York physicians drafted a bill to make euthanasia a legitimate means of what was termed "merciful release."[6] In a poll of four thousand physicians of the state of New York, 80 per cent favored mercy killing.[7] In a petition to the New York state legislature 379 leading Protestant and Jewish ministers urged the passage of a law which would permit, under careful safeguards, voluntary mercy killing.[8]

The Morality of Mercy Killing

No matter what sentimentalists may contend, euthanasia is a grave crime against the law of nature and should be called

[6] See Selwyn James, "Euthanasia—Right or Wrong?" *Survey Graphic* 37:241-43, May 1948.

[7] *Ibid.*, p. 241.

[8] *America* 80:423, January 22, 1949.

by its proper name: mercy murder. It is to be condemned for the following reasons.

1. God alone has the ownership of human life. In euthanasia the killer assumes the right of ownership over life,[9] and so the crime committed is either murder or suicide. This is the fundamental reason for the fact that euthanasia is immoral.

Some may contend that in the cases which the advocates of euthanasia envision, there is question merely of choosing the lesser of two evils, for the patient is certain to die in any event. The choice, they point out, is between a slow, agonizing death and a quick, painless death. Hence, they argue, the object of euthanasia is the diminution of suffering.

Those who favor euthanasia regard pain and suffering as evil and worthless. We shall see shortly that they are mistaken. Assuming, however, that the purpose of the mercy killer is good, one must examine the means by which he intends to accomplish his objective. It cannot be said that he is choosing the lesser of two evils. In all cases of euthanasia the choice actually lies between the following two alternatives: (1) permitting nature to run its course in producing a slow, agonizing death and (2) quickly administering a murderous blow to bring about a quick, painless death. Both these alternatives may involve evil; but in the first case the evil is physical, in the other it is moral. Moral evil is what we know as sin, and sin may never be licitly intended or committed. Murder, or the unjust killing of an innocent person, is of its very nature evil and will remain evil in every set of circumstances.

"If a dog or a horse is gravely injured so that its cure is utterly hopeless, we humanely bring it instant relief by killing it," assert those who favor euthanasia. "Should we be more cruel to our fellow men than we are to animals? Does not an incurably sick and acutely suffering man or woman deserve just as merciful treatment as a brute beast?" There is no real

[9] Some falsely assume that the killer has this right. See Foster Kennedy, M.D., "Euthanasia: To Be or Not To Be," *Collier's* 125:13, 48-51, April 22, 1950.

parity between the case of a mortally injured animal and a human being who is dying of an incurable disease. All animals were created in order to serve man.[10] A badly crippled horse or an incurably sick dog has completed its destiny in life. Once it is completely unable to serve man, its purpose in life has ended. Since it was placed in the world to serve man and to help him in accomplishing his destiny in life, it may be killed or employed in any way which accords with its purpose in life. On the other hand, a man is not permitted directly to administer a fatal blow to an innocent person, be that person himself or another. It matters not, moreover, whether the person toward whom the fatal blow is directed be eager to receive it or eager to avoid it.[11]

2. Euthanasia takes no account of man's supernatural life, disregarding the value of pain and suffering in storing up merit and in shortening one's purgatory. Advocates of euthanasia ignore Christ's words, "If anyone wishes to come after me, let him . . . take up his cross daily" (Luke 9:23). Christians believe that Christ is God and that He is our model of right living. During His life He gave us an example of suffering. The apostle St. Paul, moreover, whose writings were divinely inspired, reminds us that "whom the Lord loves, he chastises" (Hebrews 12:6).

[10] See Michael Cronin, *The Science of Ethics*, vol. II, pp. 86-92. New York: Benziger Brothers, 1949.

[11] See *Catholic Encyclopedia*, article "Homicide." See also Alphonsus Bonnar, O.F.M., *Catholic Doctor*, chap. 10, "Euthanasia and Sterilisation," pp. 105-23 (London: Burns Oates and Washbourne, 1951); Robert F. Drinan, S.J., "Euthanasia: An Emergent Danger," *Homiletic and Pastoral Review* 50:220-23, December 1949; Bernard J. Ficarra, M.D., *Newer Ethical Problems in Medicine and Surgery*, chap. 8, "Euthanasia," pp. 47-96 (Westminster: Newman Press, 1951); John C. Ford, S.J., *Mercy Murder* (New York: America Press, 1950); Gerald Kelly, S.J., *Medico-Moral Problems*, pt. 3, "Euthanasia," pp. 1-8 (St. Louis: Catholic Hospital Association of the United States and Canada, 1951); Alphonse M. Schwitalla, S.J., "Medical Opinion Concerning Euthanasia," *Linacre Quarterly* 14:16-26, April 1947; Joseph V. Sullivan, *Morality of Mercy Killing* (Westminster: Newman Press, 1950); Hilary R. Werts, S.J., "Moral Aspects of Euthanasia," *Linacre Quarterly* 14:27-33, April 1947 (also in *Catholic Mind* 45:744-50, December 1947).

3. The practice of euthanasia would greatly lessen confidence in physicians, for the patient who was gravely ill might readily fear that his physician would judge his case incurable and so administer poison to end his suffering. "By no means unimportant to consider," says Dr. Rabinowitch, "are the possible effects of legalized euthanasia upon the status of the medical profession and, thus ultimately, upon the health of the people.

"The elevated conception of the dignity and the high seriousness of the physician's calling were not easily gained. It was only after centuries of convincing proof that the sole purpose of the physician as a physician was to prolong life and relieve pain that medicine was able to advance. . . . It was only after law no more demanded infallibility on the part of the physician, nor even the highest degree of skill, knowledge and care, but only that degree of skill, knowledge and care commonly possessed and exercised by the average reputable practitioner in the locality, that it was possible for medicine to improve the accuracy of diagnosis and to better the methods of its treatment, and that came about only after one development—absolute confidence that the aim, and only aim, of the physician was to prolong life and to relieve suffering. Now there are those who would assign to the physician a duty of shortening it."[12]

On October 17, 1950, the World Medical Association, composed of national medical associations in forty-one different countries, in general assembly, adopted a resolution which called euthanasia "contrary to the public interest and to medical principles as well as to natural and civil rights."[13]

4. We may mention here a recent decision of the Holy Office. The Sacred Congregation of the Holy Office of Rome, a tribunal of the highest authority in the eyes of Catholics, was

---

[12] I. M. Rabinowitch, "Euthanasia." *Catholic Mind* 49:351-59, June 1951.

[13] The adoption of this resolution is reported in *Journal of the American Medical Association* 144:1011, November 18, 1950.

asked: "Is it legal upon the mandate of authority directly to kill those who, although not having committed any crimes deserving of death, are yet, because of psychic or physical defects, unable to be useful to the nation, but rather are considered a burden to its vigor and strength?" The congregation's answer was: "No, because it is contrary to the natural and positive law."[14]

Case 152
Euthanasia at the Request of Parents

The patient, a 2-day-old infant with severe spina bifida, is beyond medical help. At the request of the parents the physician gives it a fatal drug.

Solution. The physician is guilty of murder.

Explanation. Euthanasia is always illicit. The fact that the parents requested that the child be killed does not justify the physician, for the parents possessed no right to decree the death of their child.

Case 153
Euthanasia at the Request of the Patient

The patient, a man 56 years of age, has been wounded by a bullet in the spine. As a result of the injury he is afflicted with paraplegia, incontinence of urine and feces, and intense pain. He will probably die within a few months. The patient requests the physician to end his life and the physician complies with the request.

Solution. The physician is guilty both of murder and of formal cooperation in suicide.

Explanation. The patient has no right to take his own life and is therefore guilty of suicide. The physician, instead of attempting to dissuade the patient, approves the patient's plan and is guilty of formal cooperation in the patient's act of suicide. In addition the physician himself administers the fatal drug and is therefore guilty of murder.

Case 154
Euthanasia for the Sake of Attendants

The patient's tongue and jaws are completely replaced by carcinoma. Because of the stench and the constant drivel mixed with blood, he

[14] *Acta Apostolicae Sedis* 32:553-54, January 22, 1940.

is nauseating and repulsive to all who attend him. The physician administers a fatal drug to the patient, for, he asserts, "No one can reasonably be expected to nurse a man in such circumstances."

Solution. The physician's action is intrinsically evil and therefore cannot be justified.

Explanation. The physician's act is essentially one of murder. The fact that the patient is an intolerable burden to others does not deprive him of his right to life.

Case 155
Euthanasia by Suggestion

The patient, a woman 80 years of age, has an incurable disease that is causing her grave pain. Dr. X places at her bedside tablets of morphine. "If you take two of these, you will sleep for several hours," he tells her. "If you take all fourteen tablets, you are sure to die." He knows that the patient has been seeking some way to bring about death painlessly.

Solution. If Dr. X intended that the patient should use the pills to kill herself, he was guilty of a very grave wrong. In any case his manner of acting was gravely imprudent.

Explanation. Dr. X's act of putting the tablets at the bedside of the patient and of explaining to her the effects of various dosages is not evil in itself. Hence in some circumstances the act could be one of material cooperation only. In the present case, however, it appears that Dr. X intended that the patient should take all fourteen tablets and thus cause her death. If this was his intention, he desired her suicide, and therefore he was guilty of very serious sin.

UNNATURAL FERTILIZATION

WITHIN recent years there has been considerable experimentation with fertilization of unnatural kinds. Attempts have been made to transplant human ovaries to brute beasts for the purpose of discovering whether human ova could be fertilized by brute semen. Attempts have also been made to fertilize human ova by human semen *in vitro*.

Human and Animal Crossbreeding

It is very doubtful that human ova could be fertilized by the semen of a brute beast. The attempt to bring about this kind of fertilization is said to have been made in the past; but although it is reported that fertilization did occur, the report has not been authoritatively verified. At any rate, it has never been asserted that a living being was born of such an experiment. Apart from the grave evil involved in transplanting a human ovary into an irrational animal, the attempt to fertilize such transplanted ova with the seed of a beast would be a very grave violation of God's designs. God obviously intends that human ova be impregnated by human seed only.

The attempt to fertilize with human seed the fruit of a human ovary which had begun to function in a brute beast would also be a gross violation of the natural order of things. Pope Pius XII condemned the practice of fertilizing a woman with the semen even of her own husband unless this were but an aid to the marital act, previously had. He would certainly, then, condemn the insemination with human seed of the human ovary now residing in a brute beast, and this even though the transplanted ovary and the human semen came from two persons who were husband and wife.

During a meeting of the National Academy of Sciences in Washington reference was made to the possibility of breeding apes artificially by human semen.[15] Any attempt to do so would be worthy of condemnation as a horrifying perversion and as gravely offensive to the Creator of all things.

Ovum-Sperm Experimentation

Within the last few years physicians have attempted the experiment *in vitro* of uniting outside the woman's body a human ovum and sperm.[16] Ova were removed from a woman and exposed *in vitro* to spermatozoa. The microscope showed that, of eight hundred ova thus exposed, fertilization actually occurred in but a few. In two of the ova the three-cell stage

---

[15] See "To Breed a Brain." *Newsweek* 35:54, May 8, 1950.

[16] See John C. Ford, S.J., "Notes on Moral Theology. The Catholic Doctor." *Theological Studies* 5:511-13, December 1944.

was reached; in two others the two-cell stage occurred.[17] This study of human fertilization is no doubt regarded by some members of the medical profession as scientifically desirable; but the first question that must be looked into is the morality of the practice.

Most theologians teach that, when a human sperm unites with a human ovum in the body of a woman, a spiritual soul is at once infused into this new organism, and the resultant creature is a living person. We fully understand that the medical profession in general recognizes three stages in the development of the fertilized ovum: the ovum stage, the embryo stage, and the fetal stage. We are also aware that there is some authority for holding that the soul is not infused immediately at conception. Whether we speak of a fertilized ovum or of a fetus is merely a matter of terminology. As to the infusion of the soul, the fertilized ovum is intended by God to become a human being if it is not already one, and its destruction would therefore be at least the killing of a potential human being. It would in addition be a very grave frustration of nature. As has been explained (see page 212), if the fetus is probably a human being, any direct attack on it would be prohibited by the law of nature.[18]

If the union of a human spermatozoon and a human ovum takes place, not within the body of a woman, but outside the body, the union even *in vitro* would very probably result at once in human life. But is it permissible to bring a human being into existence *in vitro?* This fertilized ovum certainly will not grow to viability. The incipient embryo, which is prob-

[17] See John Rock, M.D., and Miriam F. Menkin, "In Vitro Fertilization and Cleavage of Human Ovarian Eggs," *Science* 100:105-07, August 4, 1944; "Artificial Fertilization," *Science News Letter* 46:99, August 12, 1944; John Rock, M.D., and Arthur T. Hertig, M.D., "Information Regarding the Time of Human Ovulation Derived from a Study of 3 Unfertilized and 11 Fertilized Ova," *American Journal of Obstetrics and Gynecology* 47:343-56, March 1944.

[18] An excellent exposition of this problem is contained in T. Lincoln Bouscaren, S.J., *Ethics of Ectopic Operations*, pp. 38-45 (Milwaukee: Bruce Publishing Company, 1944).

ably human, cannot survive for long. In uniting a spermatozoon and an ovum in this manner the experimenter is bringing an embryo (probably human) into being in a place in which it is not destined by nature to live. He is bringing it to life in unnatural circumstances which will be fatal to it. In other words, at the very moment when he is bringing it to life, he is equivalently administering to it a deathblow, and this he is under a grave obligation to avoid. Let us envision the case in which the experiment has reached so great a stage of perfection that the physician is morally certain that the fetus will reach viability. In that event his action of uniting the human sperm and ovum could not be condemned for the reason mentioned above, but it would nevertheless be illicit. Nature has ordained that the sperm and ovum be united only in the genital tract of a woman. To bring about this union outside a woman's body is opposed to nature's designs. Hence, regardless of the life expectancy of the fetus generated *in vitro,* all such experimentation is gravely illicit.

Case 156
Transplantation of a Human Ovary to a Beast

For purposes of experimentation a surgeon wishes to remove the ovaries of a female animal and to transplant one ovary from a woman into the body of this beast. When the transplanted organ begins to function, the surgeon intends to try to discover the effect which animal semen produces on the human ova.

Solution. Both the excising of the ovary for transplantation into a brute beast and the attempt to fertilize a human ovum with animal seed are gravely illicit.

Explanation. The transplanting of a human organ is licit only if the excised organ is to be placed in a human being. (See "The Transplantation of Organs," pages 139-42.) To take a woman's ovary from her for a brute beast is gravely illicit, for the ovary thus transplanted will fulfill neither its primary nor its secondary purpose. (See page 140, paragraph 1.) Its primary purpose is obviously to serve the individual woman, its possessor; its secondary purpose is to aid, not brute beasts, but other human beings. Animals were created to serve man. Man (soul, body, and parts of his body) was not made in order to serve brute beasts. But in the present case the part of the human body would actually be made to serve the animal by producing hormonal secretions. The act of taking the ovary from the woman would be an unjustifiable excision, a gravely sinful mutilation.

THE USE OF DOUCHES AFTER RAPE

WHEN a man rapes a woman, he is guilty of a gravely unjust attack upon her person. His act of injecting semen into her genital tract is obviously a violation of justice. During this attack the woman may do everything in her power to prevent the semen from entering her body, for her efforts would constitute justifiable self-defense against unjust aggression. She has certainly just as much a right forcibly to resist this attack as she has to do violence to one who is endeavoring to choke her to death.

Once the rapist's attack is ended, the semen which is within her body may be considered a continuance of the unjust aggression begun shortly before by the rapist, and therefore the woman may licitly defend herself against it. Flushing the genital tract with a germicidal solution is therefore perfectly licit for her, since it is legitimate self-defense.[19] We say that in this case the use of a germicidal douche is permitted, although it is not obligatory. Some physicians, instead of the douche, may prefer to employ curettage, germicidal powder, or other means to destroy the semen in the genital area of the violated woman. All such means may be licitly employed only for expelling the semen; they would be illicit if used in order to endeavor to dislodge a fertilized ovum or to prevent implantation of a fertilized ovum. It is true, incidentally, that conception in the case of rape is less probable because of the grave shock usually suffered by the victim.

[19] Some theologians would deny the licitness of this douche, contending that, once the act of the rapist is ended, there is no longer a continuance of the unjust aggression. See on the subject Benedictus H. Merkelbach, O.P., *Summa theologica moralis*, vol. II, p. 943, no. 1010, 3b and 3c (Paris: Desclée DeBrouwer et Cie, 1949). The opinion that is here given, however, is commonly taught, and one is safe in conscience in following it.

This right, however, ceases to exist if the rapist's semen has already impregnated an ovum. In this case a douche may not be used for the purpose of washing out the fertilized ovum. The fertilized ovum is a new human being who has every right to life.[20] To employ a douche to destroy this fertilized ovum would be directly to risk killing an innocent human being, and this would be gravely evil. The argument that the fertilized ovum is an unjust aggressor and that the woman may treat it as such is not valid. The fetus' origin was due to unjust aggression, it is true; but the fetus itself is merely the fruit of nature's act of bringing about fertilization. In no sense is the fetus itself an unjust transgressor, for it is there where nature has placed it. Hence the fertilized ovum may not be directly attacked by douche or any other means. If there is danger of destroying a fertilized ovum, the raped woman may not use a douche. The same is of course true if the victim of the rapist (for example, a married woman) was pregnant before the rape occurred. There is no one who does not understand what suffering such a ruling may involve, but to make any other ruling would be to abandon the principle that human life is always and everywhere sacred.

The raped woman, then, may licitly wash out her genital tract as long as she is destroying the rapist's semen only. The question then arises: How long after the completion of sexual intercourse would there be no danger of destroying a fertilized ovum by douching, or in other words, during what length of time after the rapist's act may the woman's sex organs be washed out because they are judged to contain semen only? The answer to this question will vary insofar as it refers to the different genital organs of the woman. The vagina may be licitly flushed with a germicidal solution at any time at all. There is no time limit that must be made in regard to vaginal douching, because at no time after the rape would washing out the vagina risk destroying a fertilized ovum. One may

[20] See pp. 191-94, where the ethician's views on this matter are explained.

safely hold that the uterus itself (but no part of the Fallopian tubes) may be licitly flushed with a germicidal solution during the first sixteen hours which immediately follow the rapist's attack.[21] Hence, if the rape occurred just after midnight, the uterus could be washed out from that time until four o'clock in the afternoon of that day. Douching the uterus during this period would not endanger a fertilized ovum, for a fertilized ovum would not yet have had time to descend into the womb. Fertilization, if it occurs, takes place at the posterior end of the Fallopian tube near the fimbriae. When semen enters the female genital organs, it moves slowly up the uterus and along the tubes. The descent of a fertilized ovum from the extremity of the tube to the uterus is very slow. Hence during the first sixteen hours after sexual intercourse it is certain that there is no fertilized ovum in or near the uterus.

Briefly, therefore, we say that in case of rape the physician may employ every possible means (within the limits of the above-mentioned periods of time) whether or not he thinks that it will prove certainly effective. It is not the part of the ethician to tell him what measures will or will not be effective, but rather to pass judgment on the licitness of measures which he knows are sometimes employed.

At times, when a raped woman is brought to the hospital, the physician wishes to douche, not only the vagina and the uterus, but the Fallopian tubes as well. When would it be licit to flush the Fallopian tubes of the victim of rape? Since the semen is judged to travel about eight inches an hour, it seems that some of it will probably reach the posterior end of the Fallopian tubes in a little over an hour. Hence, in the opinion of some medical authorities, to wash out the tubes after that

[21] If the douche is strictly limited to the uterus and does not pass, partially at least, into the tubes, it seems that it may be administered licitly even more than sixteen hours after the rape. Exactly how long after the rape the use of a germicidal uterine douche would involve no risk of harming a fertilized ovum is a question for the medical profession to answer. The answer will reveal the period of time during which the use of the douche is licit.

time would be to run the risk of killing a fertilized ovum. It is for the physician who is in charge of the case to decide during how long a period after the rape of the patient flushing out her Fallopian tubes will involve no such danger.

It no doubt happens that women who have willingly engaged in sinful sex relations at times assert that they have been raped in order to persuade the physician to administer a germicidal douche. In such a case, if a physician who knew the facts were to accede to the erring woman's request, he would be cooperating in the gravely culpable practice of artificial birth control. The physician need not, in the light of this possibility, refuse to treat any woman who claims to have been the victim of a rapist. This would not be the correct attitude for him to take. If actually the woman has been raped, she has a right to have the physician administer a uterine douche if this can be done within sixteen hours of the attack. The physician must judge each case on its own merits. As a rule there will be circumstances, such as the woman's appearance and her manner of describing the incident, which will reveal to the physician the truthfulness or the falseness of her story.

The douche which the physician uses on a rape victim may consist of any liquid which he deems best in the case. The morality of his act is obviously the same whether he employs a germicidal powder or a douche of a germicidal solution or of plain water. The age of the victim is of no moment when there is question of the morality of the act. A woman of any age, if raped, has the right to have the rapist's semen destroyed. This is true even of a married woman. A married woman, if she has been raped, may wash out the semen of the rapist.

HYGIENE DURING MENSTRUATION

I F THE use of vaginal tampons for the absorption of the menstrual discharges is medically advisable, it is as a rule morally unobjectionable. If, however, vaginal tampons are found to be injurious to one's health, they should not be used.

278

Some physicians contend that vaginal tampons do not cause injury to health.[22] Medical opinion on this matter has been summarized as follows: "Many gynecologists are opposed to the use of this type of pad for the following reasons: the dry cotton may irritate the vaginal mucosa when dragged across it; it is felt that the tampon dams the menstrual flow; many times it is handled by unclean hands; injury may occur if it is improperly inserted; and the pads are often 'lost' in the vagina, giving rise to a foul discharge. Other gynecologists apparently see no harm in their use."[23]

REFERENCES

D'Arcy, Martin C., S.J. *Pain and the Providence of God.* Milwaukee: Bruce Publishing Company, 1935.

Kelly, Gerald, S.J. "Pope Pius XII and the Principle of Totality." *Theological Studies* 16:373-96, September 1955.

Leen, Edward, C.S.Sp. *Why the Cross?* London: Sheed and Ward, 1938.

Lewis, C. S. *Problem of Pain.* New York: The Macmillan Company, 1947.

Merton, Thomas. *Exile Ends in Glory.* Milwaukee: Bruce Publishing Company, 1948.

[22] See Maurice O. Magid and Jacob Geiger, "The Intravaginal Tampon in Menstrual Hygiene," *Medical Record* 155:316-20, May 1942; Madeline J. Thornton, M.D., "The Use of Vaginal Tampons for the Absorption of Menstrual Discharges," *American Journal of Obstetrics and Gynecology* 46:259-65, August 1943; Karl John Karnaky, M.D., "Vaginal Tampons for Menstrual Hygiene," *Western Journal of Surgery, Obstetrics and Gynecology* 5:150-52, April 1943; Gerald Kelly, S.J., "Vaginal Tampons," *Linacre Quarterly* 17(no. 1):5-7 and 17(no. 4):15-16.

[23] See "Trichomonas Vaginalis." *Journal of the American Medical Association* 151:1376, April 11, 1953.

MENTAL DISEASE AND

MENTAL DEFECT

Chapter NINE

I T IS not our intention to go deeply into the subject of psychiatry. The science is advancing with amazing rapidity and new procedures and therapies are constantly being developed. A separate treatise would be required for a complete discussion of all the moral problems connected with psychiatric counseling and treatment.[1] Our purpose is not to present such a discussion, but rather to treat briefly those things that the general practitioner should know and keep in mind before he refers a patient to a psychiatrist and when he chooses the psychiatrist to whom he will refer his patient.

PSYCHIATRY AND PSYCHIATRIC PROCEDURES

ONE OF THE EARLIEST FORMS of psychotherapy was Freudian psychoanalysis. Freud taught that, hidden away in the unconscious, are strong urges which are opposed to man's conscious impulses and which strongly influence man's conscious behavior. So great is the influence of the unconscious on man's conscious attitudes and decisions that, according to

---

[1] See, for example, James H. Van der Veldt, O.F.M., and Robert P. Odenwald, M.D., *Psychiatry and Catholicism* (New York: McGraw-Hill Book Company, 1952); John B. Cavanagh, "Nervous Mental Diseases," *Ecclesiastical Review* 109:257-71, October 1943.

280

Freud, free will is weakened and at times rendered powerless. The source of man's mental disturbances, he thought, is some long-since forgotten emotional experience which wounded the soul and left a psychological scar or trauma. Because of its unpleasant nature this emotional experience was deliberately forgotten at the time it occurred, and is now the origin of the patient's difficulty. Freud was convinced that, if the cause of that emotional wound had at the time been honestly recognized and overcome, no morbidity would have resulted. His cure for the present mental disturbance consists in reviving the memory of the forgotten incident and bravely overcoming the distasteful situation. However, bringing this trouble-making memory to light is a difficult task, for the patient himself not only does not know what it is, but unconsciously endeavors to keep it secret. In order to unearth this "complex," as it is called, the analyst makes use of the following techniques: (1) word reaction, (2) life scrutiny, and (3) dream analysis. The word-reaction method consists in communicating to the patient certain stimulus words and noting his spontaneous response to them. This is judged to be effective in causing the patient to betray secrets of his unconscious memory, for the ideas which he associates with the key words are thought to reveal something of his inner life. Then the patient's entire life is, as it were, put under the microscope. He is told to let his thoughts wander freely wheresoever they will and to describe these to the analyst. It matters not how intimate the thought is or how unchaste the image which comes into his mind; he is told to recount all without the slightest hesitation or omission. He is expected to describe the beginnings and evolution of his interest in sex, his sexual fancies and fantasies, his dreams that pertain to matters of sex; and any autoeroticism, homosexuality, or other such deviation of which he has been guilty.[2] This freely rambling discussion is a thera-

---

[2] Edward A. Strecker, M.D., *Fundamentals of Psychiatry,* p. 101. Philadelphia: J. B. Lippincott Company, 1947.

peutic technique which aims at revealing the unconscious activity of the patient's mind. "Through the intimate revelation by the patient of his anxieties, worries, fears, and desires, there gradually comes, with the help of the psychiatrist, an understanding of his actions and symptoms. . . . In psychoanalysis 'transference' is . . . the reliving of the emotions of an earlier life period or of a past situation, and the unconscious refusal to accept these past actions as part of one's own doing. The patient actually passes on the responsibility for his own past acts to the psychiatrist."[3]

The dreams which the patient has described are considered to be the fulfillments of his suppressed desires, and their interpretation is judged to be an effective means of giving the analyst a clear insight into the secrets of the patient's unconscious life. During the patient's waking moments the revealing of his hidden, unconscious memories is not easy, for there is present what is called a guard or censor, whose duty it is to prevent their escape into the subject's conscious memory.

Freud was a pioneer in the field of investigating the unconscious. His psychoanalysis was the first definite effort to disclose the true nature of neurosis and to discover an effective cure. He has pointed out new problems in psychological research and has added to the scientific knowledge of some mental processes. He was the first to stress the great influence on a man's character and personality of the experiences of his childhood days. He called attention to the fact that mental treatment can actually heal various ailments of the body.[4]

The Morality of Psychoanalysis and Psychiatry

From the viewpoint of the moral law, what is to be thought of the use of psychoanalysis and psychiatry? Is there anything

[3] Robert P. Odenwald, M.D., "Psychiatry and Psychoanalysis." *Sign* 29:35-36, March 1950.

[4] See Rudolf Allers, M.D., *The Successful Error*, pp. 259-60 (New York: Sheed and Ward, 1940); Joseph Donceel, S.J., "Second Thoughts on Freud," *Thought* 24:466-84, September 1949.

in these practices which goes counter to Christian ethics? In answering these questions we must make a careful distinction between the psychoanalytic technique and the philosophy so closely associated with this technique.

"The Catholic therapist accepts in the Freudian technique the supposition that man has an unconscious as well as a conscious mind. . . . [He] agrees with Freud that mental disturbances can arise from emotional conflict and experiences that are suppressed by the patient from his consciousness, but which remain active in the consciousness as sources and the occasions of conscious mental and emotional disturbances."[5] It is not to the technique as such that the Catholic physician takes exception, but rather to the "philosophy that has been tacked on to this technique . . . [a philosophy] that is fundamentally materialistic, deterministic, and hedonistic. Freud's 'libido' theory, with its claim to a sexual origin of all nervous symptoms; his belief in the antisocial nature of the human instincts; his denial of original sin, free will, supernatural power; his regard of religion as an illusion; his replacement of the moral law with the principle of reality—these are the doctrinal and philosophic aspects of Freud's psychoanalysis that are unhesitatingly and dogmatically opposed by the Catholic practitioner."[6] If, then, the analyst is guided in his treatment of the patient by this false and poisonous philosophy of life, he will inevitably not help but greatly harm the subject. In endeavoring to cure the patient the physician must re-educate him, and it is in this process that an atheistic or amoral physician can do untold harm to his patient. "Granted a combination of a weak neurotic patient and a strong willed psychiatrist (and successful practitioners need to be strong personalities) with such a materialistic or naturalistic philosophy of life as Freud or Adler professed, we can reasonably expect that the domi-

---

[5] Robert P. Odenwald, M.D., "Psychiatry and Psychoanalysis." *Sign* 29:35-36, March 1950.
[6] *Ibid.*

nance of psychologist over patient can do irreparable harm to the latter. Moreover, if the psychiatrist does not accept the moral code of Christianity, he may give a place and interpretation to 'self-expression' in his treatment which may spell moral ruin for the individual. And it must be remembered that, however impersonal a practitioner may be in his relation with his patient, he takes upon himself the task of replacing the neurotic outlook on life by the normal, which means that a tremendous deal depends on the precise significance he gives to 'normal.' "[7]

Whether or not, then, there will be anything morally objectionable in the use of psychoanalysis and psychiatry will in practice depend not a little upon the character and the religious convictions of the physician himself. The analyst often plays the role of a father confessor, and the patient is asked to reveal to him in full detail not only sinful actions—even the most shameful—but also mere temptations which have been overcome. The physician's own way of acting during such interviews can deeply affect the patient. The latter can be influenced by the very tone of voice which the physician employs when speaking of subjects of a moral or spiritual nature, by the content and wording of the questions which he asks, by his conscious or subconscious reactions to what his investigations reveal. Some analysts go so far as to make suggestions concerning the patient's spiritual and religious life. In order, therefore, that the analyst's influence on the patient be morally wholesome, he himself must be a person of sound principles and of sincere and unimpeachable moral and religious convictions. If the one who deals with a patient in so intimate and uninhibited a manner as does an analyst were an atheist or if his philosophy of life were erroneous, he could do immeasurable spiritual harm to the patient.

[7] J. McLoughlin, "Catholic Attitude to Psychiatry," *Irish Ecclesiastical Record* 63:374, June 1944. See also Louis Beirnaert, "L'église et la psychanalyse," *Etudes* 275:229-37, novembre 1952.

The psychiatrist sets out to relieve the patient of all sense of morbid guilt. He should therefore accurately distinguish between two quite different senses of guilt: the true sense of guilt which is coupled with the performance of morally culpable actions and a pathological sense of guilt which results from a mental abnormality. Obviously the psychiatrist must beware of endeavoring to eliminate the first; he must confine his efforts to trying to rid the patient of the second.

Freud condemns some of the existing principles of Christian morality, especially those which pertain to sexual behavior. He is inclined to try to discredit, moreover, those who claim to practice sexual continence, and he assigns sexual abstinence as the cause of the mediocrity of so many inferior individuals.[8] In his *A General Introduction to Psycho-Analysis* he says: "We have found it impossible to give our support to conventional sexual morality or to approve highly of the means by which society attempts to arrange the practical problems of sexuality in life. We can demonstrate with ease that what the world calls its code of morals demands more sacrifices than it is worth and that its behaviour is neither dictated by honesty nor instituted with wisdom."[9] Jung, a most influential disciple of Freud, also finds fault with the Church's teaching on the Sixth Commandment. Although Jung broke away from Freud because of the latter's pansexualism, he did nevertheless write in an earlier work: "The 'question' that troubles the patient is . . . the 'sexual' question, or more precisely, the problem of present-day *sexual morality*. His increased demands upon life and the joy of life, upon glowing reality, can stand the necessary limitations which reality sets, but not the arbitrary, ill-

---

[8] Sexual abstinence has not interfered with the mental and spiritual development of thousands of religious men and women, of countless saints of God, and of a long list of fathers and doctors of the Church. See, moreover, the testimony of several well-known physicians (pp. 117-19) who contend that sexual abstinence is not harmful.

[9] Sigmund Freud, *A General Introduction to Psycho-Analysis,* translated by Joan Riviere, pp. 376-77. New York: Liveright Publishing Corporation, 1935.

supported prohibitions of present-day morals, which would curb too much the creative spirit rising up from the depths of the darkness of the beasts that perish."[10] Psychoanalysis employed by men such as these cannot but lead the patient astray spiritually. The first requirement, therefore, is that the practitioner accept the moral teachings of the natural law.

Psychoanalysis and psychiatry when employed by a well-instructed and practicing Christian are licitly used provided the following conditions are observed: (1) He does not give the patient to understand that unconscious motives destroy or at least appreciably lessen the freedom of decisions which he makes deliberately.[11] (2) There is a proportionately grave reason for having the patient revive dangerous memories. (3) These memories presumably will not prove for the patient a proximate occasion of sinning. (4) There is no undue stress on and investigation of matters of sex. Calling to the mind of the patient his past immoral conduct is always dangerous for the patient, especially if the memory of some types of sex sins is revived. His passions may thus be aroused strongly, and for not a few this might prove a temptation to which they would succumb. Hence there must be a sufficient reason for permitting the patient to run the risk of becoming sexually excited.

[10] Carl G. Jung, *Collected Papers on Analytical Psychology*, second edition, pp. 376-77 (London: Bailliere, Tindall and Cox, 1922). See also the statement of Jung in his *Psychology of the Unconscious*, p. 85 (New York: Moffat, Yard and Company, 1916): "The stumbling block is the *unhappy combination of religion and morality*. That must be overcome." Later, however, Jung modified this attitude.

[11] See John C. Ford, S.J., *Depth Psychology, Morality and Alcoholism*, pp. 38-43 (Weston: Weston College, 1951). See also Rudolf Allers, M.D., "Irresistible Impulses," *Ecclesiastical Review* 100:208-19, March 1939; Rudolf Allers, M.D., "Moral Responsibility of the Neurotic," *Homiletic and Pastoral Review* 42:727-33, May 1942; Rudolf Allers, M.D., "Sin and Neurosis," *Homiletic and Pastoral Review* 42:637-44, April 1942; Robert E. Britt, M.D., "Moral Limitations in Mental Disease," *Linacre Quarterly* 14:16-25, October 1947; James S. Cammack, S.J., *Moral Problems of Mental Defect* (London: Burns Oates and Washbourne, 1938); Thomas Verner Moore, O.S.B., M.D., *The Nature and Treatment of Mental Disorders* (London: William Heinemann, 1946); Pierre C. Simonart, "Imputability of the Mental Patient," *Linacre Quarterly* 14:8-15, October 1947.

If a patient is very weak and susceptible, he should not be exposed in any way to such temptations.

The Morality of Certain Psychiatric Treatments

Lobotomy consists in cutting the white nerve fibers connecting the brain with the thalamus. The operation is thought to sever the link between the emotions and the thoughts of the patient. There are several kinds of lobotomy. Prefrontal lobotomy is that in which the surgeon bores a hole through the skull in back of each temple and with a dull-edged instrument cuts through the white nerve fibers connecting the forward section of the frontal lobe with the thalamus. Transorbital lobotomy consists of inserting the instrument through the eye socket. This procedure is a blind operation, for the surgeon cannot see the interior portion on which he is doing the surgery. In topectomy the surgeon removes a wide piece of skull just over the middle of the forehead so that he may be enabled to examine the interior and see the part on which he is operating. A complete lobotomy should be avoided when fractional lobotomy will suffice,[12] for the latter limits the disturbance of the patient's personality induced by the former. It is important that the surgeon keep himself well informed in regard to the most recent progress in this field of surgery so that he can produce the most beneficial effects with the least harmful results.[13] Medical science is only beginning to obtain knowledge concerning the complexities of brain function. Lobotomy operations are experimental in character and it is extremely difficult to know in precisely what manner brain function is altered.

In performing a lobotomy the surgeon as a rule is endeavoring to reduce emotional tension in the patient. The operation

[12] See Edward K. Wilk, M.D., "Selective Cortical Undercutting." *Surgery, Gynecology and Obstetrics* 92:611-14, May 1951.

[13] We may mention by way of example the recently developed treatment by high-frequency electric needle of Dr. Everett G. Grantham of Louisville, Kentucky. See Everett G. Grantham, M.D., "Prefrontal Lobotomy for Relief of Pain," *Journal of Neurosurgery* 8:405-10, July 1951.

involves some (about 2 per cent) risk of life. Some patients have lost their sense of the moral value of their actions, but this effect is rare.

If the operation is to benefit the patient as it should, the physician must give him sufficient psychotherapy after surgery to enable him to recover some of his emotional responses.

Before performing a lobotomy it is incumbent on the physician to weigh well the good and the evil effects which, insofar as he can prudently foresee, the surgery will produce. The conditions required for the licitness of lobotomy are as follows: (1) Permission for the surgery must be obtained from the patient or from his nearest of kin. (2) The surgeon must be duly qualified to perform this delicate operation. (3) Complete lobotomy must not be done if fractional lobotomy suffices. (4) The operation is a last resort. (5) Due postoperative treatment will be given.[14] (6) The operation, so far as can be foreseen, will result in benefit rather than in harm.

The principles that were used in determining the morality of lobotomy can be applied in order to determine the morality of other types of psychosurgical treatment; for example, of hypophysectomy.

Case 157
Lobotomy on a Psychoneurotic Patient

The patient is suffering from a severe psychoneurosis. All other available remedies have been tried but have produced no satisfactory results. The physician now advises a prefrontal lobotomy. May the operation be licitly performed in this case?

Solution. As a last resort the surgeon may licitly perform a prefrontal lobotomy, provided he judges that the operation will probably produce benefit rather than harm. The explicit consent of the patient or of his guardian must be had, unless it can be reasonably presumed.

---

[14] See John McCarthy, "The Morality of Prefrontal Leucotomy," *Irish Ecclesiastical Record* 71:436-37, May 1949. See also Eugène Tesson, S.J., "La personne humaine et la chirurgie," *Etudes* 275:220-28, novembre 1952; Peter Flood, O.S.B., M.D., editor, *Ethics of Brain Surgery*, translated by Malachy G. Carroll (Cork: Mercier Press, 1954).

Explanation. To this operation may be correctly applied the principles applicable to mutilation (see pages 121-23). The surgeon's purpose is to help the patient as best he can, and there is sufficient reason for exposing the patient to the harm that could result.

Case 158
Lobotomy on a Schizophrenic Patient

In an attempt to effect the cure of a patient who is suffering from schizophrenia the surgeon severs the connecting part of the brain and other parts of the nervous system. The operation gives good hope of success, although it does bring grave danger to the patient.

Solution. This operation may licitly be performed as a last resort, provided the surgeon has good reason for believing that the good effects which probably will result counterbalance the probable evil effects.

Explanation. In this case we have an application of the principles explained in connection with mutilation (see pages 121-23). One aspect of the operation which might cause some doubt is whether or not there is present a sufficiently grave reason which compensates for running the risk involved. It is the surgeon's responsibility to decide this point. His medical knowledge should enable him to make this moral estimate.

Case 159
Lobotomy on a Violently Insane Patient

The patient, who is chronically mentally ill, is a source of danger to others because of his frequent and unpredictable outbursts of violence. The surgeon suggests lobotomy as a means of rendering the patient more manageable.

Solution. Lobotomy, if judged genuinely beneficial, may be licitly performed here.

Explanation. If the patient's outbursts of mania can be eliminated or reduced in degree of violence by the operation, this physical benefit would justify the operation. It is assumed that there is no greater hope before the operation than after it of restoring to the patient his use of reason.

Case 160
A Transorbital Operation with Probable Loss of Reason

The patient is psychotic, often suffers fits of extreme violence, and is difficult to control. There are times, however, at which the patient is evidently able to think clearly in certain fields. The surgeon desires to perform the transorbital operation which consists in severing with a sharp-pointed instrument fibers between the thalamus and the frontal lobes of the brain. This procedure will make the patient habitually tractable, but the surgeon foresees that in the present case the operation will very probably leave him permanently deprived of the use of reason. Is such surgery licit?

Solution. The operation in this case is not licit.

Explanation. Transorbital surgery on this patient would, it is true, produce pronounced physical benefits, for it would relieve him of the fits of violence and make him completely docile. A far more important consideration than these physical good effects, however, is the total loss of the patient's use of reason. Before the operation the patient had some intervals during which he could acquire spiritual merit and, if he were in the state of sin, could become reconciled with God by an act of contrition and the sacrament of penance. After the operation these spiritual benefits would be beyond his reach, for he would not be capable of a rational act. Hence the evil effects of the operation on the spiritual life of the patient far outweigh the good effects, which are merely physical benefits.

Case 161

Shock Therapy in Paranoia

The patient is suffering from paranoia. Shock treatment is indicated, but there is grave danger that this treatment may kill the patient because of his severe cardiovascular condition. Is it licit to administer shock treatment under these conditions?

Solution. If this treatment is used as a last resort and if the patient is spiritually prepared for death, the treatment is licit.

Explanation. The reason for this answer is explained on pages 259-61, where we treat of new drugs whose use involves danger of death. The morality of crymotherapy, or the freezing method, is the same as that of shock treatment.

Narcotherapy

Narcotherapy is the medical treatment in which a drug (for example, sodium pentothal or sodium amytal) is employed to reduce the patient to a state where he will freely divulge his innermost anxieties, phobias, and the like. The physician uses narcotherapy on persons who are suffering from a psychosis or neurosis in order to bring to light the source of the disorder, so that he can prescribe an effective treatment.

The morality of employing narcotherapy is the same as that of using hypnotism in the care of a patient (see pages 263-65). If proper precautions are observed and if narcotherapy will probably prove beneficial, the patient may licitly submit to its use. The physician would not of course be permitted to force the patient to take narcotherapeutic treatment, for the patient's secrets belong to him alone and he may justly refuse to permit another to probe his inner life. Even a prisoner suspected of crime need not submit to narcotherapy or the use of the so-called "truth drug." Public officials would violate his rights were they to force him to submit to this treatment. A prisoner is not obliged to betray his own guilt, nor is he under the obligation of placing himself in a state in which proof to be used against himself may be obtained by others.

It happens at times that the patient on whom the physician wishes to employ narcotherapy is not in possession of his reasoning power. The consent of such a patient's spouse, parents, or lawful guardian must be procured before narcotherapy is used. But what is to be said if the guardian were to show himself wholly unreasonable in refusing to permit the use of narcotherapy? If the patient would certainly be helped notably by the treatment, the physician from a moral viewpoint could licitly proceed in this case, for the consent of the patient himself could legitimately be presumed to be present. The physician should remember, however, that where consent is merely presumed, the patient may perhaps afterward institute a lawsuit for alleged damages. The physician should take precautions against such an event.

Since the patient's innermost thoughts may be divulged during the use of narcotherapy, those present at that time must observe professional secrecy in regard to the information thus revealed. To quiz the patient who is under the influence of a drug in the presence of a group of others (for example, physicians or medical students) is not permitted unless the patient, informed beforehand, has consented to this procedure.[15]

DIABOLICAL POSSESSION

MOST practicing psychiatrists will never encounter a case of diabolical possession. It is beyond all doubt, however, that such cases have occurred in the United States and within our own generation. Confronted with symptoms which he is forced to recognize as preternatural, the psychiatrist had best abandon the effort to effect a cure by the methods known to him and call upon the clergy for assistance, since the condition is one that can be remedied only by prayer.

It is a matter of Catholic belief that evil spirits exist and that God permits them at times to exert a certain influence on human beings, either by way of attacking their bodies from the exterior (obsession) or by inner control of the actions of the body (possession). The victim's liberty of soul always remains intact. Although the *Roman Ritual*, an officially approved book of prayers and ceremonies of the Catholic Church, mentions as probable (not certain) signs of obsession such things as speaking or understanding an unknown tongue, showing strength above one's natural capacity, revealing secrets which could not be known to the person through natural means, and like happenings, it warns against concluding too hastily that a person is possessed by the devil.[16] Many so-called cases of obsession are no doubt to be attributed to delusions, hysteria, or fraud.

HOMOSEXUALITY

AMONG the abnormal patients whom the psychiatrist will be called upon to treat, the homosexual offers an especially difficult problem. The homosexual is a person who is not only sexually attracted toward those of the same sex; he is sexually

---

[15] See Francis J. Connell, C.SS.R., "The Morality of Narcotherapy." *American Ecclesiastical Review* 113:448-49, December 1945.

[16] *Rituale Romanum*, tit. X, cap. 1.

apathetic to members of the opposite sex and in some cases may even experience a feeling of repugnance for them. The homosexual should not be confused with one who is emotionally attracted both to members of his own sex and to members of the opposite sex. Such a person is not a true invert; he is known as bisexual. Most of those who during their years of adolescence seem to be homosexual are so in appearance only, for they afterward become sexually normal. The homosexual individual will perhaps as a rule be given over to the care of a psychiatrist, but the general practitioner should be acquainted with the nature and the causes of his abnormality and should know something of the advice which would in his case usually prove profitable.

Homosexuality seems not to be altogether rare, for according to various estimates perhaps about 5 per cent of the male population of our cities is afflicted with this abnormal condition.[17] In recent reports Dr. Alfred C. Kinsey contends that there exists in the United States of America a very high percentage of sexual perversion of all kinds, and that 6.3 per cent of the orgasms occur from homosexual reactions. The reliability, however, of Dr. Kinsey's data has been strongly challenged.[18] One of the nation's leading psychiatrists, Dr. Karl Menninger of the Menninger Foundation, Topeka, Kansas, writes as follows about Dr. Kinsey's *Sexual Behavior in the Human Female:* "I was aware of serious flaws in the first volume. These were carefully pointed out by thoughtful, sympathetic fellow scientists, and I had every hope and expectation that Kinsey and his associates would make use of their suggestions and improve the research before the appearance of a second volume.

[17] See Anomaly, *The Invert,* pp. 13-14 (London: Bailliere, Tindall and Cox, 1948). Some would not agree with so high an estimate. See, for example, John F. Harvey, O.S.F.S., "Homosexuality as a Pastoral Problem," *Theological Studies* 16:97, March 1955.

[18] See Edmund Bergler and William S. Kroger, *Kinsey's Myth of Female Sexuality.* New York: Grune and Stratton, 1954.

"In this I was to be greatly disappointed. So far as I can ascertain, Kinsey appears to have heeded scarcely a word of the scholarly analyses and wise counsel of such penetrating critics as Dr. Robert P. Knight, Dr. Lawrence Kubie, Lionel Trilling and numerous others."[19]

Not everyone of course who engages in homosexual practices is a homosexual in the true sense of the term. The tendency toward homosexuality can be a permanent one or it can be of a temporary nature only. Some, surrounded for a long period by those of their own sex only, employ one of the latter as a substitute for a person of the opposite sex. However, once those of this category find themselves in normal circumstances where they associate freely with persons of the opposite sex, their sexual abnormality as a rule disappears. Many of the homosexuals, on the other hand, are constitutional, and these are difficult to cure. What is the physician to do for the pronounced invert patient who wishes help?

All homosexual practices, freely indulged in, are of course gravely sinful, for they are a grave perversion of nature. The sex organs have been given to man by nature in order that he may use them for the orderly propagation of the human race. The homosexual's use of them goes directly counter to their natural end. Before a cure of his habit is attempted the patient must first of all be convinced that this practice is of its nature evil and that it is, in no circumstances, ever justifiable. What is to be said if he argues, as many do, that nature has been unjust to him? Apart from the fact that his tendency may have been acquired and is not congenital, it can be pointed out to him that the author of nature is God, and that God, infinitely just as He is, could not possibly be guilty of unfairness or any shadow of injustice. The homosexual must frankly recognize his tendency as abnormal and endeavor to adjust his life accordingly. He can be told that very probably he is no more

[19] Karl Menninger, M.D., "What the Girls Told." *Saturday Review* 36:21, September 26, 1953.

passionate, no more strongly drawn to sexual immoralities, than the normal person. With God's help he, just as surely as everyone else, can control his conduct and avoid sin.

What advice is the physician to give the confirmed homosexual? First of all, he might urge him to cultivate a genuine sense of humor, for laughter will help greatly to prevent his becoming soured by his affliction and to lighten the hardships which he experiences. It would be well, also, if the patient endeavored to sublimate his affections.[20] Since he is excluded from normal married life, he cannot obtain the joy and satisfaction which married persons find in the family circle. He can, however, zealously devote himself to the care of the poor and the sick. In this work he will not only find contentment and deep happiness, but he will also distract his mind from his personal difficulties. He should, moreover, avoid brooding over his abnormality. He should try to cultivate self-esteem and a sense of his dignity as a child of God. He should try to shun circumstances which he knows from experience to be sexually exciting for him and should associate with wholesome-minded individuals. If he is a Catholic, he should be encouraged to frequent, as often as possible, the sacraments of penance and the Eucharist, so that he may derive from them the very effective supernatural help which they provide. It will aid him in curbing his unchaste tendencies if he practices self-denial. Cultivating the habit of giving up at times, from a spiritual motive, certain legitimate pleasure will do much to strengthen his will power and to counteract the softness of character which tends to render one more susceptible to temptations against the virtue of chastity.

May the homosexual person enter the state of matrimony? If his abnormality renders him wholly incapable of performing sexual union with a member of the opposite sex, he is of course banned from marrying because of psychic impotence.

[20] See Anomaly, *The Invert*, chap. 10, "Sublimation," pp. 117-28. London: Bailliere, Tindall and Cox, 1948.

Although most inverts entertain an utter distaste for wedlock, some do desire to enter the married state. Can marriage be regarded as a probable cure for homosexuality? It does happen at times that a homosexual man marries and does well, but, as a rule, marriage does not prove successful. The female homosexual may find it easier to adjust to married life. The physician must decide the case of each patient on its own merits. If it is only probable that the patient who is to marry is burdened with psychic impotence, he is not forbidden to marry, but he is obliged to inform his fiancée of this possible defect.

STERILIZATION OF THE UNFIT

STERILIZATION was discussed somewhat briefly in Chapter Six, pages 171-73. We were there concerned solely with the sterilization, for medical reasons, of normal persons. Here we are concerned chiefly with the sterilization of mental defectives and criminals; but in order that the presentation may be comprehensive, we will summarize all that is to be said concerning sterilization, no matter what its purpose.

Sterilization, as the word is here used, means the mutilation or treatment of the body in such a manner as to produce loss of the power of begetting or of bearing children. It consists in rendering the faculties of generation unfruitful and is accomplished by means of surgery, X ray, or drugs. There are three quite different kinds of sterilization: remedial, contraceptive (in which is included eugenic), and punitive. These types of sterilization must be carefully distinguished one from the other, for the morality of all three is not the same.

Remedial Sterilization

Remedial sterilization (called by some therapeutic) means a sterilizing operation which is indicated as necessary for the patient's health. By "indicated as necessary" we mean that the health of the patient can be safeguarded in no other way than by this procedure. "Necessary for the health of the patient" means that the condition of the patient's body here and now is such that, unless the organs of generation are either wholly or partially excised or sprayed with X ray, the patient will suffer grave consequences because of the pathological state of these organs. It is the removing of a diseased organ and not the suppression of the generative function itself which is the means used to safeguard the patient's health. If the uterus of a patient is found to be cancerous, the act of surgically removing the uterus is called *remedial sterilization.* In this operation there is sterilization, for the mutilation brings about in the patient's body the loss of the power to bear children. It is remedial, for the operation is necessary to protect the patient against the ravages of cancer. In the same way the operation of removing testes, ovaries, or Fallopian tubes which are dangerously diseased is called remedial sterilization.

The reason justifying remedial sterilization is quite clear. The whole body is obviously more precious than any one of its parts; hence if it becomes necessary to sacrifice one of the parts in order to preserve the whole, the action taken is licit. No one will deny that it is far preferable to preserve the body, even at the cost of a hand, an appendix, or a gall bladder, than to permit the whole body to become poisoned and to die.

At times mothers are warned by their physicians that another pregnancy will very probably cause their death. "Since surgeons consider more than two or three of such operations [caesarean sections] hazardous for the mother, they often recommend tying off the tubes at the time of the final delivery," says Dr. Clarence J. Gamble.[21] A directly sterilizing operation, however, is never justifiable because a future pregnancy may jeopardize the mother's life. The form of sterilization (called tubectomy) which is mentioned by Dr. Gamble is but another form of artificial birth control. The tying off or cutting of the Fallopian tubes is not required by, nor intended

[21] Clarence J. Gamble, M.D., "Why Fear Sterilization?" *Hygeia* 26:22-23, 60, January 1948.

to aid, the *present* state of the patient's health. It is directed toward preventing her from conceiving *in the future*. It thus is intended to safeguard her against a danger which another pregnancy will supposedly create for her.

No type of operation, then, the purpose of which is directly contraceptive can be said to be remedial. Surgeons must be on their guard against the false teaching on this matter which is found in medical publications of good repute. In the eighth edition of *Williams Obstetrics*, for example, we read: "In the case of unintelligent women of the lower classes suffering from active tuberculosis, renal disease, serious cardiac lesions and certain other conditions . . . the mere induction of abortion, and the injunction to avoid the possibility of future pregnancies, are not satisfactory; as a large proportion of such patients soon become pregnant again, . . . we hold that in such patients it is justifiable to follow the abortion by a *sterilizing operation*."[22] The reason for condemning as immoral all such operations as these is explained in the discussion of artificial birth control on pages 156-61.

Contraceptive Sterilization

Contraceptive sterilization is an operation the direct aim of which is to suppress either temporarily or permanently the generative function. Sterilization of the reproductive organs is not infrequently resorted to, because of economic or social reasons, as an effective form of artificial birth control. But perhaps one reads more often of the direct sterilization of healthy organs for eugenic purposes; that is, for the avowed purpose of "improving the race."

Eugenic Sterilization

Eugenic (a type of contraceptive) sterilization means a sterilizing operation which is performed to prevent the patient

---

[22] Henricus J. Stander, M.D., *Williams Obstetrics*, eighth edition, p. 1119. New York: D. Appleton-Century Company, 1941.

from propagating subnormal offspring. It may be rightly termed contraceptive sterilization. The eugenists teach that certain physical or mental defects and certain evil tendencies are either directly transmitted by parents to the child or at least are acquired by the child through its early environment. Some eugenists recommend the sterilization of the insane, the dipsomaniac, the tubercular, the blind, and the badly deformed. "Most frequent of all," states Dr. Gamble, "is the need to prevent children from being born to parents whose reproductive cells carry well defined inheritable defects. . . . Sterilization of feebleminded parents is perhaps the most important of all— prescribed for both the protection of the patient, who is unequal to the exacting task of parenthood, and for the child."[23]

Eugenists endeavor to justify the practice of eugenic sterilization on the following grounds.

1. Defectives are a source of disease, misery, and crime to their fellow citizens, and so the state is justified in using sterilization to prevent these undesirable members of society from coming into the world. Only healthy citizens make for the good of the state.

2. Defectives are a great burden to taxpayers, who must provide institutions for their care. Sterilization would eliminate the necessity of such taxes.

To eugenists who thus argue the righteousness of their cause, we admit that their objectives are very praiseworthy, but we ask: "What of the means you advocate for accomplishing these objectives?" Promoting a healthy citizenry and lessening the taxpayers' burden—these are good *ends,* but the *means* through which eugenists would achieve them are evil.

The state does not have supreme power over its citizens, but only such power as is conformable with the accomplish-

[23] Clarence J. Gamble, M.D., "Why Fear Sterilization?" *Hygeia* 26:22-23, 60, January 1948. For the opinion of some who in certain cases favor eugenic sterilization see James F. Donnelly, M.D., and Frank R. Lock, M.D., "Indications for the Sterilization of Women," *Bulletin of the American College of Surgeons* 38:97-102, May-June 1953.

299

ment of its end. The state has the right to punish adequately and even to execute duly condemned criminals. This power is necessary for accomplishing the purpose of its existence, the maintaining of peace and right order in the community. But the state has no right to kill or to mutilate an innocent man. To give the state such a right would be to empower it to use one human being as it willed for the benefit of others—a thing contrary to natural justice. The individual as such is antecedent to the state by priority of nature, and so certain rights of the individual are prior to those of the state. Life and bodily integrity are given man before he enters society, and he does not lose the right to them because he becomes a member of society. Every citizen, then, has from the natural law an inalienable right to life and bodily integrity. The law may interfere with this sacred right only when a man has, through some serious crime, submerged it in the higher right of the state to punish evildoers. Now, because a man is mentally defective or physically diseased, he is not therefore guilty of any crime. Hence the state may not punish him because of his misfortune. The state may not mutilate an innocent citizen.

We quote that scholarly pontiff, Pius XI, on the subject of eugenic sterilization:

"Public magistrates have no direct power over the bodies of their subjects; therefore, where no crime has taken place and there is no cause present for grave punishment, they can never directly harm, or tamper with the integrity of the body, either for the reasons of eugenics or for any other reason."[24]

As for the power of sterilizing the unfit, civil authority never had this power over that natural faculty of man and can never legitimately possess it. Direct eugenic or contraceptive sterilization, therefore, is never licit. No reason imaginable can be adduced to justify this practice. No church official nor any other human authority is empowered to grant an excep-

[24] Pius XI, *Christian Marriage.* In *Five Great Encyclicals*, pp. 96-97. New York: Paulist Press, 1939.

tion to this rule, for eugenic sterilization is prohibited by the law of nature. To employ sterilization to try to rid the human race of the mentally deficient, of morons, imbeciles, and idiots, is to use an evil means to accomplish what, according to some at least, is a praiseworthy end.[25] And this is never permissible, no matter how praiseworthy the end may be.

Even if sterilization were allowed, however, it would not prove successful in purifying the race to any great extent. We shall here record some of the findings of authorities in this matter. These data show us the expected results of sterilization, interpreted in a very favorable light. Some very highly esteemed authorities would deny that even the physically good effects here mentioned, comparatively insignificant though they be, would *certainly* follow.

About 50 per cent of the cases of feeblemindedness arise from nonhereditary causes. Mental deficiency can be traced in many instances to injury which the child suffers before birth, during delivery, or after birth. This 50 per cent would in no wise be affected by sterilization.

The remaining 50 per cent of the cases may be attributed to hereditary causes. Feebleminded offspring come from two sources: from feebleminded parents and from normal parents who are carriers of feeblemindedness. If all feebleminded parents were prevented by means of sterilization from procreating children, the procreation of feeblemindedness by the second group would not be affected. H. S. Jennings, an authority in this field, says: "Individuals are very different in their gene combinations, and consequently the offspring usually have combinations very different from those of their parents. They may therefore differ from their parents in many of their characteristics. From vigorous and efficient parents may be pro-

[25] Some might well argue that the presence of these defectives among us is not an unmixed evil, since their care can aid greatly in bringing out the latent noble qualities of those who attend them and since their care can provide rich opportunities for the practice of works of mercy.

duced offspring that are weak and inefficient. From defective parents may be produced offspring that are normal."[26] Very many of those whom physicians consider to be altogether normal are actually carriers of genes which will produce mentally defective children. Science has no way of discovering, before the defective offspring is born, who these "carriers" are. J. B. S. Haldane, one of the older geneticists who is still highly respected, voiced a number of years ago an opinion on this point which later research has served only to confirm. He said: "I think that the following proposition would be accepted by most biologists: 'It is never possible, from a knowledge of a person's parents, to predict with certainty that he or she will be either a more adequate or a less adequate member of society than the majority.' In a very few cases, it is true, we can predict with certainty that a given unborn child, if legitimate, will have a certain physical defect. Thus two albinos probably always produce albino children. But our knowledge of the heredity of psychological characters, desirable or otherwise, is insufficient to make predictions of this kind. We can, of course, make statistical predictions. But we do not, in my opinion, know enough to accord rights to any individual, or to deprive him or her of any rights, on the basis of ancestry only."[27]

Of the cases due to hereditary causes only a small fraction come from feebleminded parents. Sterilization of this fraction would not appreciably reduce feeblemindedness in the generations to come. Tredgold, still recognized as an authority on the subject, brought out this point a number of years ago. He says: "It is necessary to emphasize, however, that even if every defective in existence were to be sterilized, this would not eliminate mental defect, as is sometimes thought; or even very appreciably reduce its amount. . . . The chief source of mental

---

[26] H. S. Jennings, *Genetics*, p. 298. New York: W. W. Norton and Company, 1935.

[27] J. B. S. Haldane, *Heredity and Politics*, pp. 93-94. New York: W. W. Norton and Company, 1938.

deficiency is not defective parents, but parents who come of psychopathic stocks and who are 'carriers' of mental defect."[28] Tredgold's opinion is not only still accepted by geneticists, but is perhaps accepted even more unreservedly than it was accepted in the past. Wallin says: "The tendency with the passing years has been to attribute fewer cases [of mental defect] to heredity."[29]

Dunn and Dobzhansky confirm this opinion. They say: "Most of the recessive genes we might want to eliminate occur in hidden form in heterozygotes, in people who do not show them at all, instead of in homozygotes who could be identified and whose reproduction might consequently be prevented. . . . Mental diseases present a human problem even more serious than blindness. Here again, a certain proportion of cases have little or nothing to do with heredity. Cases attributable to defective heredity are of many kinds which can be more or less easily distinguished by a specialist and are almost certainly due to different genes. Each gene is rare if its frequency is computed for the total population of the country. This is a great difficulty which advocates of sterilization do not always take account of. For defects which are rare, or caused by recessive genes which show only in certain environments, or dependent on two or more recessive genes present in the same individual, very little is accomplished by sterilizing even all the defectives in a single generation. To be sure, if a sterilization program is continued for many generations, the defect will become even-

---

[28] A. F. Tredgold, *A Textbook of Mental Deficiency,* sixth edition, p. 520 (Baltimore: William Wood and Company, 1937). See also Anthony Barnett, *The Human Species: A Biology of Man* (New York: W. W. Norton and Company, 1950). Mr. Barnett says: "Just as mentally defective parents can have normal children, so can normal parents have mentally defective children. Indeed, most defective children have normal parents. It follows that eugenic measures can do little to prevent the appearance of mental defectives; and that, if all defectives were sterilised or otherwise prevented from breeding, this would prevent the production of many more normal children than of defectives" (p. 126).

[29] J. E. Wallace Wallin, *Children with Mental and Physical Handicaps,* p. 238. New York: Prentice-Hall, 1949.

tually less common than it was to begin with. The process may, however, take centuries or even millenia."[30]

At its annual meeting of 1935 the American Neurological Association accepted and approved a report on eugenic sterilization that had been prepared by a committee headed by Dr. Abraham Myerson. Nothing has occurred since the report was drafted to render necessary any substantial change in its findings. The committee laments the fact that, largely because of the failure to provide control groups, most studies of the inheritance of mental defect are inadequate and inconclusive. It says: "It is obvious to us that investigation of the problem of inheritance, especially of the psychiatric conditions, has been haphazard and often inexact . . . and it well may be that no complete scientific approach is possible in the present state of our knowledge or rather of our ignorance."[31] Because of our lack of knowledge we cannot say who, if any, could well be sterilized: "Very little prediction can be made in a complete way as to the results of sterilization of the feebleminded themselves, nor could there possibly be, in the present state of our knowledge, any selection of individuals who themselves are not feebleminded to sterilize for the prevention of feeblemindedness."[32] A program of sterilization might cause society

[30] L. C. Dunn and Theodosius Dobzhansky, *Heredity, Race and Society*, pp. 88, 92-93 (New York: The New American Library of World Literature, 1954). See also Curt Stern, *Principles of Human Genetics* (San Francisco: W. H. Freeman and Company, 1949). What the author says in Chapter 24, pages 525-27, of a recessive genotype applies to feeblemindedness. Hence the table on page 526 justifies us in affirming that it would require 68 generations to reduce the number of feebleminded persons from 100,000 to 10,000, that it would require 216 generations to reduce the number of feebleminded persons from 10,000 to 1,000, and that it would require 634 generations to reduce the number of feebleminded persons from 1,000 to 10. This is substantially confirmed by Amram Scheinfeld, *The New You and Heredity*, p. 548 (Philadelphia: J. B. Lippincott Company, 1950), although Scheinfeld requires fewer generations to reduce the number of feebleminded persons to one tenth of what it is at present.

[31] Abraham Myerson, M.D., and others, *Eugenical Sterilization*, p. 181. New York: The Macmillan Company, 1936.

[32] *Ibid.*, p. 131.

to lose far more than it gained. The report says: "When one studies the histories of the men of genius as given by Lange-Eichbaum, one is impressed by the fact that many valuable members of society, worth more to it than the cost of maintenance of all state institutions put together, would have been lost if sterilization laws had been enacted on a compulsory basis a few centuries ago."[33] Despite all these facts, however, the committee does say, with what appears to be some reluctance, that voluntary sterilization may be "considered" in the case of a limited number of diseases. It gives no approval to enforced sterilization.

There is also evidence indicating that the offspring of mental defectives tend to be superior in intelligence to their parents. The genes for serious mental defect seem to tend to eliminate themselves. These and other facts concerning the inheritance of mental defect are now so well known that eugenic sterilization is no longer advocated by the well-informed as a means of eliminating feeblemindedness or of appreciably reducing its incidence. We do have, however, strong advocates of what might be called protective sterilization. It is argued that, when parents are morons or when families have a history of mental deficiency, the chances that their children will be morons are greatly increased; that mentally defective parents are usually incapable of maintaining homes in which children can grow up in a wholesome manner and develop into good citizens; that many of our worst crimes, especially rape and rape followed by murder, are committed by feebleminded individuals; and that, even though sterilization did nothing to improve the minds of the next generation, it would at least prevent the birth in this generation of children who upon maturing would in many cases become scourges of society. There is undoubtedly truth in what is thus said, but it does not follow that eugenic or protective sterilization is ethically justifiable. Fundamental principles remain unchanged, and the individual

[33] *Ibid.*, p. 172.

still retains his rights. We are not free to prevent or correct an evil by committing another evil. Evil may not be done in order that good may follow. The end does not justify the means.

Punitive Sterilization

Punitive sterilization is a sterilizing procedure performed on criminals as a penalty for their crimes. A certain type of criminal, for example, the habitual sex offender, is in some places punished in this manner.[34] The licitness of this operation is disputed by moralists. Strong arguments are alleged both for and against the licitness of punitive sterilization.

The arguments for those who defend the operation are as follows. The state has the right to decapitate for grave crime, and so it has the right to inflict on a grave offender a lesser punishment, mutilation. Sterilization is a real punishment, for it deprives the criminal of a physical good, his corporal integrity and the precious power of begetting or bearing children.

Those who condemn the operation as illicit argue as follows. Sterilization is not a real punishment, for there is little if any suffering involved. Besides, it offers the culprit an opportunity for wanton indulgence with no possibility of undesired consequences. A penalty may be inflicted only if it is deemed efficacious to prevent subjects from violating the law. Sterilization is not efficacious in this. Today criminologists agree that sterilization is not an effective penalty.

The conclusion here proposed is as follows. Theoretically the state may sterilize criminals if sterilization is a genuine punishment. In practice, however, a sterilizing operation (for example, a double vasectomy) which leaves the sex organs otherwise intact seems clearly to encourage the sex offender in his crime rather than to deter him. Hence such punitive sterilization for sex crimes seems to be illicit.

[34] For a short and authoritative account of the sterilization laws in this country see Edgar Schmiedeler, O.S.B., *Sterilization in the United States* (Washington: National Catholic Welfare Conference, 1943).

306

Case 162

Assisting at a Sterilizing Operation

Dr. X, an intern at the State Hospital, is assigned to assist Dr. Y in a sterilizing operation of an adult female. Dr. Y will perform the surgery itself, but Dr. X will be expected to assist him by applying retractors and hemostats and in performing similar actions. Dr. X is aware of the fact that the patient's Fallopian tubes are in a normally healthy condition and that the sterilization is clearly eugenic. He is convinced that such operations are immoral, but he would find it extremely difficult to refuse the assignment.

Solution. If Dr. X cannot refuse to give this type of assistance without grave hardship and if his helping Dr. Y would not cause scandal, he may licitly accept the assignment.

Explanation. Cooperation in this case on the part of Dr. X would be licit for the following reasons. The actions exacted of Dr. X are not in themselves evil. Dr. X does not desire the evil action of Dr. Y. His cooperation is, moreover, not essential to the accomplishing of Dr. Y's action, for Dr. Y would undoubtedly find another physician to help him in case Dr. X could not be had. It is true that Dr. X is obliged in charity to refrain from lending such material cooperation, but this obligation ceases when he cannot refuse without proportionately grave difficulty to himself.

REFERENCES

Bruehl, Charles P. *Birth-Control and Eugenics,* chap. 13, "Church and True Eugenics," pp. 200-17. New York: Joseph F. Wagner, 1928.

Cammack, James S., S.J. "Confessor and/or Psychotherapist." *Clergy Review* 18:290-303, April 1940.

Davis, Henry, S.J. *Moral and Pastoral Theology,* vol. II, chap. 6, sec. 8, "Mutilation and Sterilization," pp. 156-66. London: Sheed and Ward, 1949.

Diamond, J., S.J. "Pre-frontal Leucotomy." *Clergy Review* 36:231-40, October 1951.

Donceel, Joseph, S.J. "Second Thoughts on Freud." *Thought* 24:466-84, September 1949.

Gest, John B. "Legal Status of Sterilization Laws in the United States." *Ecclesiastical Review* 91:401-11, October 1934.

Harvey, John F., O.S.F.S. "Homosexuality as a Pastoral Problem." *Theological Studies* 16:86-108, March 1955.

Kelly, Gerald, S.J. *Medico-Moral Problems,* pt. 3, "Lobotomy for Pain Relief," pp. 29-32. St. Louis: Catholic Hospital Association of the United States and Canada, 1951.

Lehane, Joseph B. *Morality of American Civil Legislation concerning Eugenical Sterilization.* Washington: Catholic University of America Press, 1944.

McCarthy, John. "Psychosurgery and Medico-Psychological Therapy." *Catholic Encyclopedia,* vol. XVIII (Supplement II). New York: Gilmary Society, 1951.

McCarthy, Raphael C., S.J. "Common Ground for Psychiatrists and Priests." *Linacre Quarterly* 14:1-4, October 1947.

McFadden, Charles J., O.S.A. *Medical Ethics,* second edition, "Eugenic Sterilization," pp. 277-98. Philadelphia: F. A. Davis Company, 1949.

McLoughlin, J. "Catholic Attitude to Psychiatry." *Irish Ecclesiastical Record* 63:371-76, June 1944.

Michaels, Peter. "Christian Abnormal Psychology." *Integrity* 1:2-44, January 1947.

O'Brien, Patrick V., C.M. *Emotions and Morals.* New York: Grune and Stratton, 1950.

O'Doherty, Eamonn. "Religion and Psychology." *Catholic Mind* 49:739-44, November 1951.

Rosenheim, Frederick, M.D. "Religion and Psychiatry." *Catholic Mind* 45:462-64, August 1947.

Schmiedeler, Edgar, O.S.B. *Sterilization in the United States.* Washington: National Catholic Welfare Conference, 1943.

Schwitalla, Alphonse M., S.J. "Sterilization." *Catholic Encyclopedia,* vol. XVIII (Supplement II). New York: Gilmary Society, 1951.

Stern, Karl. *The Third Revolution: A Study of Psychiatry and Religion.* New York: Harcourt, Brace and Company, 1954.

Sutherland, Halliday, M.D. *Laws of Life,* chap. 7, "How Heredity Is Transmitted," pp. 108-22; chap. 8, "Sterilization of the Unfit," pp. 123-43. New York: Sheed and Ward, 1936.

Tonquedec, Joseph de. *Les maladies nerveuses ou mentales et les manifestations diaboliques.* Paris: Beauchesne et Ses Fils, 1938.

Uffenheimer, M.D. "Anxiety and Fear." *Catholic Medical Guardian* 17:122-35, January 1940.

White, Victor. "Analyst and the Confessor." *Commonweal* 48:346-49, July 23, 1948.

THE PHYSICIAN AS COUNSELOR

PHYSICIANS who have gained the confidence of their patients can expect to be asked on many occasions for their advice. We are thinking here of those normal patients who sincerely desire further information on matters pertaining to marriage and family life, and not of those neurotics who at almost every visit fret their physician with stories of domestic difficulties that had best be referred to a clergyman or a psychiatrist. Persons belonging to the latter class can often be helped only at the cost of an excessive amount of time, if they can be helped at all. Those belonging to the former class can not only be helped, but have some sort of right to expect to receive help from their physician.

The physician, however, cannot be expected to advise his patients in matters that do not fall within his own professional field. It is not his part to offer advice on how his patients should invest their money, how much insurance they should carry, what make of car they should buy, and other things of a similar nature. The physician may have very sound ideas on such matters; but if he gives his patients the benefit of his opinion, he is acting as a friend and not as a physician. It is quite different if patients ask their physician whether, in view of their health, temperament, and character it is wise for them to marry; what their attitude toward having children should be; how they should give sex instruction to their children; and other things of a similar kind. These are matters on which the physician, because of the special training that he has received, can speak with authority.

As a matter of fact, churches and schools are more and more frequently calling upon physicians to counsel individuals and groups of individuals on problems pertaining to marriage, the care of children, and the correction of undesirable sex habits in children. It is a privilege and an honor for a physician to be asked to render public service of this kind. The purpose of this chapter is not, of course, to supply him with any of the medical knowledge that he needs, but solely to discuss certain matters in which moral issues are involved.

ADVICE TO THOSE ENGAGED TO BE MARRIED

IT OFTEN happens that the physician is consulted in his professional capacity by those who are engaged to be married. On such occasions he has a valuable opportunity of imparting to them information and advice which will aid them greatly in adjusting themselves to the new life which they will soon begin. Some physicians make it a practice to impress on young couples the fact that married life cannot be happy if it excludes all thought of God or if it is marked by notable selfishness.[1] They remind their youthful patients that all during their wedded life they must continue to cultivate their love for each other by external marks of affection.

Fitness To Marry

Physicians are well aware of the fact that among the qualities that are desirable in a partner in marriage a very important one is physical fitness. A woman should be reasonably certain that the man whom she intends to marry will be able to fulfill his duty of supporting her and the children who may be born to her. A man whose physical or mental disability would pre-

---

[1] Fulton J. Sheen, *Three To Get Married*. New York: Appleton-Century-Crofts, 1951.

vent his living up to his new obligations should not enter the state of matrimony. A person's right to marry is not an unlimited one. The licit exercise of this right is conditioned by one's ability to fulfill the duties which are involved in this state of life. Every husband has the grave duty to provide for the temporal needs of his dependents. This task, however, could be performed for the husband by another. Hence if his parents or some other relative or friend were to guarantee the adequate maintenance of himself, his wife, and his future family, even a helpless cripple could licitly marry.

The Mentally Unfit

Because they cannot give a valid consent to the matrimonial contract, idiots and lunatics are mentally unqualified to marry. Defective consent could be an invalidating circumstance in all cases, too, where one of the parties does not have the use of reason at the time when he is attempting marriage. Hence infants cannot marry, nor are men or women who are completely intoxicated or who are hypnotized capable of giving a valid consent while they are in that state. Although persons with a low mentality can validly marry if they can reason sufficiently well to understand what the true purpose of marriage is, it is preferable in most cases for them to remain single. If both parents are feebleminded, their children would, ordinarily speaking, be deprived of proper care and training.

If an individual is a confirmed drunkard or a drug addict, he should not marry, for he could not fulfill the obligations of married life. If he is dominated by his evil habit, he will be unable to support his wife and family in decency. He will, moreover, cause untold heartache and trouble to his spouse, and will be a pernicious influence in the lives of his children. A woman should beware of marrying such a man in order to bring about his reformation. If he will not correct his sinful life for her sake before marriage, when his love for her is strongest, he will certainly not reform later. If such a one promises to amend his ways, he should be obliged before marriage to prove the seriousness of his desire and the efficacy of his good resolution. He can demonstrate this by means of a period of probation.

A man or woman, therefore, who cannot lead a reasonably normal life should not marry, for he or she would be the source of great unhappiness to the other spouse. Men and women who have a violent and uncontrollable temper would bring grave discord into the family circle and would be unable properly to perform the task of rearing their children. Those who are afflicted with emotional instability or who are inveterate gamblers fail as a general rule to make a success of their marriage.

The Physically Unfit

May a person marry if he is afflicted with a dangerous and contagious disease? In answering this question we must make a distinction between what pertains to the validity of such a marriage and what has reference to its licitness. Neither the natural law nor the ecclesiastical law invalidates the marriage of those who have some contagious and dangerous disease. A leper, for example, can marry validly. The same is true of a syphilitic whose disease is active and highly infectious. The licitness, however, of these marriages is a different matter. One who has a disease such as syphilis in the active stage must either reveal his condition to his fiancée or refrain from marrying. If he were to marry without first manifesting his secret affliction to the other, he would be guilty of a grave violation of justice. His act would be seriously sinful because in this contract he would be fraudulently imposing on his bride a seriously defective object; namely, his diseased body.

If a person with a dangerous and contagious disease were to marry, he would transmit the affliction to his spouse and perhaps to his offspring too. In the event that the syphilitic husband infected his wife without her knowing of his disease, he would be acting unjustly toward her. If she knew of the danger to her health from marital relations with her husband, and in spite of this consented to the marriage act, no injustice would be done.

If one has been infected with syphilis, he should not marry until there is certain proof that the germs of the disease are dead. If the patient has been free for two or three years from all signs of syphilis, this will as a rule mean that he has been cured. Recently discovered methods are said to effect a permanent cure within a comparatively short time. In all cases, however, one should be guided by a competent physician who can, through his own experience and through medical tests, authoritatively pronounce on the presence or the absence of the disease. *Now A Matter of weeks or months at the most.*

Hereditary Defects

Those defects are called hereditary which are transmitted to the child by the parents' reproductive cells. Experience has demonstrated the fact that certain physical abnormalities are passed on to children by their parents. Some examples of these are blindness and other serious defects of the eyes, deafness, and hemophilia. There is good reason for believing that, at least in many cases, some diseases (for example, epilepsy) are inherited. Tuberculosis, most forms of cancer, and diabetes are *There is a marked tendency to inherit this predisposition* not looked upon as hereditary. If, however, one parent has tuberculosis, some authorities believe that the child may inherit susceptibility to that disease. Hence if such a child were to be exposed to tuberculosis, he would be more likely to contract *T. B. is not a medical fact* it than a person both of whose parents were healthy. In the case of diabetes and most forms of cancer, it is doubtful whether even the predisposition to these diseases is transmitted by generation.

The probability, or even the certainty, that his children will be defective does not deprive a person of the right to marry. In many instances it would be preferable if he did not enter into marriage; but if he does marry, the marital contract is both valid and licit. Pius XI has made the following observations on this point:

"Although often these individuals are to be dissuaded from entering into matrimony, certainly it is wrong to brand men with the stigma of crime because they contract marriage, on the ground that, despite the fact that they are in every respect capable of matrimony, they will give birth only to defective children, even though they use all care and diligence."[2]

The Rh Factor

The Rh factor, an element in man's red blood corpuscles, takes its name from the Rhesus monkey, in whose red corpuscles a similar element was discovered. Those in whose blood this element is found are known as Rh positive. Those in whose blood this factor is not present are termed Rh negative. If Rh positive blood finds its way into the blood stream of some Rh negative person, the latter develops what is called a sensitivity to Rh positive blood. This sensitization is not harmful to the Rh negative person himself; but if, already thus sensitized, he receives more Rh positive blood, there can be evil effects. This sensitization can occur in any Rh negative person after a transfusion of Rh positive blood, and it can be brought about in an Rh negative pregnant woman by an Rh positive fetus. Probably only one Rh negative mother in every twenty-five or more is sensitized by the child in her womb.[3]

If a wife is Rh negative and her husband is Rh negative, or if she is Rh positive and he is Rh positive, there is nothing to fear. If, however, the wife is Rh negative, the husband Rh positive, some of their offspring may be diseased. The first child of this couple will usually be normal, but some of the later children may be affected with erythroblastosis fetalis, a

[2] Pius XI, *Christian Marriage.* In *Five Great Encyclicals,* p. 96. New York: Paulist Press, 1939.
[3] See *Journal of the American Medical Association* 132:10-11, September 14, 1946 and 133:577, February 22, 1947.

disease which destroys the red blood cells. It is not at all certain that the second, third, or fourth child will be affected adversely, for possibly the husband is heterozygous, by which is meant that one of his parents was Rh positive, the other Rh negative; and so the fetus may be Rh negative. Even if the second fetus is Rh positive, the mother may not have been sensitized by her first Rh positive child. Blood transfusions, moreover, may perhaps offer a happy solution to difficult Rh problems.

There are several problems connected with the Rh factor which concern the moralist. Some of these problems relate to those who are contemplating marriage, and some to those who are already married.

Before Marriage. Is it, for instance, licit for an Rh positive man to marry an Rh negative woman? There is no law that forbids such persons to marry. If, moreover, marriage takes place and mother and child are given adequate medical care, there should be no great difficulty. Hence incompatibility in regard to the Rh factor should not cause a couple to hesitate about entering marriage. *further, only 5% of such couples actually develop trouble with Rh.*

The Married. Once such a couple is married, the marital act will never become illicit because of the danger of producing babies that are stillborn or gravely diseased. Even though the couple were certain (and they cannot have certitude) that any fetus which was conceived would be seriously defective or would die within a short time, they would nevertheless be permitted to perform the marital act as often as they desired. If defective offspring resulted, their deficiency would be due to nature and not to any fault of father or mother. It is better, moreover, that the child, though defective, be brought into being than that it never have had existence.

Births. Is it permissible for the physician to hasten the birth of a child to protect it against erythroblastosis? Premature delivery of a viable child is licit when the good to be hoped for equals or outweighs the probable evil effects.

315

Artificial Insemination. If the wife is Rh negative and the husband Rh positive, would it not be advisable, in order to insure healthy offspring, that the wife be artificially inseminated with the semen of an Rh negative donor? The answer is that the insemination of a woman with the semen of one who is not her husband is never permissible. (See "Artificial Insemination," pages 150-55.)

Cousin Marriages

Is it in general advisable for relatives to intermarry? For a Catholic the answer to this question will depend upon whether the matter is being considered from the viewpoint of church law or from the viewpoint of science. The Church forbids her subjects to marry within certain degrees of kindred. Catholics may not, without a dispensation, marry those who are either their first or second cousins. As to the desirability of cousin marriages from the standpoint of genetics, scientific authorities accept the following as reasonably well-established effects of inbreeding.

If two persons—for example, cousins—who have common ancestors were to marry each other, this would bring about a union of two lines of heredity which are much alike. In the children born of such a union would be present a similarity of those characteristics which are of an hereditary nature. Such characteristics are the qualities—good or bad—which are transmitted to the children by their forebears. If, however, a particular trait has not shown itself in the three previous generations of the child's progenitors, it is not considered hereditary. When the common ancestors of the parents of the marriage partners have been blessed with desirable dominant qualities, the offspring of the present marriage are apt to receive in double measure a share of good traits. If, however, the common ancestors have undesirable recessive qualities, the children may receive in double measure a portion of undesirable characteristics. Hence from the biological viewpoint the

316

intermarriage of relatives is good if both parties are carriers of desirable qualities; it is bad if they are carriers of defects.

From the social viewpoint cousin marriages are to be disfavored because they deprive the parties of the advantages which would be theirs if they took nonrelatives as life partners. Marriage with a nonrelative brings one into a new family circle, and this will result in an extended range of friendship. When one finds himself thus in a different family group, he is obliged to adapt himself to new situations and to make many new mental adjustments. Intimate association with persons whose habits of life, points of view, ancestry, and so forth, are not the same as those in one's own family circle tends to dissipate narrowness of outlook and to broaden one's character.

Attitude toward Children

The physician will prove himself to be a true friend of those who are about to be married if he prudently reminds them of the innumerable blessings which children bring to married couples. Experience teaches that, during the first months of marriage, the young couple will as a rule overflow with ardent love for each other and will be much enamored of their new life. After about a year the novelty of marriage tends to wear off, and each begins to realize that the other has certain defects—defects which may be quite irritating. The burdens of life together then begin to make themselves felt, and the husband and wife find that their hearts are not so perfectly united as they were during the honeymoon. If at this time a baby is born to them, it will serve as a golden link of love between husband and wife. The child will bind them together more firmly, for each will see in the baby a reflection of his own personality and of the personality of his spouse. The young husband and wife will be thrilled by the realization that the child is the flower of their mutual love and that it has been formed from their own flesh and blood. Their parenthood will render their affection for each other far more solid than it was before. It will bring to them a more complete sense of their mutual responsibilities and will foster in them a spirit of un-selfishness, both toward each other and toward their offspring. The privilege which they have had of sharing in the task of creating a living child will be for them a lasting source of joy and gratitude toward God. God has deigned to permit them to be coauthors with Him in the fashioning of a human being who is gifted with five magic senses of the body and with wonder-stirring powers of the soul. This child is destined to live eternally in heaven, where he will for endless ages be pro-foundly grateful to his parents. Reflecting upon these thoughts, the young couple cannot fail to appreciate more deeply the beauty of their married life and the happiness which parent-hood normally engenders.

Because there is nothing which husband and wife can share so fully and so lastingly as their own offspring, children tend to unite their parents more deeply and more permanently. One would expect, then, that a marriage which is blessed with children would be more likely to succeed than a childless marriage. As a matter of fact, experience confirms this judg-ment. Recently gathered statistics indicate that, the greater the number of children a couple has, the stronger is the marital bond. Divorce between parents of large families is rare, and the number of divorces and separations increases proportion-ately as the number of children in the family diminishes. In one such survey we find that 20 per cent of the divorcées had only one child and about 57 per cent of them had no children at all.[4]

Children should be regarded as a source of great spiritual benefit to parents. The years of care which children require

---

[4] Harold A. Phelps, *Contemporary Social Problems*, p. 478 (New York: Prentice-Hall, 1947). Data gathered from records of seven thousand Catholic marriages on the point of breaking up between 1943 and 1948 indicate that the exclusion of children by one or both of the parties accounted for the break-down of two thirds of the marriages. See John L. Thomas, S.J., "Marital Failure and Duration," *Social Order* 3:24-29, January 1953.

call for innumerable sacrifices and whole-souled generosity on the part of the parents. In conscientiously performing their task of providing for their offspring from babyhood until the age of majority, the father and mother will undoubtedly experience notable spiritual development, for rearing a normal family calls for the exercise of many virtues. It demands from the parents a long period of unselfish devotion to the best interests of their children. The father and mother will have to give up many pleasures and to endure many discomforts. During long years they must stand in constant attendance upon their helpless children to minister to their needs. They will see the little ones, whom they love so dearly, visited with various afflictions and sicknesses, and they cannot escape being harassed with anxiety and burdened with heavy sorrow. They must exercise unruffled patience in the day-after-day training which they give to their growing offspring. They must be ready with prudent guidance and constant vigilance to tide them over the difficulties of childhood and adolescence. This unselfish solicitude and generous sacrifice are conducive to the acquisition of holiness. By fulfilling their God-given task properly, parents enjoy the rich opportunity of growing in virtue and of acquiring a rich store of merit.

Another benefit which children bring is that they help their parents to remain young in spirit. Parents are inclined to relive their own youth in their children. The father and mother of a large family are mingling continually with the young. They are sharing their experiences, talking of things which interest the children, watching games, listening to their companions. All this tends to produce a rejuvenating effect upon an adult. Even when old age sets in, the aging couple are spared the loneliness which often makes this period of life so difficult to endure. By their loving and generous care and by their cheerful and refreshing presence, the children will bring much solace to their parents and will brighten the dullness of the often uneventful days of the autumn of life.

From the viewpoint of material advantages alone, large families are beneficial. Parents are benefited by numerous off-spring. Moreover, the children derive definite advantages from being members of a large family. The only child is often greatly handicapped because he lacks the educative influence of brothers and sisters. The companionship which the children of a large family provide for one another affords invaluable training in dealing with various personalities. The give-and-take of such associations helps toward a character development which is wholesome and well balanced. Living with brothers and sisters trains the child to adapt himself to difficult situations, to make allowances for the reasonable wishes of others, to adjust his conduct to the needs of varying circumstances. As a child habitually acts at home, he will behave outside the family circle; and so it is clear that home life is a preparation for the child's activities outside the home. He will later have to contend with the peculiarities and foibles of all sorts of persons in business and in his social life, and the experience gained by association with the various members of the family group will aid him in accommodating himself to whatever situations he may later encounter.

Some parents give as their reason for not wanting more than one or two children that they wish to provide for these few offspring more advantages than would be possible if the family were a large one. It should be clear from what was said in the preceding paragraph that this reason is unsound. It is true that not a few husbands and wives sincerely believe, in their ignorance, that it is preferable for the sake of the child to have a small family, but the common reason for limiting offspring to one or two is unadulterated selfishness. The parents wish to be left free to give their time to amusements, sports, social activities, and travel. Such mothers are not long held down by domestic cares. Such fathers need not spend their money on the costly rearing of a large family, but can enjoy the luxuries which otherwise they would be obliged to forgo.

Husbands and wives should beware of allowing themselves to be deceived in this very important matter. They should not come to a decision without having carefully weighed the reasons which, in their case, favor or make undesirable a large family. They should form their judgment independently of the "planned-parenthood" propaganda so widespread today.

Spacing Children

It is evident from what has been said that large families are a most singular benefit both to the parents and to the children. There is, however, no obligation for a husband and wife to have as many children as possible. Is it not, as a matter of fact, preferable from the viewpoint of health for a couple to avoid having numerous offspring? Do not modern medical authorities urge parents to "space" their children so that there will be a lapse of several years between the successive births? If lengthy intervals occur between the coming of babies, is this not more conducive to the health of the mother and to that of the offspring? Scientifically speaking, should there not be a period of rest of two or more years between births? An affirmative answer to all these questions would unhesitatingly be given by the promoters of planned parenthood and by the propagandists of artificial birth control. Recent scholarly studies, however, have proved false the doctrine of these contraceptionists. Science has established the fact that, from a medical viewpoint, an interval of two or three years between births is not necessarily desirable. Dr. Nicholson J. Eastman of Johns Hopkins University has published findings with regard to (1) the mother's health and (2) the effect on the baby which we may summarize as follows:

1. The longer the period of rest there is between pregnancies, the greater is the possibility that the mother will suffer some form of blood poisoning. When the interval between births is from one to two years only, she has the greatest hope of escaping such infections. *based on pre-Antibiotic statistics —. The statement is absolutely without foundation today.*

321

2. The interval of one to two years between births is at least as favorable to the health of the baby as longer intervals would prove to be.[5]

GIVING FORMAL MARITAL INSTRUCTION

SINCE the physician often deals with those who are already married or who are soon to marry, his advice is sought about many problems that occur in married life. The physician should be qualified to impart to parties soon to marry the necessary pertinent facts about the marital embrace. He should be acquainted with the morality of the practice of rhythm. He should have a clear concept of the intrinsic evil of artificial birth control. The morality of these practices is fully discussed on pages 156-61, 163-67.

There are two types of marital instruction which the physician may be called upon to give: group instruction and individual instruction. The two differ in content, and therefore we shall treat them separately.

Group Instruction

Group instruction on the physical details of sex should not be given to those who are below college age.[6] The physician may be invited to address a Pre-Cana Conference about the physical side of marriage. (Pre-Cana Conferences, so called because it was at Cana that Christ and His Mother attended the wedding feast, are conferences under the auspices of the Catholic Church for those who are not yet married. Cana Con-

---

[5] Nicholson J. Eastman, M.D., "The Effect of the Interval between Births on Maternal and Fetal Outlook." *American Journal of Obstetrics and Gynecology* · 47:445-66, April 1944.

[6] In their annual statement for the year 1950, issued on November 17, 1950, the Roman Catholic bishops of the United States protested strongly against sex education in the classroom ("The Child: Citizen of Two Worlds." In *Our Bishops Speak*, pp. 161-69. Milwaukee: Bruce Publishing Company, 1952). In 1942 the Catholic bishops of England and Wales had taken a similar stand. See J. Leycester King, S.J., *Sex Enlightenment and the Catholic*, p. 35, n. (London: Burns Oates and Washbourne, 1948).

ferences are for the benefit of the married.) This group is made up of young men and women who are about to be married. Even though the physician is speaking to those who are somewhat mature, he must be on his guard against describing intimate details that would prove for some at least a source of temptation. There is no necessity of exposing any of the audience to the danger of sinning by a sexually exciting lecture. Complete sex instruction should be given the person who is soon to marry, but its more intimate side should be reserved for a private conference.

In the Pre-Cana Conference lectures the following points should be explained. With the exception of the matter that is mentioned in nos. 1, 2, 10, and 12, it is preferable that the lecture be given separately to each sex.

1. The psychological differences that exist between men and women.[7]

2. The importance of premarital chastity both from a moral point of view and from a psychological point of view. The natural law imposes on the couple a grave obligation to refrain from sexual relations before their marriage. Several studies have brought to light the fact that those marriages are the happiest in which neither party has been guilty of any previous sexual experience.

3. Attention should be called to the fact that it is of importance that husband and wife have a clear knowledge of the sexual anatomy of both the male and the female. Lack of accurate knowledge regarding the sex organs will prove a decided handicap and may even occasion injury during the performance of the marital act. In a manner that is sufficiently detailed, the physician should explain separately to those of each sex the anatomy of man and woman.

4. The nature of the marital act should be simply explained as the joining of the male and the female sex organs so that the

[7] See Edwin F. Healy, S.J., *Marriage Guidance*, pp. 19-25. Chicago: Loyola University Press, 1948.

semen is spilled into the vagina. The manner in which the ovum is fertilized should be briefly outlined.

5. The physician should mention the difference which is normally present between the male and the female attitude toward the marriage act. In the husband the physical side predominates; in the wife the emotional and spiritual side. In the man the sexual urge is as a rule stronger than in the woman and asserts itself more frequently.

6. The married couple should cultivate self-control regarding the marital act. It will be necessary at times to practice continence—for example, during sickness and after childbirth—and both should prepare for such enforced abstinence.

7. Sexual adjustment is very gradual and in some cases requires months and even years. Unselfishness must be the rule. Each should seek primarily not one's own but the other's pleasure. The husband especially must be gentle and considerate in the marital relations.

8. Mention should be made of the possibility of miscarriage. In case of miscarriage the fetus should be carefully baptized, regardless of its age, provided it is not certainly dead.

9. The physician can point out the many advantages of breast feeding both with regard to the health of the child and with regard to the problem of spacing children.[8] It should be mentioned that the mother has an obligation to suckle her child unless she has a good reason for not doing so. The mere inconvenience involved would not excuse her from this duty.

[Apt to be a source of guilt in those who fail — Today bottle fed babies are as well nourished as Breast fed.]

10. Artificial birth control is not only a grave moral evil; it is even medically a very undesirable practice. Each act of frustrating nature is a grave offense against God. Artificial birth control tends to foster neurotic conditions in the wife.[9]

[8] See Alexis Carrel, M.D., "Breast Feeding for Babies," *Reader's Digest* 34:1-7, June 1939; John F. Cunningham, M.D., *Textbook of Obstetrics*, p. 449 (New York: Grune and Stratton, 1951).

[9] Raoul de Guchteneere, *Judgment on Birth Control*, pp. 113-72 (New York: The Macmillan Company, 1931). See also Jules Paquin, S.J., *Morale et médecine*, pp. 267-342 (Montréal: L'Immaculée-Conception, 1955).

[Note! Today all premature babies are placed on bottles for the very reason that it is safer (easier to estimate the nutritional intake)]

11. Rhythm and basal body temperature as a means of spacing children may be described. The physician should explain that neither of these may licitly be used to avoid having children unless there is present a justifying reason for their use. The group should be informed that these methods prove useful at times as an aid in bringing about pregnancy in wives who are eager to have children.

12. A premarital physical examination of both parties is to be recommended. This examination is intended to disclose any conditions which might interfere with marital happiness. In this category may be placed such conditions as the general ill health of either party, incipient tuberculosis, an abnormality of the sexual apparatus, a venereal infection, and so forth. In many cases where some such unfavorable condition is present, the party himself does not know of its existence. The medical examination will acquaint him with any physical defect which he has, and he can then apply a suitable remedy before marriage. Each of the parties should, prior to the marriage, acquaint the other with the state of his health. There seems to be no obligation for one to reveal the fact that there has been insanity in his family history unless the other asks explicitly about the matter.

Is a young man or woman whom the physician finds to be sterile under the obligation of revealing this defect to the future spouse? In answering this question one must distinguish between sterility which has been artificially produced and congenital sterility. If the sterility has been artificially produced (for example, by means of an operation), charity obliges one to make known this defect. The reason is that after marriage, when this condition is discovered, the other spouse will be gravely offended at the deliberate silence about so important a matter, and that this may cause a serious breach between the husband and wife. If one is congenitally sterile, he has in general no obligation to reveal this condition to his fiancée. Most of those who are so afflicted are ignorant of their defect. If before marriage one party happens to discover that he is congenitally sterile, the other need never know that he had knowledge of this defect before the wedding, and so there would be from this source no danger of marital discord. If, however, the congenitally sterile person knows that his intended spouse greatly desires children, or that the fact that he knew of the defect before marriage will later become known to his spouse, charity requires him to make known his defect.

The physician would do well to recommend that those who are engaged to be married subscribe to *Marriage-Preparation Service*, published by the University of Ottawa.[10] This service consists of a correspondence-school course of printed instructions which treat of the many problems that arise in married life. The physician might also call the patient's attention to *Marriage Guidance*, a book intended to explain both the remote and the immediate preparation for marriage and the obligations of husband and wife toward each other and toward the offspring with which God may bless them.[11]

Individual Instruction

The individual instruction of those who are soon to marry should include the following points:

1. The party should be told of the necessity of cleansing the whole body and especially the genital organs prior to engaging in the marital act. Carelessness in this matter may not only lead to offending the marriage partner, but to infecting the genital tract of the wife.

2. The first act of sexual intercourse must be performed with great care and gentleness, so as to avoid causing undue pain and to provide against injury which might be caused by any roughness in fitting together the organs.

[10] The Catholic Centre, University of Ottawa, 1 Stewart Street, Ottawa, Canada.

[11] Edwin F. Healy, S.J., *Marriage Guidance*. Chicago: Loyola University Press, 1948.

3. The physician should explain the nature of love play and its great utility, especially in regard to the wife. The wife requires a large measure of love play before her organs are ready for coitus. The husband should see that the wife experiences an orgasm.

4. The various positions in which the marital act can take place should be described and the advantages or disadvantages of each should be made clear. *doubt This?*

5. The physician should mention what might be consid- *best To simply make clear The. basis for successfull mutual development of Technique* ered to be normal frequency of sexual relations in the lives of married couples. He should explain the undesirable effects of too-great frequency and the norm for judging when the marital act is indulged in excessively.

6. The couple should be warned about the dangers of performing the marriage act during the last months of pregnancy and soon after childbirth.

7. To the bride-to-be should be explained the ordinary indications of pregnancy and the advantages of prenatal care under the guidance of a physician. She might be told something about the period of gestation and be given the assurance that childbirth today carries with it little danger. No mention should be made of frightening or offensive abnormalities in regard to either parturition or offspring.

During the instructions the physician might permit the one whom he is counseling to discuss the matter being treated, and he would do well to reply in sufficient detail to any questions which are asked. It is advisable that the physician make sure that the patient's attitude toward the marital act is a wholesome and Christian one.

It has been found to be distinctly beneficial to give the party, at the conclusion of the instructions, a publication which contains the information useful for the bride and groom so that they can study it before the honeymoon. He would do well to warn them about keeping such reading matter strictly to themselves and about the danger of leaving it where it might be seen by those for whom it would be harmful. The young couple might also be warned against placing too great emphasis on the purely physical aspects of marital love. Spiritual love alone is part of the essential foundation of a truly happy marriage.

MARRIAGE RIGHTS

E ACH partner to a marriage is obliged to respect the rights which the other has in regard to the marital act. St. Paul says: "The wife has not authority over her body, but the husband; the husband likewise has not authority over his body, but the wife" (1 Corinthians 7:4). By virtue of the matrimonial contract both spouses have equal rights in this matter. This is explicitly stated in ecclesiastical law (Canon 1111). The obligation to participate in the conjugal act when one is asked by the other to do so is as a rule a grave one, provided the other requests his marital rights seriously and lawfully. To "request seriously" means that one is in earnest and is not trifling. When the request does not imply a demand, but is made only by way of suggestion, it is not said to be a serious request. It merely expresses a preference and does not aim at exacting the payment of what is strictly due. To "request lawfully" means that one is within his rights when he requires his partner to participate in the marriage act. There are times when one partner is freed from the obligation of acceding to the other's request for the marital act, even though the demand be made seriously. The following circumstances excuse one from the duty of participating in the marital act.

1. If the other is insane or completely intoxicated. Only a request which is a human act can induce the obligation of complying with it. A human act is one which is deliberately performed by a person possessed of the use of reason. A man or a woman who is insane or completely intoxicated is incapable of a human act. The spouse may accede to the request of the marriage partner who is in such a condition as this if he

chooses to do so, but is equally free to refuse to participate in the act.

2. If the other intends to perform the act in a sinful way. Here there is never an obligation to cooperate with the other in his sin, and in certain cases there would be a grave duty to refuse to participate in any way in the act.

3. If the act would cause one grave harm. This condition might be verified if, for example, the other has at the time a highly contagious disease.

4. If one spouse has certainly been guilty of adultery. In this case the innocent marriage partner need never again perform the marital act.

In order to safeguard the health of a pregnant wife and that of the child, it is preferable in ordinary cases that marital relations be discontinued about two months before the expected birth of the baby and that they be not resumed until at least six weeks after childbirth. If there would be no danger to either wife or child, greater liberty is permitted, and the parties may follow the counsel of the physician.

Physicians are sometimes asked about pregnancies in the case of married women who have given birth to stillborn babies only. The fact that all their children have been stillborn need not dissuade husband and wife from having more children. Although their offspring may be born dead, the mothers are in no way accountable for this misfortune. It is better, moreover, for these children to be called into being than never to have existed at all. The parents should of course spare no effort to have such infants baptized while they are still alive; but if the babies die before baptism can be administered, they will enjoy forever a natural beatitude.

SEX TRAINING OF CHILDREN

THE physician may be consulted by parents concerning the advisability of informing their children about matters of sex and about training them in the virtue of chastity. Safeguarding the virtue of chastity in one's children is a most important task, and one that requires intelligent planning. Parents know that their children will sooner or later meet with strong temptations against the virtue of chastity and that these temptations are often most alluring. Unless the child is solidly fortified against these attacks, which are often sudden and persistent, he will succumb to them. The task of the parent is twofold: to give the child a general preliminary training that will prepare him to live a pure life and to convey the necessary specific information at the proper time.

Preliminary Training

It is now acknowledged, even by authorities outside the Catholic Church, that complete sex information of an anatomical and physiological nature provides no guarantee whatsoever that an individual will avoid sexual irregularities. On the contrary, it may only excite morbid curiosity, inflame the passions, and suggest the performance of actions that should be avoided. Of far greater importance than mere information is the development of an ideal and of the strength which God has made possible to those who use the spiritual helps provided by Him. The wise Catholic parent, therefore, begins to prepare his child to be chaste from his earliest years. Observance of the following six points will aid parents in preparing their offspring to face the trials and temptations that they will inevitably meet.

1. Inspire in the child a love of purity. Describe the beauty of this virtue in such a way that the child will become enamored of its radiant splendor. Show him how it ennobles the one who cultivates it and makes him more Christlike. Recount to the child stories of the saints whose lives reflected a spotless purity. Mention the eternal reward in store for those who keep their souls unsoiled. Point out, on the other hand, the ugliness and degrading character of the opposite vice, and try to create in the child a genuine disgust for impurity. Let him know that

this sin causes grave sorrow to the Sacred Heart of Christ and that it can only too easily lead to the everlasting fires of hell.

2. Inculcate the habit of mortification. Many sins of impurity are committed because the sinner's will is weak. A good protection against violations of chastity is a strong will. A will is not made strong in a few days or weeks. It must be trained constantly over a period of years. Acts of self-denial are an effective means of strengthening the will, and a child will be greatly benefited if he practices acts of penance from a supernatural motive; namely, in order to please God and to show a willingness to make genuine sacrifices for Him. Parents should foster in their children the desire to perform little acts of mortification, such as abstaining occasionally from choice foods that are served at table, deliberately interrupting a story or radio program at an interesting part, forgoing a movie, and so forth.

3. Keep the child occupied. The idle child is more apt to be tempted to sin than the busy one. Hence it is advisable to see to it that the child is constantly engaged in work, play, reading, hobbies, or some other similar occupation that will absorb his attention.

4. Urge frequent reception of the sacraments. In order to remain chaste amid the many seductive influences of the world, supernatural help is essential. The ordinary channel of grace is the sacraments. The youngster should be convinced of the surpassing value of the sacraments of penance and the Eucharist in helping one to ward off evil. By means of the frequent reception of the sacrament of penance (1) the young person acquires a more thorough realization of those circumstances which are a source of spiritual danger for him, (2) his will is strengthened by the sacramental graces against future falls, (3) carelessness and indifference toward sex offenses are prevented from arising, and (4) incipient evil habits are destroyed under the guidance of a prudent confessor. One should go regularly to the same priest to confession, so that he may

become acquainted with one's spiritual needs. By means of the frequent reception of Holy Communion (1) the passions are diminished in intensity, (2) the soul is strongly fortified against grave sin, (3) the soul is purified of many venial faults and will be stained with fewer in the future, (4) the temporal punishment due to one's sin is abolished wholly or in part, and (5) the soul is enriched with sanctifying grace which will increase its reward in heaven.

5. Protect the child against evil companions and evil reading. A large percentage of those who sin against chastity can in great part blame their downfall on the evil conversation, suggestions, or example of friends or acqaintances. Parents should exercise prudent surveillance over the persons with whom their child associates. Evil reading often proves to be an occasion of sin for the young.

6. Win the child's confidence. Much of a child's difficulty in sex matters is caused by the fact that he has no one to consult about his doubts. Parents should induce their offspring to confide in them in all things. They should never appear shocked or angry at any of their child's confidences, no matter what the nature of these may be.

Formal Sex Instruction

The instruction of children on matters of sex is a task which most parents today are inclined to neglect. This negligence may be traced to various causes. Perhaps the principal reason for their failure is that parents do not know how to impart this knowledge. If their own knowledge is adequate, they may because of excessive sensitiveness (fostered perhaps by an unchristian attitude toward sex) feel too much embarrassed were they to discuss these subjects with their children. Another reason that prompts parents to refrain from all sex instruction is that they wish to "keep the child innocent." The instruction of which there is question here means the imparting to another knowledge of the "facts of life." The "facts of life" are four; namely, (1) the origin of babies, (2) the sex differences between male and female, (3) bodily changes that occur at the age of puberty, and (4) the marital act.

To reveal too much about sex to a child is a grave error, for it will foster a premature ripening of his sexual instincts and will fill his mind with phantasms of a troublesome nature. He will as a result experience temptations with which he is not sufficiently prepared to cope. Pius XI warns that sex instruction, if given to the child prematurely and in too great detail, will prove dangerous:

"In this extremely delicate matter, if . . . some private instruction is found necessary and opportune . . . every precaution must be taken. Such precautions are well known in traditional Christian education, and are adequately described by Antoniano cited above, when he says: 'Such is our misery and inclination to sin, that often in the very things considered to be remedies against sin, we find occasions for and inducements to sin itself. Hence it is of the highest importance that a good father, while discussing with his son a matter so delicate, should be well on his guard and not descend to details, nor refer to the various ways in which this infernal hydra destroys with its poison so large a portion of the world; otherwise it may happen that instead of extinguishing this fire, he unwittingly stirs or kindles it in the simple and tender heart of the child.' "[12]

Again, pointing out that sex instruction which stresses the physical side alone is to be condemned, Pius XI says:

"Another grave danger is that naturalism which nowadays invades the field of education in that most delicate matter of purity of morals. Far too common is the error of those who with dangerous assurance and under an ugly term propagate a so-called sex-education, falsely imagining they can forearm youth against the dangers of sensuality by means purely nat-

[12] Pius XI, *Christian Education of Youth*. In *Five Great Encyclicals*, p. 56. New York: Paulist Press, 1939.

ural, such as a fool-hardy initiation and precautionary instruction for all indiscriminately, even in public."[13]

Of parents' duty to give instruction Pius XII says:

"With the discretion of a mother and a teacher, and thanks to the open-hearted confidence with which you have been able to inspire your children, you will not fail to watch for and to discern the moment in which certain unspoken questions have occurred to their minds and are troubling their senses. It will then be your duty to your daughters, the father's duty to your sons, carefully and delicately to unveil the truth as far as it appears necessary, to give a prudent, true and Christian answer to those questions, and set their minds at rest. If imparted by the lips of Christian parents, at the proper time, in the proper measure and with the proper precautions, the revelation of the mysterious and marvellous laws of life will be received by them with reverence and gratitude, and will enlighten their minds with far less danger than if they learned them haphazard, from some unpleasant shock, from secret conversations, through information received from over-sophisticated companions, or from clandestine reading . . . Your words, if they are wise and discreet, will prove a safeguard and a warning in the midst of the temptations and the corruption which surround them."[14]

When Should Sex Instruction Be Begun

To delay too long the giving of instruction to the child in matters of sex is unwise, for every child, sooner or later,

---

[13] *Ibid.* See also Kilian J. Hennrich, O.F.M.Cap., "Sex Education in Public Schools," *Homiletic and Pastoral Review* 42:645-52, April 1942; Hierarchy of England and Wales, " 'Sex Education,' a statement issued by the hierarchy of England and Wales," *Catholic Mind* 42:460-61, August 1944; J. Leycester King, S.J., *Sex Enlightenment and the Catholic* (London: Burns Oates and Washbourne, 1948).

[14] Pius XII, "Allocution to a Concourse of Women of Catholic Action, November 26, 1941," *Clergy Review* 22:136, March 1942. See also Hierarchy of England and Wales, " 'Sex Education,' a statement issued by the hierarchy of England and Wales," *Catholic Mind* 42:460-61, August 1944.

becomes curious about sex differences. This is a natural inquisitiveness, and the child has a right to know the truth insofar as he is ready to receive it. If he is not enlightened on these questions, he will be incited to make a morbid search for the desired knowledge in dictionaries and among friends of his own age. Eventually the child will obtain information in some way or other, and his parents cannot prevent it. Parents can see to it, however, that their child is not left to his own blundering pursuit of this knowledge. Many boys and girls read risqué magazines, objectionable newspaper accounts, and questionable stories merely because of their desire to learn something about sex. Thus their quest for this information is unduly prolonged and lasts perhaps for years, their ideas of sex are unclear and distorted, and they fail to acquire the reverential attitude which they should have toward sex. They learn to look upon it as something that is dirty or impure, and do not have a true appreciation of the noble function that it has in the plan of God.

Ignorance exposes boys and girls to the danger of contracting immoral habits without realizing the sinfulness of such actions. They are of course guilty of no formal sin in this; but later, when they come to know the true malice of the habit, it may prove extremely difficult to put an end to this evil way of acting. Moreover, ignorance in these matters lays a young person open to seduction on the part of older persons. This is especially true in the case of girls. Ordinarily speaking, they desire to be loved and are inclined to accept from male friends kisses and embraces as mere signs of affection. If a girl knows nothing of the inflammable nature of the passions, she may innocently permit actions which can suddenly and gravely jeopardize her virtue.

Premature and too-long-delayed sex instruction are both to be condemned. When, then, should this information be imparted to the child? The rule is this: Instruct the child insofar as ignorance may harm him. A child of eight obviously does not need the same amount of knowledge as a youth of sixteen. A sheltered child will not require as much as one who is exposed to the influence of immoral acquaintances. The object of the one who gives the instruction should be to communicate to the young person sufficient information to satisfy his present curiosity and needs. Instruction should tend to decrease, not to increase, his interest in sex.

The parents' instruction should begin by explaining to the little child the origin of babies, and it is not completed until a son or daughter who is about to be married attains a full knowledge of marital rights and privileges. In some instances a child may begin to ask about these matters when he is but three years of age. His questions should be answered frankly but without too great detail. Ordinarily children seek information on sex before they are six or seven years old. In cases in which the child does not ask spontaneously, the parents should arrange opportunities for him to make inquiries. This can be done by mentioning subjects which will suggest such questions to the child.

Who Is To Give Sex Instruction

Which one of the parents should impart sex information to the children? To answer this question we must make a distinction. When the child, either boy or girl, is small the mother seems to be best fitted for this task. Besides, since she is with the child during the whole day, she will most probably be the one who is present when the questions come into his mind. When a child approaches puberty he becomes more prone to the stimulation of the passions, and it is preferable that sex instruction to a child of his age be given by one of the same sex. The father, therefore, should instruct his son when the latter reaches the age of about thirteen; the mother should instruct the daughter. One is reminded of what Pius XII says in his allocution to Catholic mothers in the passage already quoted on page 334. "It will then be your duty to your daughters, the father's duty to your sons, carefully and delicately to unveil the truth."

How Sex Instruction Is To Be Given

The sex talk should be given in a manner that is clear, free from embarrassment, and satisfying. Parents should avoid using words the meanings of which are not well known to the child. Technical expressions and obscure phrases will do more harm than good, for they mystify and befuddle the child. Moreover, one should not recite to the child a passage of an author which he has memorized. He should use his own words and his own ways of expressing the thought, for otherwise his instruction will sound stilted and preachy, and will lack the conviction which is here so desirable. One's manner of stating the facts should be as unemotional and matter-of-fact as possible. There should be no evidence of embarrassment, for embarrassment on the part of the parent will react on the child and will cause him also to become embarrassed.

Embarrassment can in most cases be avoided if one stresses the sublimity of the sex function. One should remind himself that sex holds a very important and sacred place in God's plan of the universe. Little embarrassment will be experienced by the normal parent who begins these instructions at the proper time and continues to give them periodically as the child's needs increase. If one finds himself becoming nervous during the talk, he might restore his calmness by a temporary digression or interruption. If a parent believes that he cannot discuss this matter with his child without suffering noticeable embarrassment, he should ask another to give the instruction for him. He should, however, make certain that his substitute is well qualified and that he will not impart false or sinful ideas.

What Is To Be Told?

The questioning child should be told the truth about matters of sex, but he should receive only that measure of truth which he needs to know at the time. The stork story or the cabbage-patch fiction should not be employed in order to explain the origin of babies. When a child asks his mother the question, "Where do babies come from?" the mother might answer something like this: "Babies come from the hand of God. They grow under their mother's heart like a rose on a rosebush. They remain inside the mother until they are strong enough to live outside, and then they are born." When the child grows older he will ask the parent: "What is the difference between boys and girls?" To answer this question the mother might give a development of the following thoughts.

"God is of course all-powerful. That means that He can do anything. He could, then, create boys and girls in the same manner in which He created the angels or Adam and Eve. He created the angels by directly drawing each of them into existence by His own hand. They had no father or mother. God Himself also directly created Adam and Eve. Taking up some earth, He Himself formed and molded it into a human shape, into the body of a man. Now, God is infinitely wise and infinitely holy and infinitely powerful. It is clear, then, that every part, every line, every member, every organ of that body was the choice of God Himself, who is immeasurably wise and holy and powerful. Therefore every part and member and organ of that body was sacred. Then God breathed into that human shape a living, glorious soul and in that moment there was created the first man, Adam.

"From the body of Adam God then took a part and formed and fashioned it into another human shape, into the body of a woman. Now God, who did this, is infinite wisdom, infinite holiness, and infinite power. Therefore every part, every line, every member and organ of this body was the express choice of infinite wisdom and holiness and power. We must conclude that every part and member and organ of this body was sacred. Into this body God then breathed a gloriously beautiful soul, vibrant with life, and there was created the first woman, Eve.

"Eve was like Adam and was unlike Adam. She resembled Adam in this way. She had a soul that was gifted with the wonderful powers of memory, understanding, and free will; she possessed a body with its five magic senses of sight, hearing, smell, taste, and touch. Like Adam, she had been created by God, and like him, she was intended to go to the everlasting home of heaven. She was unlike Adam physically. She was weaker, more delicate, and more refined of form. Her body was not the same as man's. Its shape was different. Its skin was smoother. Woman's voice was of a higher pitch. Woman, then, has certain qualities which man lacks and man has certain qualities which woman lacks, and it is because of the differences that man and woman are attracted to each other and are destined by God to help each other in life.

"God in His infinite goodness gave Adam and Eve a most precious gift; namely, that of helping Him to create other human beings like themselves, the glorious privilege of bringing into the world babies who were destined to live forever in heaven. He placed in the body of Eve female cells of life and in the body of Adam male cells of life. According to God's plan, when the male cells of life met the female cells of life, a new human being was created, a tiny baby took up his nesting place under his mother's heart. These cells of life are located in the parts of the body which are called the genital organs. It is obvious, then, how sacred these genital organs are. They must always be treated as something sacred. No one should ever joke about them, nor touch them without a justifying reason, nor expose them without necessity."

The physical development which occurs in the bodies of boys and girls at the age of puberty should be clearly explained, and the youngster should be informed about the natural phenomena which accompany this growth toward maturity. In order to protect him or her from spiritual harm the manner in which the male seeds of life meet the female cells of life—namely, by the union of the genital organs—may be

339

explained to the child who is approaching puberty. The young person should be told that this act is called sexual intercourse or the marital act. It is termed the marital act because it may licitly be performed only by a man and a woman who are married to each other. For an unmarried boy or an unmarried girl to be guilty of such an act is a grievous offense against God, and one which can, moreover, diminish the happiness of their future marriage, since they would then have a shameful action to conceal. Since everyone is subject to temptation, young persons should pray often for the help of God to preserve their virtue.

Adolescent girls should be informed of the marked difference between a boy's reaction to sexual stimuli and that of a girl. Sexual stimuli are actions or objects which tend to arouse venereal pleasure. Examples of these are unchaste touches, the sight of a scantily clad person of the opposite sex, indecent pictures, and lewd conversation. Because God intended man to be the more active partner in the sex relationship, He made man's passions more readily excitable. Hence a boy may be strongly aroused sexually by a stimulus that leaves a girl unmoved. It often happens that an adolescent girl will permit a boy to engage in actions which she regards as innocent marks of affection, though actually they awaken the boy's passions. Girls should be warned against providing boys with the occasion of sin and against the dangers to their own virtue that may result from carelessness in this matter.

We recommend the following as informative reading material suitable for the age levels mentioned.

For Physicians and Parents

Bruckner, P. J., S.J. *How To Give Sex Instruction.* St. Louis: The Queen's Work, 1937.

King, J. Leycester, S.J. *Sex Enlightenment and the Catholic.* London: Burns Oates and Washbourne, 1948.

Lord, Daniel A., S.J. *Some Notes for the Guidance of Parents.* St. Louis: The Queen's Work, 1944.

For Boys between 7 and 18 Years of Age

Listen, Son. Chicago: Franciscan Herald Press, 1955.

For Girls between 7 and 18 Years of Age

Mother's Little Helper. Chicago: Franciscan Herald Press, 1955.

For Boys and Girls between 10 and 12 Years of Age

Juergens, Sylvester P. *Fundamental Talks on Purity.* Milwaukee: Bruce Publishing Company, 1941.

Lord, Daniel A., S.J. *Pure of Heart.* St. Louis: The Queen's Work, 1928.

For Girls 12 Years of Age

Growing Up. Chicago: Benziger Brothers, 1939.

For Boys and Girls between 16 and 18 Years of Age

Kelly, Gerald, S.J. *Modern Youth and Chastity.* St. Louis: The Queen's Work, 1943.

For Engaged Men and Women

Marriage-Preparation Service. The Catholic Centre, 1 Stewart Street, Ottawa, Canada.

Wayne, T. G. *Morals and Marriage.* New York: Longmans, Green and Company, 1936.

For Married Persons

Fundamentals of Marriage. The Catholic Centre, 1 Stewart Street, Ottawa, Canada.

MASTURBATION

IT HAPPENS at times that the physician discovers, either through a confession made to him or through the examination of the sex organs, that the patient is afflicted with the habit of self-abuse. In such cases, what is the physician's attitude to be? Does he have an obligation of attempting to correct the patient, even if the latter does not request him to do so? In the event that the patient does appeal to the physician for assistance and that the physician is endeavoring to cure the patient of this way of acting, what means could he employ to insure success?[15]

It should be clearly understood, in the first place, that self-abuse is a grave violation of the law of nature. The generative organs were given to man in order to accomplish, in the married state, the propagation of the human race. The unmarried person has no right to set in motion the sexual organs either in a natural or unnatural way. Masturbation consists in the direct stimulation of the sex organs outside sexual intercourse. This self-stimulation may be physical (effected by means of an instrument, the hands, movements of the body, and so forth) or it may be psychic (effected only by means of evil imaginations or unchaste desires). The act of directly stimulating the sexual organs in this manner defeats the very purpose for which God gave them to man. The directly intended misuse of the procreative faculty is a moral fault or sin because it constitutes a perversion of a natural faculty. The perversion consists in setting the generative apparatus in motion and at the same time endeavoring positively to prevent it from accomplishing the purpose or end for which it exists: the procreation of offspring. This misuse of the procreative faculty is gravely sinful, for it is the perversion of so noble and important a faculty. This faculty is obviously noble and important, for on its proper use depends the survival of the human race. Moreover, each misuse of the mature generative faculty can involve a frustration of life itself. It is evident that such frustration is seriously wrong.

The conscientious physician, therefore, should realize that there is cause for concern when a patient is found to be afflicted with the habit of masturbation. He should be ready to give whatever help he can in order that the patient may successfully overcome this evil practice. The extent of the physi-

---

[15] The problem of self-abuse is discussed scientifically in Baron Frederick von Gagern, M.D., *Problem of Onanism,* translated by Meyrick Booth (Cork: Mercier Press, 1954).

cian's obligation spontaneously to point out to the patient the moral fault which masturbation involves depends upon the circumstances of the case. If the patient, obviously ignorant of the sinfulness of the habit, is religious-minded and would presumably welcome enlightenment on the morality of the practice, the physician must in charity reveal the sinfulness of masturbation. If, on the other hand, there is adequate reason for believing that the patient would resent receiving such instruction, the physician may remain silent.

There is no doubt about the fact that one who has long been addicted to the practice of abusing his body will probably find a quick cure difficult. There are many things, however, which a physician may suggest that might prove helpful. A complete physical examination of the patient may reveal some contributing cause of the vice. In the male a tight foreskin may bring about frequent excitation of the penis and thus unduly fix the patient's attention on this organ. A long foreskin with but a small opening may create difficulties, for a small residue of urine is apt to collect near the opening and produce an itching sensation that leads the person to rub the genitals. In the female adhesions about the clitoris favor self-abuse. Minor surgery can remedy these abnormal conditions.

The following points may be of some help to the physician whose patient wishes to overcome the habit of masturbation.

Proper Sleep. The patient should sleep alone and on a fairly hard bed. The covering should be light and the room well aired. Heavy blankets will produce too much warmth in the body and this condition prepares the way for the excitation of the genitals. If the bedroom is poorly ventilated, the patient readily becomes lethargic and he will be then less apt to resist sexual stimulation.

Bathing. The patient should keep the sex organs clean. He should carefully rid the folds of skin around the genitals of all smegma, for the latter can produce itching. A cold bath followed by a brisk rubdown is to be recommended.

343

Exercise. General tenseness of the body helps to excite sexual desires and tempts the patient to seek relief in masturbation. Vigorous exercise, regularly taken, will diminish the nervous tension. Patients who most often abuse themselves in bed at night just before they go to sleep should be urged to make sure that they are physically fatigued when they retire. A moderate amount of exercise is recommended.

Avoidance of Idleness. Introspection fosters in the masturbator temptations to practice this vice, and idleness opens the way for introspection. Hence the patient should endeavor to keep himself occupied all day long. While trying to fall asleep at night, he could hold a rosary in his hands and pray very slowly. A deliberately languid manner of drawing out the words of the prayers will tend to induce sleep.

It has been found that masturbation is most frequently indulged in by persons who are depressed, discouraged, or lonesome. The patient should be urged to engage in social activities and to gain the friendship and respect of others. Participation in these activities will counteract his inclination to loneliness and will divert attention from himself.

Developing Will Power. The habitual masturbator's will is weak, at least in regard to temptations against the virtue of chastity. To prepare the patient to overcome the tendency to yield to such seductive influences, his will must be strengthened. The process of strengthening his will might be initiated by his practicing acts of self-denial for the purpose of cultivating the virtue of chastity. He should be inspired with the strong and sincere desire to rid himself of a shameful habit and employ, to this end, acts of mortification which may win him God's help and develop his powers of resistance. Let us suppose, for example, that he desires to perform some pleasing action which is wholly legitimate and that he deliberately refrains from doing so. This act of consciously denying to himself some pleasure gives him an increase of power over his natural inclinations. It tends to strengthen his will. Such actions by

344

which his will power is increased need not be of much importance in themselves. Little things will prove effective. If the patient smokes, he could forgo smoking for a few hours, or even for a whole day, or a whole week. If he is accustomed to enjoy the radio or television frequently, he could omit one or other program which he finds entertaining. He could give up a movie occasionally. Where the distance is not too great, he could walk instead of riding. Such means, though perhaps almost insignificant in themselves, serve to give the patient more effective dominion of his passions and prepare him to resist when he is assaulted by strong temptations.

Avoidance of Erotic Stimuli. The patient should be persuaded to avoid, insofar as he can, anything that tends to excite his passions. There are of course some sights that will prove troublesome but which he cannot avoid. He must beware of all reading, pictures, movies, and radio and television programs which are suggestive or sexually stimulating. He should examine his life to discover special circumstances which in the past proved dangerous for him, and he should resolve to avoid these in the future.

Quick Distraction. The temptation to masturbate arises in many cases from an unchaste image that stimulates the passion. To rid oneself of this image is to subdue the temptation. Hence the patient, when assaulted by evil imaginations, should endeavor at once to divert his attention to some wholesome thought. One mental picture can expel another. If the patient vividly portrays to himself a clean, interesting incident, this will drive out the seductive image. If the new picture excites laughter, disgust, anger, and so forth, it will as a rule prove effective, for any of these emotional reactions will tend to quiet the sexual excitation.

The physician should do what he can to convince the patient of the desirability of overcoming the vice of masturbation. To this end the physician might emphasize the manliness and nobility which characterizes the chaste person and point out the fact that failure to control one's sex appetite debases and enslaves. He might also mention how, in so many cases, the habit of self-abuse diminishes one's self-respect and robs one of interior peace.

In order that the physician be of genuine help, he must inspire in the patient genuine confidence that he can be cured completely. Patience and understanding are very necessary in this matter. The patient should be informed that numberless persons who were once strongly gripped by this evil habit have successfully overcome it entirely, and that his passions are not any stronger than those of thousands of other persons who successfully keep them in check.

If the patient is a Catholic, the physician would do well to persuade him to go frequently to the sacraments of penance and the Eucharist. It should be pointed out to him that there is a great advantage in having a regular confessor who will become acquainted with his particular difficulties and proffer effective guidance. Whether the patient is a Catholic or not, he should be encouraged to pray for God's help in his efforts to overcome his evil habit.

Parents may have occasion to consult their physician about their child's tendency to practice self-abuse. When they discover their child playing with his genital organs, they should be warned against manifesting anger or undue excitement, for this will impress the incident unduly on the child's mind. Besides, he is in all probability completely ignorant of the evil of his actions. The parents should refrain from making frightening threats and from administering severe corporal punishment. Some forms of chastisement do the child much more harm than good and should be sedulously avoided. "Sending a youngster to bed in punishment for some misdeed has, aside from other disadvantages, often the effect that he masturbates, having nothing else to do and replacing the worry over his humiliation with something which to him affords gratification; often, as a matter of fact, it is this type of punishment which gives to the child the first impetus to perform the act. The same is true of forcing a child to retire long before he is ready for it or letting him remain in bed in the morning unoccupied for a long time."[16] The first point that the parents should make clear to the child is that the sex organs are delicate, that they are sacred, and that they should not be touched unnecessarily. The mother should see that the child's clothing does not fit too tightly and thus cause local irritation of the genital parts. It is well to keep the child in surroundings that are pleasant and cheerful. During the day he should not be permitted to remain unoccupied for long, since idleness will provide him with an occasion for indulging in self-abuse.

Masturbation and the Very Young Child

At times the physician will be asked by a parent, especially by a young mother, what can be done to cure a child three or four years of age of the habit of masturbation. Because of the extreme youthfulness of the child the case presents special difficulties. The physician should point out to the parent that the young child is not guilty of conscious wrongdoing. Although it is true that he is not aware of the evil nature of his actions, the actions are nevertheless actually against the law of nature, and the mother has the duty to endeavor to dissuade her child from engaging in such a practice. If, moreover, the child is not corrected, he may contract a habit which will be very difficult to break later when he comes to realize its sinfulness. The parent should not become angry when she notices the child masturbating, nor look upon him as exceptionally bad. Most children are said to experiment in this way with their genital organs. The question is how best to overcome the habit, and it is not easy to provide a satisfactory answer.

When the mother first notices that the child is touching his genital parts without necessity, she should quietly inform him

[16] L. Kanner, M.D.; A. Meyer, M.D.; and E. A. Park, M.D., *Child Psychiatry*, p. 402. Springfield: Charles C. Thomas, 1935.

that that part of the body is very sacred and must be treated with reverence. She might impress upon the youngster the fact that God does not wish him to touch the genitals unless it is necessary. Should she sharply command the child not to touch that part of his body? Much will depend on the character of the individual child. One child will respond well to one type of treatment; another to a different procedure. A sharp command may make one child resentful and eager to repeat the bad action as soon as he can do so without being observed. Another will accept the impressive command as final and will give up the practice once and for all. The mother will know from her experience with the child in regard to other things what his probable reaction to a sharp command would be. She should make allowance for the difference in personality that exists in various children. She should beware of making grave threats and of punishing excessively.

ADOPTED CHILDREN

WHEN a couple realizes that they are unable to have offspring of their own, they would do well to consider the merits of adopting one or more children.[17] The tendency of childless couples is to grow self-centered. Adoption would turn their attention away from themselves and keep them busy with the many tasks required in caring for the child. The pouring out of their love on the youngster, the making of sacrifices for him, the supervising of his physical and mental development, would broaden their own characters and increase their happiness. Adopted children are not so desirable as one's own, but they are an excellent substitute. If husband and wife intend to adopt a child, they should not wait too long before doing so. Once they are somewhat advanced in years and settled in their

[17] See, however, Joseph B. Doyle, M.D., "The Role of the Gynecologist," *Linacre Quarterly* 21:40-44, May 1954. Dr. Doyle, an internationally known specialist on infertility, contends that a very large percentage of childless couples could have children if they would seek proper medical aid.

348

habits of living, it is difficult for them to adapt themselves to the changes in their lives which a child will bring.

Adoption entails the exercising of many of the corporal and spiritual works of mercy, for the adoptive parents provide their young charge with food and drink, with clothing and shelter. They care for him in sickness and in health. They instruct him and guide him and comfort him and pray for him. The atmosphere of the home in which they rear him could not be provided in an orphanage. The adopted child ordinarily receives the same name as that of his adopted parents. He looks upon them as father and mother, and becomes in all things one of the family.

As to the advisability of letting the child know that he has been adopted, the best general rule seems to be that the child should be so informed. Since adoption is a public fact, the child will in all probability learn of this fact sooner or later. If he hears of the adoption from a source outside the family circle, he may resent having been permitted by his "parents" to be deceived in so important a matter. If he is to be informed, it should be done when he is very young, so that he will accept the fact with no unfavorable reaction.

When parents have had one child and are unable to have more, adoption may prove a blessing. As we have said above, an only child labors under great disadvantages, for he is deprived of the salutary influence of brothers and sisters. His parents are very apt to spoil him with too much attention and to be too ready to yield to his wishes. Adopted children are accepted by one's own children without question and are treated without objectionable discrimination.

The placing of a child in a home is today surrounded by many safeguards. The adoptive parents present themselves to a reputable child-placing agency. The agency will then investigate the couple's social background, their personalities, their sense of responsibility, their health, stability, and so forth; and if these prove satisfactory, the child is given into their care for a period of probation. Once the couple is fully approved, the legal formalities of adoption are completed. Catholic orphanages and hospitals, the United States Children's Bureau, and other agencies provide information regarding the adoption of children.

THE CARE OF THE AGED

Old age often brings with it many trying ailments and inconveniences. A person who is well advanced in years not infrequently feels that he is isolated from those with whom he dwells. Although for many years he contributed richly to the welfare of the members of his family by wholesome example, sound advice, cheerful companionship, and financial aid, he may now be given the impression that he is looked upon as useless and that he is an unpleasant burden upon those around him. A few years ago he was perhaps very active; now he has nothing with which to occupy his time. Much loneliness may come into his life because his physical infirmities tend to make association with him less attractive to others.

The physician will have to care for many aged persons, and he should take a genuine interest in such patients. Motivated not only by professional duty but also by the virtue of charity, he should apply his skill in an effort to lighten their burden. In this effort he will make use of whatever the rapidly advancing science of geriatrics has to offer. He should endeavor to keep alive their interest in the things around them. Perhaps he could at times suggest some appropriate occupational therapy. To the religious-minded he can point out the singular spiritual value of this period of their life, for it can be of notable help to them in preparing their souls for the life after death and it affords a rich opportunity for acquiring supernatural merit. The physician, as a rule, will be highly respected by those who surround the elderly person, and by both his words and his example he can bring others to realize that true Christians do not regard the aged as either useless or burdensome.

It usually happens that the aged person is being cared for by his children. The physician may find occasion prudently to remind the children that they have the obligation of showing their parents both internal and external affection, and that this duty endures all through their lives. Children must manifest toward their parents genuine respect and fitting deference in their language as well as in their conduct. This duty of filial reverence arises from the fact that this man and this woman are one's father and mother; it does not depend on the presence of the good qualities which parents ordinarily possess. Hence, in regard to this obligation of the child, it matters not whether one's parents have become objects of disgrace, are leading lives of sin, or are burdened with many faults which make them difficult to live with peacefully. They still retain their right to reverence from their children. Even children who are over twenty-one years of age and those who are married must acknowledge their parents' lifelong right to affection and reverence. Adult children, too, would offend against this obligation by heaping on their parents contempt, ridicule, or insult and by unjustly threatening them.

The use of forceful language in regard to one's parents, however, need not in all circumstances imply disrespect. Sharp words employed merely to persuade an aged person to do what is best for him would involve no lack of reverence. Old persons are at times inclined to engage in conduct which would cause them serious injury. In such cases strong words or reprimands and effective brusqueness used to prevent a parent from injuring himself by such a way of acting would not be blameworthy.

The physician, because of his experience, is well aware of the problems which exist in regard to the care of the elderly, and because of his specialized training he can do much to improve the care that is being given. He may rightly be looked to for leadership in suggesting and promoting measures for the efficient, tactful, and sympathetic help of the aged. His cooperation is expected in fostering in adults a fitting attitude toward their aging parents and in actively participating in public projects for the benefit of those who are advanced in years. The physician is as a rule a man of public influence in his community, and the example of his sympathetic and solicitous attitude toward old people cannot but have a wholesome effect on others.

Physicians, if their previous experience has not made it necessary for them to learn about institutions and rest homes in their own area that care for the aged, will know where to turn to obtain this information. If their patients who need to be institutionalized are Catholics, they can inquire either of the chancery office or of the Catholic Charities.[18]

REFERENCES

Bacon, Selden D. "Excessive Drinking and the Institution of the Family." In *Alcohol, Science and Society* (Yale Summer School of Alcohol Studies), pp. 223-38. New Haven: Quarterly Journal of Studies on Alcohol, 1945.

Bradford, Elizabeth. *Let's Talk about Children.* New York: Prentice-Hall, 1947.

Cooper, John M. "Near-Kin Marriages." *Ecclesiastical Review* 87:136-48, 259-72, August, September 1932.

Daley, Edmund F., M.D. "Medical Aspects of Marriage and Child-Bearing." In *Family Today,* pp. 88-95. Washington: Family Life Bureau, National Catholic Welfare Conference, 1944.

"Doctor Needs Cana." *Linacre Quarterly* 16:21-29, January-April 1949.

Etteldorf, Raymond P. "Approach to Sex Education." *Family Digest* 1:21-24, February 1946.

Fleege, Urban H., S.M. *Self-Revelation of the Adolescent Boy.* Milwaukee: Bruce Publishing Company, 1945.

Giminez, V., S.J. "Training the Emotions." *Catholic Mind* 43:612-17, October 1945.

[18] For material on the problems of old age see Robert T. Monroe, M.D., "Medical Problems of Old Age," *New England Journal of Medicine* 240:57-60, January 13, 1949; Max Jacobson, "Old Age Is Your Problem," *Reader's Digest* 57:46-50, November 1950.

Haley, Joseph E., C.S.C. "Instructing to Purity." *American Ecclesiastical Review* 111:428-38, December 1944.

Hierarchy of England and Wales. "'Sex Education,' a statement issued by the hierarchy of England and Wales." *Catholic Mind* 42:460-61, August 1944.

Hunt, Raymond J., O.M.I. "Our 'Emotionally Unfit.'" *Catholic Mind* 43:543-46, September 1945.

Into Their Company. New York: P. J. Kenedy and Sons, 1932.

Jellinek, E. M. "Heredity of the Alcoholic." In *Alcohol, Science and Society* (Yale Summer School of Alcohol Studies), pp. 105-14. New Haven: Quarterly Journal of Studies on Alcohol, 1945.

Jessine, Sister Mary. "Our Children Need Sex Education." *America* 85:376-78, July 14, 1951.

Metropolitan Life Insurance Company. "Marriage and Long Life." *Statistical Bulletin* 18:7-10, February 1937.

———— "The Married Live Longer." *Statistical Bulletin* 24:5-6, July 1943.

———— "Why Married People Live Longer." *Statistical Bulletin* 22:4-7, November 1941.

Popenoe, Paul. "Consanguineous Marriages." *Journal of Heredity* 7:343-46, August 1916.

———— "Marriage of Kin." *Scientific Monthly* 17:427-34, November 1923.

Toomey, John A., M.D. "Learned Doctor Speaks." *Family Digest* 2:35-36, September 1947.

Wilson, Margery. *How To Make the Most of Wife,* chap. 8, "Married Men Really Do Live Longer," pp. 157-75. Philadelphia: J. B. Lippincott Company, 1947.

Chapter ELEVEN

Few things that the physician can do will go farther toward gaining the respect and confidence of his patients, and especially of patients who are critically ill, than a reverential attitude on his part toward religion and a willingness to assist his patients in discharging what they consider to be their obligations. Self-interest alone should therefore prompt the physician to do what he can in this respect, but a still better and stronger motive is the desire to practice the virtue of charity. It is religion that strengthens men and women to live virtuously, to accept as from the hand of God the illnesses that befall them, and to prepare themselves to face the judgment of God when death comes. It is therefore an act of charity to assist patients in receiving the spiritual ministrations that they need and desire.

While there may be occasions when the physician can speak of religious matters in his office—for example, if a disturbed or discouraged patient can well be encouraged to pray with confidence for God's help—our principal concern is with patients who are ill at home or in hospitals and who should receive the sacraments of the Church. In addition to these patients we have the very large number of newborn infants who are in danger of death and who should therefore be baptized. Those who are ill at home or in hospitals receive the sacraments of the Eucharist and extreme unction, in preparation for which they receive the sacrament of penance. Occasionally, if they wish to enter the Church, they receive the sacrament of baptism. The sacraments concerning which it is well for the physician to have some information are baptism, the Eucharist, and extreme unction.

It is not our purpose to discuss these sacraments as would be done in a treatise on theology, but rather to tell the physician what he needs to know concerning them. Since the physician himself can in case of necessity administer baptism, he will need to know more concerning this sacrament. As regards the Eucharist and extreme unction, it will be sufficient if he knows enough to answer intelligently the questions that may be asked and to conduct himself in general in such a manner as to show that he is well informed as to what should be done. Some few things may be said for the purpose of giving the physician a better and helpful understanding of the reasons because of which his Catholic patients attach such importance to these sacraments.

BAPTISM

THE word baptism is derived from a Greek word which means a washing or cleansing. The spiritual cleansing of man through baptism is distinguished according to the three different ways in which it produces grace. There are three kinds of baptism: the baptism of blood, the baptism of desire, and the baptism of water.

Baptism of Blood

Baptism of blood is the act of martyrdom of an unbaptized person. Martyrdom consists in willingly submitting to death inflicted out of hatred of Christ or of His teaching. In the early Church many persons who were preparing for baptism but who had not as yet been baptized became martyrs. Among these martyrs, despite the fact that they were not old enough to accept death willingly, are included the male children two years and under, known as the Holy Innocents, who were massacred by King Herod.

Baptism of Desire

Baptism of desire is an act of perfect love of God made by one who has not yet received the sacrament of baptism. This love must be prompted by God's grace and must be founded on supernatural, not merely natural, motives. When we speak of an act of perfect love of God we do not mean that this act must be exceedingly intense or that it must partake of the holiness of an act of love in some great saint. We mean simply this, that the act of love proceeds from a perfect motive rather than from an imperfect motive. One's motive is perfect if he loves God because God is infinitely perfect in Himself and to be esteemed and obeyed in preference to everything else that exists. One's motive is imperfect if he elects to obey and worship God as God desires because he will be subjected to severe penalties if he refuses to do so.

Anyone who places God first in his scale of values and who is prepared to do whatever God requires of him must have at least an implicit desire of baptism. He may never have heard of baptism, or because of his upbringing he may even have false ideas concerning its necessity; but if he saw clearly that God desired him to be baptized, he would present himself for baptism. Without this willingness he could not be said to have perfect love of God. The act of perfect love of God will moreover in very many cases, if not indeed in the majority of cases, take the form of perfect sorrow or contrition for one's offenses against God.

The baptism of desire is sufficient for salvation, and the reason is that God in His goodness will not cast off anyone who sincerely seeks to serve Him, no matter how erroneous some of his ideas may be. The baptism of desire, however, does not make one a member of the Church nor does it entitle him to receive the other sacraments.

These facts concerning the baptism of desire have a two-fold significance for the physician. In the first place, they will guide him in deciding what he is free to do in the case of an unbaptized adult who is about to die in the state of unconsciousness. Such a person may and in general should be baptized, but conditionally, as we shall explain later. In the second place, knowledge of the effects of the baptism of desire will sometimes make it possible for the physician to offer comfort to the survivors of a patient who has resisted their efforts to lead him into the Church. His refusal may have been due to ignorance or prejudice for which he should not be blamed and which is not incompatible with the baptism of desire.

Baptism of Water

Baptism of water is the sacrament of spiritual rebirth by the ablution of the body with water and through the invocation of the most holy Trinity. It produces a rebirth, for by infusing into his soul the new life of sanctifying grace it makes the recipient a child of God. Moreover, the sacrament of baptism gives the new Christian the title to certain actual graces which he will need for maintaining his baptismal innocence. It takes away original sin and it remits all the actual sins, both mortal and venial, of which the recipient may have been guilty, provided he has at least imperfect sorrow for them. The debt of all temporal punishment for sin is canceled if the person baptized has at least attrition, or imperfect contrition, for all his sins. If his sorrow does not include his venial sins, these remain after baptism and the temporal punishment for them still awaits him. Baptism of water, unlike baptism of desire and baptism of blood, is a sacrament and imprints on the soul its sacramental character. This sacramental character is an indelible mark or seal which is the badge of a special dignity.

Baptism is the most important of the sacraments because it is necessary for salvation. No one can be saved unless he has received baptism of water, of desire, or of blood. Baptism of desire and baptism of blood include the desire for baptism of water. If one, then, is not martyred and does not have perfect love of God, he cannot reach heaven except through the saving waters of this sacrament. A baby, for example, is incapable of baptism of desire. If he dies without baptism, he will never see God. It does not follow that he is condemned to a place of punishment and suffering. He will live in a state of great natural happiness, but he will be excluded from the intuitive knowledge of God and from that participation in God's divinity which are reserved for those who have been raised to a supernatural state by baptism. We will not attempt here to give an explanation of what is called the beatific vision, but will content ourselves with saying that it is the desire of parents and of others to make this beatific vision possible for infants in danger of death which causes them to go to such lengths to provide for their baptism.

Because Catholics realize the very great importance of the sacrament of baptism, they readily recognize their obligation to administer it in the circumstances described above. There can also be an obligation on the part of those who are not of the Catholic faith to baptize dying infants. Everyone has a duty in charity to come to the assistance of another person who is in extreme need. The fetus or infant is in extreme spiritual need if he is dying without baptism or if he is in danger of so dying. Everyone, therefore, no matter what his religious convictions may be, shares in the duty of coming to the assistance of such an infant. It must of course be recognized that some persons simply cannot see the existence of such an obligation and that others not only deny its existence but would consider themselves guilty of moral fault were they to act according to this teaching. As we have mentioned above, each individual must follow the promptings of his own conscience. If his conscience tells him that so to act would be morally wrong, he should of course avoid that course of action. Hence those who are convinced that baptizing a dying infant would be illicit would be guilty of no moral fault in refraining from this act. If a non-Catholic physician has no conscientious objection in this matter, perhaps he might say to himself: "I suppose that the baptism could possibly help. Just as I would use any remedy which offered a chance of life in a desperate case, so I will use this baptism in the hope that it may do some spiritual good for the child." He might remember, too, how very much his action would please parents and near relatives of the infant, who see in baptism an inestimable blessing.

The Water To Be Used in Baptism

The water to be used in baptism is natural water, by which is meant whatever in the common opinion of men is considered to be real water. Water which is found in ocean, lake, river, well, or spring is certainly true natural water. Ice, hail, and snow constitute water if melted. Rain, dew, and distilled water likewise fulfill the definition of true water. Water remains water even if it is muddy, old, or stagnant.

The physician who is called upon to perform a baptism in a home or hospital will under ordinary circumstances find water readily available. It might therefore seem useless for us to say anything concerning liquids that might or might not be considered water, but the reader should remember that we are seeking to make this section a manual for use in emergencies as well as under normal conditions. Emergencies arise constantly. The water supply in a home or hospital may be temporarily cut off. On the battlefield, in cases of train or airplane wreck, after fires, hurricanes, and tornadoes, and in other similar situations it can easily happen that no natural water, or what we would ordinarily call drinking water, is immediately available to the one who wishes to baptize. He may then seek desperately to find some substitute which it is proper for him to use, and he should know what it would be altogether out of order for him to use and what he is free to use with certain restrictions in case of necessity.

Among the liquids that he might think of using but that he is not free to use are fruit and vegetable juices, wine, oil, strong coffee, amniotic fluid, and any secretion of the body, such as saliva or perspiration. The use of any of these would make the baptism certainly invalid. There might be a reasonable doubt concerning tea, weak coffee, beer, and the sap of plants, and these may be used (1) if undoubtedly true water cannot be had, (2) if it is a case of emergency, and (3) if baptism is conferred conditionally. An emergency is considered to exist if there is danger that the person will die without baptism unless he is baptized at once. It is licit under such circumstances to baptize with something that is doubtfully valid because one should do everything possible to confer a sacrament so eminently important. One baptizes conditionally by prefixing to the words of the formula of baptism the words "If you are capable." These words are understood to cover all possible contingencies: If you have not been baptized before; If you can be baptized on this part of your body; If (in the case of an adult dying in the state of unconsciousness) you would wish to be baptized; If you are capable of being baptized with what I am forced to use.

In uterine baptism the physician may, if he wishes, add one one-thousandth part of bichloride of mercury or of some other disinfectant to the water which he is to use.[1]

The Method of Conferring Baptism

In baptizing one should proceed in the following manner. The head of the person to be baptized is tilted forward and turned somewhat to the side. It is well to place a receptacle under the head in order to catch the used baptismal water. The one who is baptizing then slowly pours the water over the recipient's forehead or temple and at the same moment pronounces the formula "I baptize you in the name of the Father, and of the Son, and of the Holy Ghost." The word Amen is not

[1] Decree of the Holy Office. *Acta Sanctae Sedis* 34:319-20, August 21, 1901.

part of the formula and should not be added, but its addition would not render the baptism invalid. The words should be audibly enunciated, but there is no necessity that they should be said in so loud a tone that they can be heard by others. It is essential that the words be pronounced while the water is being poured. There must be no interval, however slight, between the pronouncing of the words and the pouring of the water. If one pours the water and only when this is finished begins to pronounce the words, the baptism is doubtful. The reason is that in this case it is not certain that there is a moral union between the matter and the form. It is very important that one always remember that the pouring of the water and the pronouncing of the words must be simultaneous. This does not mean that they must last exactly the same length of time. It is sufficient for the validity of the sacrament if at least some of the words of the formula are being spoken while the water is being poured.

It is the head which must be baptized, for the head is the principal part of the body. If the water ran off the hair of the head and did not flow along the scalp, the baptism would probably be invalid, and therefore the person must be baptized again conditionally. In order that the baptism be certainly valid, the water must wash the head. Baptism on the hair is doubtful, for it is doubtful whether the hair can be considered part of the head. If one baptizes on a large scab on the head and the water flows over this part alone, the baptism is clearly valid, for the scab is undoubtedly part of the head. If the water were to touch only the head covering, a scarf, silk handkerchief, or ribbon, which the recipient was wearing, the water would not wash the skin and the baptism would not be valid. Baptism should not be administered to a part of the head which is covered with vernix. This cheeselike matter is extraneous to the infant and may be likened to a layer of dirt or to a caul. The physician should wipe the head clean of vernix or any other such substance before baptizing.

361

Baptism which is administered on the shoulder, the breast, the back, or the lower part of the body is doubtfully valid. If, however, the head of the person cannot be reached, one should baptize him on the part nearest the head on which the water can be poured. In such circumstances, when through necessity baptism has been administered on any part other than the head, it must be repeated conditionally on the head if this is at all possible. Baptism on the umbilical cord of an infant seems to be almost certainly invalid; but if no other part can be reached, the umbilical cord may licitly be baptized conditionally. In a sense it is a part of the infant, since it belongs to him; but it may be aptly termed a merely temporary lifeline. There is some slight probability that baptism on this cord would be valid.

In many hospitals the newborn baby is rubbed down with oil, and the question arises whether baptism administered to an infant whose head has been oiled would be valid. In deciding this question we must distinguish as follows. (1) If the oil has been applied recently (for example, within twelve hours), there would be a film of oil over the infant's skin. Hence the water applied in baptism probably would not wash the skin, and so the baptism would be doubtful. (2) If the oil had been applied to the baby more than twelve hours before, it would be at present absorbed by the skin. The skin might now appear oily, but the oil would not create a new surface. The baptism, then, would be valid. In practice, the physician would do well to wipe the forehead of an oiled infant with cotton and pour the water of baptism on the spot thus cleansed.

The Baptism of Fetuses

Any living person who has not already been baptized is capable of receiving the sacrament of baptism. The life of a fetus begins at the first moment of conception, and so according to the more common teaching it becomes at that time a living human being. Consequently fetuses which are but a few weeks old may and should be baptized if they are born alive prematurely.[2] They are to be considered as probably still living unless general putrefaction has set in, for general putrefaction is the only certain sign of death. It is important that mothers, nurses, and physicians keep this clearly in mind, for the eternal life of a baby may depend on their remembering and acting upon this teaching. At times it happens that infants regarded for hours as stillborn are revived and live for many years. Hence, even though the newborn infant is apparently dead, he should be baptized, provided the body has not corrupted. In case the immature fetus, when born, is enclosed in the amniotic sac, it is advisable to baptize in the following manner. Place the fetus in a basin of warm water, tear open the enveloping membranes, and at once pronounce the words, "I baptize you in the name of the Father, and so forth." While this formula is being recited the fetus should be raised out of the water and submerged again, in order that the amniotic fluid may be washed off and that the water may touch the fetus. If there is any doubt whether the infant is alive, the formula should be: "If you are capable, I baptize you in the name of the Father, and so forth." If what is born is a shapeless mass of flesh, but there is some probability of its being a human fetus, it should be baptized conditionally in the same way.

At times there is danger that an infant may die before it is born, and consequently, unless it receives the sacrament of baptism where it now is, it may be deprived forever of the sight of God. In such a case the infant should be baptized conditionally in the mother's womb. Nurses and physicians should

---

[2] Canon 747 states: "Care should be taken that all abortive fetuses, at whatsoever time they are born, be baptized absolutely, if they are certainly alive; conditionally, if doubtfully alive." Baptizing conditionally means baptizing under a condition; for example, "If you are capable." Baptizing absolutely means baptizing unconditionally; that is, without prefixing any condition to the words of the form. Hence the form for conditional baptism is: "If you are capable, I baptize you in the name of the Father, and of the Son, and of the Holy Ghost."

be sure to learn the method of baptizing a baby before it is born. The fetus in utero might be baptized in the following manner. The physician procures a fine syringe and fills it with plain water. After the os uteri is partially dilated, the syringe is introduced through the vagina into the os so that it touches the body (if possible the head) of the fetus. If the membranes (that is, the amnion, chorion, and decidua) still enclose the fetus, a small aperture should be made in these and through this the syringe is passed. The physician then ejects the water so that it washes part of the fetus and at the same time pronounces the words of baptism, "I baptize you in the name of the Father, and of the Son, and of the Holy Ghost." In an emergency, when a syringe is not available, a sponge soaked in water can be employed. The administration of baptism would be successful only if the os uteri can be entered. If there is no dilation of the os, baptism cannot be validly administered in utero. Because it is not certain that a child still in utero is capable of receiving the sacrament, it is to be baptized under the condition "If you are capable."

There are cases in which the baptizing of an immature infant in the womb of a dying mother might cause an abortion. If the infant is viable—that is, if it can live outside the mother's womb—one should proceed with the baptism. But let us suppose that the child is not yet six months old and that consequently, if it leaves the womb, it will certainly die. Is it lawful in such circumstances to confer the sacrament? In this case one should, if possible, administer the baptism so as not to risk causing an abortion. If, however, there is no other way of providing for the spiritual welfare of the child, it seems that one may baptize such a fetus while it is in the womb, even though this act of baptizing will result in an abortion. Here some would apply the principle of the twofold effect.[3] The act of baptizing the child is a good one. From it result two effects;

[3] See Benedictus H. Merkelbach, O.P., *Quaestiones de embryologia et de ministratione baptismatis*, pp. 62-63. Liége: La Pensée Catholique, 1928.

namely, the child's spiritual salvation and the child's loss of temporal life. The good effect is not produced by means of the evil effect, for even though the bad effect did not result, the good effect would be produced. It would not, however, be licit to produce an abortion in order that the infant may be baptized, for this would be to perform an intrinsically evil act. Evil may not be done that good may result. The end does not justify the means.

If a child has been baptized in the womb and then is born alive, he must be baptized again, but conditionally: "If you are capable, I baptize you, and so forth." The reason is that, since baptism in the womb is only probably valid, the child when born is probably not yet baptized effectively. One must therefore always make certain by rebaptizing that the sacrament is conferred.

There are difficult parturitions during which there is grave danger that the infant will not be fully delivered before its death. In such a case the child should be baptized on the part of its body which emerges; for example, on the head, the foot, or the hand. This baptism should be absolute if it is the head which is baptized, but only conditional if any other part is baptized. Afterward, if the baby survives the birth, it should be rebaptized conditionally unless it was baptized upon the emerging head. (See Canon 746.)

The Baptism of Abnormal Infants

Medical history records cases of infants who were physically quite abnormal. Some babies had several heads; others had one head but two bodies. It is important to know what one should do with regard to conferring baptism on infants of this kind. The procedure to be adopted is the following.

1. If there are *two heads* and *two bodies*, one should baptize *both heads* absolutely. The reason is that in this case there are certainly two separate human beings present. The celebrated Siamese twins, Eng and Chang, had two heads and two

bodies. Everyone readily concedes that these twins were two distinct individuals.

2. If there are *two bodies* and only *one head,* one should baptize *the head* absolutely and then baptize *both bodies* conditionally ("If you are capable, I baptize you, and so forth"). The reason is that it is difficult to ascertain which body belongs to the single head. If one were to baptize the head and only one of the bodies, he would run the risk of baptizing both the head and the body of one baby and of allowing the headless body of the other baby to go unbaptized.

3. If there are *two heads* and *one body,* one should baptize *one head* absolutely and then baptize the *other head* conditionally ("If you are capable, I baptize you, and so forth"). The reason is that it is doubtful whether there are two individuals here, and so the second head is baptized conditionally to provide against the possibility that it is the head of a second person.

4. A *double-faced* fetus should be baptized on one forehead absolutely; then on the other forehead conditionally.

5. If there is merely *a headless body,* one should baptize it conditionally ("If you are capable, I baptize you, and so forth"). Even though this mass of flesh has no chest, but only part of the torso and legs, it should be baptized thus, for there is some probability that it is a living human being.

The Baptism by Catholics of Non-Catholic Infants

Catholic teaching stresses the fact that, without the parents' consent, baptism may not be conferred on non-Catholic infants who are in no danger of death. The reason is that the natural law imposes on parents the duty, and so gives them the right, to provide adequately for their children. It is their responsibility to procure, according to the promptings of their consciences, what is necessary for the physical and spiritual welfare of their offspring. Hence they have the right to supervise the religious instruction and care of their children. Unless, then, the parents give their consent, it is not licit to baptize their child if the child is in no danger of death.

If the Catholic position is different in regard to infants who are in danger of death, it is not because the Church seeks in any way her own gain or that she wishes to impose her will on others. The infant in danger of death will in all probability not live, and therefore the Church is not acting with the idea of increasing her membership. Her only desire is to help the infant obtain eternal happiness. Many non-Catholics, whatever their religious affiliations, would wish their child to be baptized in such circumstances. If it should happen that the parents object most strongly to this action, the infant should nevertheless be baptized.

If one were thus to administer the sacrament against the express wishes of the parents, he would not be violating their natural rights. The dying child is in extreme spiritual necessity, and only the conferring on it of baptism can withdraw it from that necessity. The child has the right that no one interfere with his being aided in this extreme necessity, and this right of his prevails over his parents' natural right to supervise his care. Ordinarily speaking, then, every dying child who has not as yet achieved the use of reason should be baptized whether the parents are willing or not. In case it is foreseen that the parents would not consent to the baptism, the sacrament should be administered secretly. If, however, it is impossible to baptize the child secretly and the parents refuse their consent, one should let the matter rest. The reason is clear. If a Catholic openly baptized a dying child against the express wishes of the parents, this act would redound to the harm of the Church. The parents would spread the news of the baptism conferred on their child despite their protests. This story might alienate many from the Church and hinder its normal growth in the community. Consequently, in order to safeguard the common spiritual good, one should in such circumstances refrain from administering the sacrament.

Danger of death means any circumstance in which death is imminent from whatsoever source. The danger which threatens may be serious sickness (pneumonia, cancer), the forces of nature (a stormy sea, an earthquake, a tornado), the hazards of a war zone (presence in a town being bombed), an impending major operation (excision of goiter, gall bladder, or prostate gland). The danger need not be certain. It is enough if there is a well-founded probability of such danger. If there are grounds for believing that such danger is probably present, there is sufficient reason for administering baptism. One may and should, for example, baptize a non-Catholic child who has not reached the age of reason, who has tuberculosis, and who in all probability will not die for several years, provided it is probable that he will die before attaining the use of reason. If any child one or two years of age will probably die before he reaches the age of seven, it is licit to baptize him, even though his non-Catholic parents know nothing about the baptism and even though they are opposed to it.

The Baptism of Dying Adults

The physician—and the same is true of all lay persons—may administer baptism only in an emergency, by which we mean that the patient will probably die before a priest can arrive. Just as the physician may baptize infants under these conditions, so he can baptize adults.

The dying adult may be either conscious or unconscious. One may licitly baptize a dying adult who is conscious provided he desires to receive the sacrament, has sorrow for his sins, and is sufficiently instructed in the truths of the faith. But what of a dying adult who has lapsed into the state of unconsciousness? If such a person probably has elicited the desire for baptism and has sufficient sorrow for his grave misdeeds, there is no difficulty. He may and should be baptized conditionally ("If you are capable, I baptize you, and so forth"). Very likely he has fulfilled these requirements if he has shown himself well disposed toward the Church and has led a moral life. If on the other hand a person has never shown any inclination to become a Christian nor given any indication of repentance for his seriously sinful life, may he, while dying and unconscious, be baptized conditionally? It would seem that the essential requisites are certainly lacking; nevertheless, because there is some slight probability that the required dispositions are present, one may baptize him under the condition, "If you are capable, I baptize you, and so forth." In brief, then, one should remember this rule: It is licit and even preferable to baptize conditionally every dying unbaptized adult who is unconscious, whether he appears to be an impenitent sinner who neither believed in God nor thought of becoming a Catholic, or whether his identity is totally unknown.

The Minister of Baptism

Any man, woman, or child can validly administer the sacrament of baptism provided he or she has the use of reason. This includes even enemies of the Church and those without faith. Except in danger of death, however, no one but a priest may administer this sacrament licitly.

If there are several lay persons present when baptism must be administered in an emergency, a man should be chosen in preference to a woman, and anyone is to be selected in preference to the parents of the one to be baptized. The reason for giving first preference to a man and not to a woman is that the usual minister of the sacrament is a priest, who must be of the male sex. The Church selects anyone in preference to the parents because she wishes to avoid multiplying relationships between parent and child. Between the child and its father and mother there is the relationship resulting from natural birth. If father (or mother) baptized his (or her) own child, an additional relationship between the baptized and the baptizer would arise from his (or her) being the author of the child's spiritual regeneration.

This order of preference in administering baptism may be altered for a good reason. If, for example, the only man who is present is not sure of the proper method of baptizing, a woman who is well instructed in this matter should be chosen as the minister. Moreover, if circumstances are such that the presence of a man would be less becoming, a woman may licitly administer the sacrament.

Godparents

Even in an emergency baptism such as a physician might confer there should be at least one godparent or sponsor. The sponsor should be a baptized person at least thirteen years of age, and should be one who is not excluded by church law as unacceptable for sponsorship. This means in general that the sponsor must be a Catholic in good standing. Moreover, neither the father, mother, nor spouse of the one to be baptized may be the sponsor. The sponsor, however, need not be of the same sex as the infant who is being baptized, but there should not be two male sponsors for a baby girl nor two female sponsors for a baby boy. There should never be more than two sponsors. While baptism is being conferred the sponsor should lay his hand lightly on the shoulder of the one being baptized. The sponsor assumes an obligation of looking after the religious education of the infant should he live and should his parents fail to do so. Baptism may be conferred without a sponsor if it is difficult or inconvenient to find or use one.

Case 163
Double Conditional Baptism

The patient, a woman at term, is admitted to the delivery room. Examination indicates that the fetus is large and hydrocephalic. Fetal heart tones are present. A trocar is inserted into the cranium and 750 cc. of fluid are drained off. The physician baptizes the fetus in utero. Three hours later a living child is spontaneously delivered. It is spinabifida and is again baptized. Did the physician act properly in thus baptizing twice?

Solution. The physician was correct in baptizing the fetus conditionally in utero and in administering a second conditional baptism after the delivery of the child.

Explanation. All baptisms in utero should be conditional, since it is not certain that an unborn child is capable of receiving baptism. The baptism after delivery should likewise be conditional because the child may or may not have already been validly baptized. In both cases the words "If you are capable" should be prefixed to the formula of baptism.

Case 164

Baptism of a Catholic Infant by a Protestant

Dr. H, a Protestant, has just delivered a Catholic patient of an infant who shows no signs at all of life. The mother is under anesthesia and cannot be questioned. No priest is available. Dr. H hesitates to baptize the infant, thinking that a Catholic mother might object to his doing so.

Solution. If Dr. H judges that the infant is actually alive, he should baptize him absolutely. If he judges that it is only possible that the infant may be alive, he should baptize him conditionally.

Explanation. Dr. H need have no scruples concerning the propriety of administering baptism to the infant of a Catholic mother. His baptism is certainly valid provided he intends to administer baptism according to the mind of the Church and uses the correct rite as explained on pages 360-61. The mother would not wish her child to be deprived of baptism. If the mother because of ignorance or prejudice should object later to his action, Dr. H might tell her that any priest would say that he should have acted as he did.

Case 165

Baptism of a Well-Intentioned Adult

The patient, an unbaptized non-Catholic, has been friendly to the clergy and has sent his children to a Catholic school. Moreover, he has been honest in business, faithful to his wife, and religious-minded. Finding him unconscious and at the point of death, the physician baptizes him conditionally.

Solution. The physician acted properly.

Explanation. The patient is evidently desirous of doing his duty, and his failure to be baptized was due to ignorance or to procrastination. Since it is not known, however, that he ever expressed a wish to be baptized, he should be baptized conditionally.

371

Case 166
Baptism of a Prejudiced Adult

The patient, a Quaker 78 years of age, has from childhood been faithful in the practice of his religious duties and enjoys a spotless reputation in the community. For some reason, however, he is bitterly hostile toward the Catholic Church. He is now unconscious and about to die, and the physician wonders whether it is proper to baptize him.

Solution. The patient should be baptized conditionally.

Explanation. It may be assumed that the patient's prejudices are due to misunderstandings. While evidently unprepared to do what the Church says he should do, he is certainly prepared to do what God wishes him to do. He therefore has the necessary dispositions for the reception of baptism. Since there is room for some doubt in the matter, he should be baptized conditionally.

Case 167
Secret Baptism of the Child of Hostile Parents

The child, 2 years of age, is dying at home of leukemia. The physician has suggested that the child be baptized, but the parents have expressed violent opposition to the idea. The physician, seizing an opportunity when no one else is in the sickroom, quickly baptizes the child.

Solution. The physician acted properly.

Explanation. The child is in a state of grave spiritual need. The lack of baptism would affect him for eternity. His right to receive baptism takes precedence over his parents' right to supervise his care. The baptism should be administered absolutely, since as the case is described there is no doubt that the child is capable of being baptized. In such cases the physician, if he never finds himself alone with the child, can place on the child's forehead a piece of cotton well soaked in water, compress it so that some water trickles along the skin, and quietly pronounce the words of baptism.

Case 168
Refraining from Baptizing because of Circumstances

The physician is a Protestant of strong religious convictions. He has suggested to the parents that the dying child be baptized, only to discover that they are irrevocably opposed to the idea. Rendered suspicious by his suggestion, the atheistic parents never leave him alone with the child and watch his every move. The physician then decides that it is best under the circumstances for him to refrain from attempting to baptize the child.

Solution. The physician acted prudently and properly.

Explanation. It was impossible to baptize the child secretly. The physician's attempt to baptize would probably have been interrupted. Even though he knew, however, that he could succeed in his attempt, it would be better for him not to make it. The parents would become still more antagonistic to religion and would have talked to others about the matter. As a consequence a hostile attitude toward baptism would be fostered and spiritual harm to members of the community would result. This spiritual harm would probably outweigh the spiritual harm done to the child by denying him baptism.

Case 169
Conditional Baptism on the Foot

The physician, summoned to the scene of an accident, finds a passenger pinned under the wreckage. So far as the physician can judge, the passenger has been fatally injured. The passenger asks the physician to send for a priest so that he may be baptized, but the priest would almost certainly not arrive in time. The physician, finding that he is unable to reach any other part of the body, conditionally baptizes the passenger on the foot.

Solution. The physician acted properly.

Explanation. With death at hand the physician was qualified to confer baptism. Since he could not reach the head, it was proper for him to baptize on any other part of the body that he could reach. If later he was able to reach the head, he should rebaptize conditionally, since the first baptism was only doubtfully valid.

THE EUCHARIST

THE purpose of this material on the Eucharist is to call the physician's attention to certain points of Catholic practice, so that he may better understand the actions of his Catholic patients, and, when occasion offers, enlighten them regarding privileges with which they may not be acquainted.

The Meaning of the Eucharist

The Eucharist is the sacrament of the body and blood of Christ under the species or appearances of bread and wine for the spiritual refection of souls. In the Eucharist Christ is really present in every part and remains present until that part has corrupted. The act of receiving the Eucharist is known as Communion or Holy Communion; when the Eucharist is received by one who is about to die it is called Viaticum, which word in Latin means provision for a journey.

Christ remains present within the recipient after Communion until the gastric juices of the stomach have changed or, as is said, corrupted the appearances of bread. Since the gastric juices function differently in various individuals and since even in the same individuals they function differently according to different circumstances, it is not possible to say definitely for how long a time Christ is present. The following, though not certain, is perhaps as accurate an estimate as can be given.[4]

1. In a healthy person the species may remain incorrupt perhaps for a half hour or more if he takes no food after Holy Communion, but the host is soon corrupted if he takes a meal after Holy Communion.

2. In a sick person the species may remain unchanged for several hours.

This point regarding the corruption of the species has practical importance when there is question of the use of gastric lavage. Except in case of urgent necessity it would be gravely sinful to use gastric lavage after Holy Communion as long as there is probability of expelling the sacred species.

The Eucharistic Fast

The law of the Church (Canon 858) prescribes that one who wishes to receive Holy Communion be fasting from mid-

---

[4] These statements are based on the common teaching of moralists up to the present time. Recent experimental tests, however, indicate that the complete dissolution of the ingested host occurs much more rapidly than was formerly believed. See Eugene G. Laforet, M.D., and Rev. Thomas F. Casey, "Medical Aspects of the Holy Eucharist: A Physiological and Canonical Study," *Linacre Quarterly* 22:11-17, February 1955. The problem is basically a scientific one. Whatever is scientifically established as fact should of course be followed.

night. By the term "fasting from midnight" is meant that no food or drink is consumed from the time of the previous midnight of the day when Holy Communion is received. The new law of the Church,[5] however, makes one general and important exception in this matter, for it now decrees that any quantity of plain water may be taken without violating the fast. The reason for the prescribed fast is the safeguarding of reverence toward the Holy Eucharist. Since, however, this law is purely ecclesiastical in origin, the Church undoubtedly has the power to relax or to abrogate the law just as she sees fit. Ever eager to promote the spiritual welfare of all her children, she has judged it wise actually to modify this law. The exceptions which will interest the physician concern (1) those who are in danger of death and (2) the sick. We shall now discuss these important exceptions to the general law of fasting.

Privileges Granted Those in Danger of Death

Those who are in danger of death from whatsoever cause are by ecclesiastical law (Canon 858, 1) released from the obligation of the Eucharistic fast. This danger need not be certain. If it is probably present, one is not bound to fast. The threatened danger may arise from any cause whatsoever. The source of the danger may be, for example, gangsters, a judicial death sentence, blood poisoning, a grave wound, and so forth. One who is in danger of death may use this dispensation even if he could with no inconvenience fast before receiving Holy Communion, for the law unconditionally excuses him from the fast. To fast when this would cause him no marked inconvenience would nevertheless be praiseworthy.

Privileges Granted Those Who Are Sick

The law of the Church permits a certain relaxation of the strict fast in favor of the sick. The "strict fast" means the

[5] See the apostolic constitution *Christus Dominus* of January 6, 1953. In *Acta Apostolicae Sedis* 45:47-56, January 16, 1953.

abstention from all food and drink, water of course being permitted. If one is sick and if his sickness would cause a moderately grave inconvenience in the observance of the strict fast, he may with his confessor's consent take medicine and liquids. No alcoholic drink, however, no matter how small the quantity, is permitted. The patient may take medicine and liquids as often and in as large a quantity as he wishes. There is in this no limitation of time, and therefore he may continue taking the medicine and liquids up to the moment immediately before receiving Holy Communion. The word medicine, although it excludes anything of an alcoholic nature, includes pills, tablets, jelloids, syrups, and everything else, whether it be solid or liquid, as long as it is medicine in the technical sense of the term. The word liquids includes everything that partakes of the nature of drink or liquid food. In this category are included tea, coffee (even with cream and sugar), ginger ale, fruit and vegetable juices, cocoa, milk, malted milk, milk shake, eggnog, raw eggs, syrups, broth, creamed soup, and soup into which are mixed small particles of bread or crackers.[6]

EXTREME UNCTION

IN SPEAKING of extreme unction we will confine ourselves to those things which it is helpful for the physician to understand. Our purpose in saying something about its effects is to give the physician a better appreciation of the reasons because of which their Catholic patients attach such importance to the sacrament.

The Nature and Effects of Extreme Unction

Extreme unction may be defined as a sacrament by which the gravely ill are strengthened through the anointing and the prayer of the priest. It is called extreme unction because it is the last sacred anointing which the Christian receives. The

[6] See John C. Ford, S.J., *New Eucharistic Legislation*, pp. 74-84. New York: P. J. Kenedy and Sons, 1953.

first unction is had in the sacrament of baptism, the next in confirmation, and the final one is received at the end of one's life. Like the other six, this sacrament was instituted by Christ to care for a particular need of the faithful. The effects of extreme unction are as follows.

1. It imparts sanctifying grace and the actual graces which are peculiar to this sacrament. These graces are special helps to fortify the sick person against the many severe temptations which may occur at the time of death. These temptations may include despair of God's mercy, resentment because of the injuries suffered during life, lack of resignation to God's will, and other temptations to which the individual is peculiarly subject. When a patient is so ill as to be in danger of death, it is more difficult for him to resist temptation because of the weakened condition of his body.

2. It remits all unforgiven sins, both mortal and venial, if the sick person has at least imperfect contrition for them. If a dying Catholic adult is unconscious and in the state of mortal sin, extreme unction will remit his sin provided he is sorry for his sins, even though he does not regain consciousness before he dies. As long as he has at least attrition or imperfect sorrow for his grievous faults, extreme unction will, by restoring his friendship with God, enable him to reach heaven.

3. It takes away the remnants of one's sins. These "remnants" consist of the weakness of will and the spiritual sloth which are contracted from past sins and of temporal punishment due to one's sins.

4. It helps the patient to accept with resignation the pain, inconvenience, and anxieties attendant upon his sickness. We know that the sick often tend to chafe under their sufferings and to cry out against God for sending them so much pain and sorrow. Extreme unction provides them with the light and strength to overcome such inclinations.

5. It restores health to the body if that is most conducive to the sick person's eternal salvation. Some physicians, even though they are not Catholics, make it their custom to summon a priest at once whenever they are called to attend a Catholic patient who is gravely ill.

Since extreme unction so richly benefits the dying, one may judge how important it is not to risk depriving a sick person of this sacrament. One should not wait until the patient has lapsed into unconsciousness, for the spiritual fruits are much greater when the recipient realizes that he is receiving the sacrament. Moreover, if before summoning the priest one waits until the patient is hopelessly beyond recovery, he is preventing the sacrament from producing one of its not infrequent effects; namely, the cure of the recipient. Many a time this sacrament has brought about changes in the patient's physical condition which were quite remarkable and could not be satisfactorily explained by physicians in a natural way.

Giving Warning of Death

The physician is obliged to warn the patient or his near relatives of the danger of death, so that the dying person may arrange his spiritual and temporal affairs. In the case of Catholic patients his warning will prompt the relatives of the sick man to call a priest to administer the last rites. If they fail to do this, the physician himself should summon the priest. He should gently inform the non-Catholic patients of their danger of dying and remind them that they may soon find themselves in God's presence. The physician would do well if he tried to excite in the patient sorrow for the faults which he committed during his life.

The obligation of warning the patient, which is one of charity, would not exist in the following circumstances: (1) if the warning would cause the physician serious inconvenience; (2) if the warning is entirely unnecessary (because, for example, the patient is already well aware of his condition); (3) if the warning would prove useless (because the patient would ignore it completely); (4) if the warning would prove harmful (because it would deeply disturb a patient who is already well prepared to die, or would drive the patient to despair or risk his committing suicide). When the obligation to warn exists the physician must inform the patient at once if death may come within a short time (for example, within a few days). If, however, death is not imminent and if the patient at present is not in a good mood to receive such news, the warning may be postponed until a more suitable time. If withholding the information does not interfere with his preparation for death, there is no necessity of describing the source of the danger of death to the patient.

The physician who wishes to aid his dying patients spiritually will find that they will be much helped by a card containing a few simple prayers prepared by Monsignor Markham. This card for the sick and dying, acceptable to both Catholic and non-Catholic, costs but a few cents and is available not only in English but in twenty-four foreign languages.[7]

Because they fear that the administration of extreme unction will frighten the patient and make his condition worse, the relatives of a dying person at times delay too long before calling a priest. This fear is for the most part unfounded. Well-instructed Catholics realize that if their condition is somewhat grave, they have a right to the special aid of this sacrament. Instead of unduly exciting the sick man, extreme unction often enough brings him peace and calmness. If in an extraordinary case the physician believes that his patient would become unduly alarmed, he should inform the priest of this apprehension. The priest will administer the sacrament in a manner so as to prevent any such undesirable reaction.

Who May Receive Extreme Unction

It is well for the physician to know who may receive extreme unction, for otherwise he may cause himself embarrass-

[7] Copies may be obtained from Sisters of the Poor of St. Francis, St. Clare Convent, Hartwell, Cincinnati 15, Ohio.

ment by suggesting that extreme unction be given in cases in which it cannot be given. In order to be capable of receiving this sacrament one must fulfill three conditions.

1. He must be baptized. The recipient must be baptized because baptism is the gateway to the Church. The physician may of course safely assume that all his Catholic patients have been baptized.

2. The recipient must be capable of committing sin, though it is not required that he should actually have committed any sin. Children who are not yet able to reason and those who have been insane from birth are incapable of sinning and therefore cannot receive extreme unction. The physician should be on his guard against suggesting that a very young child be given extreme unction. If a distraught mother should ask whether she had not better call the priest to give the last sacraments, the physician can make a good impression by explaining why extreme unction cannot be given.

3. The recipient must now be dangerously ill. It is not sufficient that the recipient be in danger of death, as might happen when a city is being bombed in time of war or when a tornado is approaching; he must be in present danger of death from *sickness*. By sickness is understood in this connection, not only the commonly recognized serious illnesses, but also old age, wounds and injuries sustained in war or in accidents, electric shock, and difficult childbirth.

It is obvious that one who is in danger of death must be still alive and not already dead. It is therefore of very practical moment for the physician, since he may often be in a position in which he should or should not suggest that a priest be called, to keep in mind the facts concerning apparent death as opposed to true death.

Since a dying man may still be alive after the usual tests indicate that he is dead, it is uncertain at what moment death actually occurs. In some cases, for example, though the heart has ceased to beat, massage will bring back its activity. The lungs may fail to function any longer, but nevertheless the patient is sometimes still capable of being revived. Medical journals give instances of those who were restored to life after apparently being dead for many hours. Fetuses, for example, and newborn infants have been judged to be dead, only to be revived five or six hours afterward.[8] There is on record the case of a hospital nurse who took a lethal dose of morphine and veronal. She swallowed the poison on the evening of October 27, 1919, and wandered about the streets until, unconscious, she fell to the pavement. When she was found the next morning the body was deathly pale. There was no pulse, no respiration, no heartbeat. The trunk and limbs were partially stiff and there was complete absence of reflexes. The body was sent to an undertaking establishment and placed, just as it was, in a coffin. Fourteen hours afterward a lawyer came to identify the body. The coffin was opened and it was noted that the girl's cheeks were blue. There was a slight movement of the head and there were present faint heart sounds. The patient was at once sent to a hospital and on November 3, seven days after the attempted suicide, she was well on the road to complete recovery.[9]

For how long a period after a person takes his last breath or after his heart stops is he to be considered as probably still alive? We must distinguish between those whose death was preceded by a protracted illness and those who were in good health until overtaken by a fatal accident. During their sickness those of the first category usually suffer a general weakening of their bodies and the progressive destruction of their vital organs. When the heart or the lungs finally fail, their physical structure is too debilitated to survive for long, and death soon occurs. With the second class, however, when the fatal blow

---

[8] See Austin O'Malley, M.D., *The Ethics of Medical Homicide and Mutilation*, pp. 83-91. New York: Devin-Adair Company, 1919.

[9] See "The Apparently Dead," *Catholic Medical Guardian* 6:83-84, July 1928. See also Juan B. Ferreres, S.J., *Death, Real and Apparent in Relation to the Sacraments* (St. Louis: B. Herder Book Company, 1906).

came their vital organs were strong and vigorous, and so these organs will usually continue to function for some time after death seems to be present. The period, therefore, during which the patient is merely dead in appearance varies with different patients. As long as there is any probability, even slight, that true death is not as yet present, the victim should be given the sacrament of extreme unction conditionally.

The only certain sign of death is the general putrefaction of the body. General putrefaction is manifested by the appearance on the skin of blisters and elevations of a dark green color. The rule regarding the administration of extreme unction, then, is this: The patient may and should be anointed unless general putrefaction has begun. If there is doubt about the presence of general putrefaction, the patient should be anointed conditionally. A safe norm for judging when extreme unction may licitly be administered is the following. The patient may be anointed (1) within one hour after apparent death when death results from a long-drawn-out infirmity (tuberculosis, cancer, and the like); (2) within four hours after apparent death when death results from a sudden accident (lightning, drowning, fire, wounding, hemorrhage, apoplexy, asphyxiation, cholera, and the like).

This time norm merely indicates the amount of time after apparent death before general putrefaction usually begins. In a particular case, if the general corruption of the body has not as yet begun at a time beyond these limits, extreme unction may be licitly administered. Even in cases of protracted illness the final cause of death is at times a sudden straining, a fall, or some other accident. Apparent death then comes before the organs have been worn out.

Even if a person is apparently dead, his friends and relatives should summon a priest to minister to him. When one is about to leave this world it is important that he be spiritually fortified in every way possible. A man who is now unconscious and who will not regain the use of his senses before death may be in the state of mortal sin. If he has at least attrition for his faults, extreme unction will restore him to God's friendship. If such a person were to die without the sacraments, he would never reach heaven. One should, therefore, remember that a dying man's eternal salvation may depend upon the cooperation of those who are attending him in his last illness.

Case 170
Administration of Extreme Unction after Apparent Death

Mr. N, a Catholic businessman, has been killed instantly by a train. He is taken to the nearest hospital and pronounced dead. A nurse who recognizes him sends for a priest to administer extreme unction.

Solution. The nurse acted properly.

Explanation. In cases of death from accident it is licit to administer extreme unction within four hours after apparent death. While it is very probable that real death has occurred, there is some possibility that life is still present. Even a slight possibility is sufficient to justify the administration, conditionally, of extreme unction.

Encouraging the Faith of Patients in Prayer

The usual way in which diseases, broken bones, and other bodily ailments are cured is through the use of natural remedies and the aid of qualified physicians. These are the ordinary means which are available for the care of our health, and God intends us to make use of them. There is, however, no reason for asserting that the Author of nature cannot, if He so wills, make use of extraordinary methods of cure. He is omnipotent and can interfere with the habitual way in which the physical cause of a thing reacts. Anyone with a correct concept of God must believe in the possibility of miracles. Technically a miracle is defined as a fact, perceivable by the senses of the body, which cannot be achieved by a natural cause and which must be due to God's extraordinary intervention.

The physician should acknowledge at least the possibility of miracles, and, given adequate proof in a particular case, admit its actuality. There have been, and still are, cases of seemingly wondrous cures in which a prudent analysis of the facts made it clear that the alleged miracles were due to fraud or hysteria or perhaps even to diabolic influence.[10] Some genuinely miraculous happenings, however, have occurred, which careful scientific investigations have proved that the Author of nature alone could have produced. The fully documented testimony of a group of highly qualified physicians, Catholic and non-Catholic, on this point is incontestable.[11] Many miracles are recorded in the Old Testament and many in the New Testament.[12] For those who, like the Roman Catholics, believe that the Bible is the word of God Himself and therefore that it cannot assert as true what is false, the scriptural proof is sufficient to establish the fact that true miracles are possible.

The physician will therefore not smile condescendingly if his gravely ill patients and their relatives and friends pray that health may be restored through a miracle. In His infinite wisdom God does not work miracles too frequently, yet He does work them. There is also good reason for believing that God often answers prayers by causing the physician's therapies to be more effective, yet not in such a way that the cure must certainly be attributed to God's intervention rather than to the care of the physician. The physician should be happy when he finds his patients praying for their recovery and should encourage them to do so when the occasion seems opportune. If

---

[10] See Herbert Thurston, S.J., *The Physical Phenomena of Mysticism,* edited by J. H. Crehan, S.J. (Chicago: Henry Regnery Company, 1952). This is a very exacting scientific analysis of curious happenings such as stigmatization, bodily elongation, levitation, luminosity, and the like which have often been associated with holy persons and which have been judged by not a few to be miraculous.

[11] See Prosper Gustave Boissarie, *Heaven's Recent Wonders* (Cincinnati: Frederick Pustet Company, 1909); Bruno F. de Grandmaison, *Twenty Cures at Lourdes* (St. Louis: B. Herder Book Company, 1920). For a recent report of well-qualified French physicians on the cures at Lourdes see Peter Flood, O.S.B., M.D., editor, *New Problems in Medical Ethics,* pp. 147-246 (Cork: Mercier Press, 1953).

[12] In the Old Testament see 4 Kings 6:5-7; Daniel 3:24. In the New Testament see Luke 24:39-43.

faith in the power of prayer did nothing else, it would increase a patient's courage and confidence; and this is something which should be earnestly desired by every physician who believes that all disease is to some extent psychosomatic.

CHURCH LAWS

THE Catholic Church has framed certain laws for the spiritual welfare of her members. In order to insure the performance of their obligation of worshiping God, she prescribes the hearing of Mass on Sundays and holydays of obligation. In order to foster the spirit of penance, she has established laws regarding certain days on which the use of meat is forbidden or on which only one full meal may be taken. The Church, however, is not unreasonably exacting in her demands; and therefore, if the observance of any of these ecclesiastical laws would involve a moderately grave inconvenience for one of the faithful, she excuses him from the obligation. For this reason, then, the sick and the convalescent who would find it difficult to fast or to attend Mass on Sundays or holydays are excused from the observance of these laws. If fasting would cause one severe headache, dizziness, or notable insomnia, he is excused from the law. Patients, moreover, who require a meat diet for their recovery need not observe the abstinence prescribed for Fridays, ember days, and certain vigils.

The Physician's Right To Declare a Patient Excused

In not a few instances a Catholic patient will consult his physician about the advisability of his fasting, abstaining from meat, or attending Sunday Mass. If the physician judges that the fulfilling of the obligations imposed by these laws would constitute a serious inconvenience for the patient, given the latter's present condition, he may inform the patient that he is excused for the time being from these church precepts. On the one hand, the physician should not magnify a slight sickness into an excusing cause in order to favor the patient, for this would be dishonest; but on the other hand, he must avoid being too severe in his judgments.

Priest Patients

The physician will at times have the care of priest patients. Sick priests also are of course included in what was said on page 385 regarding those who are excused from the laws of fasting, abstinence, and the hearing of Mass on Sundays and holydays. The church law, however, imposes on priests an additional obligation, that of reciting every day a certain portion of a book which is called the Breviary. The fulfillment of this obligation, which is termed that of the Divine Office, requires about one hour's time each day. For his own information, it is well for the physician to know in which circumstances the priest is excused from the obligation of reciting the Breviary.

A priest need not recite the Divine Office if this (1) would prove to be a moderately grave hardship; or (2) would involve a severe strain on his eyes; or (3) would probably produce a general weakening effect. If a patient is confined to bed because of his weakened condition, he is excused; or (4) would probably cause pain or headache severe enough to prevent his fulfilling his ordinary duties; or (5) would delay ridding the patient of his fever; or (6) would probably bring on periods of grave pain (because, for example, of the position required for reading the Office); or (7) would expose the patient to the danger of a relapse or of catching cold.

Even if the patient is able, during a great part of the day, to read newspapers, magazines, and books, he might still be excused from the Breviary, for the latter requires greater attention and therefore tends to fatigue the reader. The reading of light matter such as newspapers brings little strain and has a recreative effect.

A patient who is convalescing from a grave ailment is excused from the obligation of the Office for some days, in order that he may fully recover his normal strength. Much depends, of course, on the disposition of the particular patient, for some, because of their enfeebled constitution, are more readily weakened than others.

The physician will probably discover that priests as a class are men of independent judgment who are sometimes not quite so tractable as other patients. For this reason and also because of their piety they frequently insist on saying their Office or on celebrating or at least attending Mass when their physical condition makes this highly inadvisable. In such situations the physician may gain little by merely insisting that he be obeyed. It is better for him to tell his patient that he will pray better and for more years and that he will celebrate Mass more frequently if he takes proper care of his health. The physician may also tell his patient that he has a duty to his flock, who will be the better served the more quickly their pastor recovers his health. He may ask him what he himself would tell a mother who by failing to take proper care of her health was endangering the welfare of her children. Arguments such as these will frequently produce a far better effect than the dogmatic issuance of orders which are resented.

It should be noted that, in all these cases, the physician is not *dispensing* a patient from a church law. The power to dispense belongs only to church authorities. What the physician does is to declare that the patient is *excused*. Catholic teaching makes it clear that the Church's laws concerning fasting, abstaining, attending or celebrating Mass, and saying the Divine Office are not meant to bind when serious inconvenience or injury to health would result. A patient may decide for himself that he is excused and often does so decide when seriously ill. Patients, however, sometimes hesitate to decide in their own favor and seek the counsel of someone competent to advise them. In matters pertaining to health the physician is more competent than anyone else. In expressing his judgment he says, first of all, that the patient is *free* to take advantage of the exemption. Whether or not the patient is *obliged* to take advantage of the exemption is another matter. The patient is obliged in conscience (see pages 60-63) to use ordinary means for the preservation of his health. If the physician thinks that failure to use the exemption would result in such serious harm that the patient would be at fault morally, he is free to say so.

Case **171**

Declaring a Patient Excused from Sunday Mass

The patient, an adult male, is convalescing at St. Mary's Hospital from an attack of influenza. The physician tells him that he may go home on Sunday afternoon but advises him not to go to the hospital chapel on Sunday morning for Mass. Is the physician justified in assuming that this patient need not attend Sunday Mass?

Solution. If the physician believes that attending Mass would be injurious to the patient's health, he may licitly pronounce him excused from the obligation of attending Mass.

Explanation. There are some circumstances involved in attending Mass which might exert a bad influence on a patient's health and impede his convalescence. The evil effect might be foreseen from the fact that he would have to be with a large number of others in the chapel, or that the chapel was too cold or drafty, or that the strain of sitting up for so long a period would prove weakening—any of these, or some similar condition could constitute a reason that would suffice to release the patient from the duty of hearing Mass on Sunday or a holyday of obligation.

Cremation and Burial

The law of the Catholic Church (Canon 1203) not only requires that the bodies of deceased Catholics be buried, but it expressly forbids their cremation. Even the bodies of immature fetuses, of whatsoever age they may be, are as a rule to be buried. These fetuses were living human beings, and therefore their bodies should receive fitting burial.

There is of course nothing about burning human corpses which is considered to be evil of its very nature; but in order to inculcate in the faithful due respect for their bodies as

388

temples of the Holy Ghost and as instruments through which one can reach heaven, the Church commands her subjects to inter the bodies of deceased Christians. An additional reason for this command is to offset the teachings of certain enemies of religion. Some of these endeavor to spread the practice of cremation in order to destroy belief in the immortality of the soul and in the resurrection of the body at the Last Judgment. Even from the viewpoint of the civil government, cremation is not desirable, for it makes judicial exhumation impossible. In cases of crime, cremation destroys toxic salts and alkaloids such as morphine and eliminates all trace of violence. Postburial examinations of the body of the deceased have in the past saved innocent persons who were under suspicion and brought about the conviction of the guilty.

With regard to the disposal of dead fetuses, the general rule is that, if the parents of the fetus are Catholic, it should be buried. It may, however, be burned in the following cases: (1) if cremation is necessary in order to avoid the danger of contagion; (2) if the cost of burial would be far more than the parents can afford; (3) if the legal formalities required for burial would cause much inconvenience or loss of time; (4) if burial, because of the required death certificate, would create the risk of revealing the sin of an unmarried mother. The reason that in the above-mentioned circumstances the fetus may be cremated is that the law which prescribes Christian burial is of purely ecclesiastical origin. If, then, in a particular case its fulfillment would involve grave inconvenience not intrinsic to the law, the law would cease to bind the subject. In some states, however, the civil law requires that any fetus which is over five months of age be buried. In not a few places a charitable organization (for example, St. Vincent de Paul Society) will, if the parents of the child cannot do so, defray the expenses which proper burial involves. The practice of preserving fetuses in jars for educational purposes is licit provided no irreverence or desecration is intended.

The church law demands the interment not only of the entire body of the deceased; but it requires the burial of even notable parts which have been excised from living persons. A member of the body which is of notable size and which is recognizable as a part of a human being must be buried. If, however, the amputated member is small (for example, a finger, an ear, an eye, or a female breast) or if it is no longer recognizable as a part of a human being (for example, a leg or an arm so badly crushed that it is but a mass of flesh and bone), it need not be buried. Internal organs such as the appendix, a kidney, the spleen, the uterus, an ovary, the stomach, need not be buried. What is here said applies to the parts of cadavers that have been dissected in medical schools, but the parts that should be buried may be cremated if burial would involve too great inconvenience.

REFERENCES

Arendzen, J. P. *What Becomes of the Dead?* "Limbo of the Children," pp. 145-61. St. Louis: B. Herder Book Company, 1925.

Barry, David. "Warning the Sick of Approaching Death." *Ecclesiastical Review* 63:126-34, August 1920.

Bouscaren, T. Lincoln, S.J. *The Canon Law Digest*, vol. I, pp. 564-66. Milwaukee: Bruce Publishing Company, 1934.

—— and Adam C. Ellis, S.J. *Canon Law*, pp. 602-03. Milwaukee: Bruce Publishing Company, 1946.

Devlin, William. "Cremation." *Catholic Encyclopedia*, vol. IV, pp. 481-83.

FitzGibbons, Gerald H., S.J. *Spiritual First Aid Procedures.* St. Louis: The Queen's Work, 1950.

Hassett, Maurice M. "Eucharist." *Catholic Encyclopedia*, vol. V, pp. 572-90.

Heinz, Gerald. "Effects of Extreme Unction." *Homiletic and Pastoral Review* 40:1227-32, August 1940.

Joyce, G. H., S.J. *Question of Miracles.* London: Manresa Press, 1914.

Kelly, Gerald, S.J. "Disposal of Amputated Members." *Linacre Quarterly* 15:51-55, July 1948.

Kelly, Gerald, S.J. *Medico-Moral Problems,* pt. 3, "Adult Baptism," pp. 36-45. St. Louis: Catholic Hospital Association of the United States and Canada, 1951.

—— *Medico-Moral Problems,* pt. 2, "Should the Cancer Patient Be Told?" pp. 7-9. St. Louis: Catholic Hospital Association of the United States and Canada, 1950.

—— "Should We Baptize Dying Adults?" *Review for Religious* 4:49-59, January 1945.

Labauche, L. *Three Sacraments of Initiation,* "Eucharist," pp. 169-500. New York: Benziger Brothers, 1922.

Lewis, C. S. *Miracles.* New York: The Macmillan Company, 1947.

McAllister, Joseph B., S.S. *Emergency Baptism.* Milwaukee: Bruce Publishing Company, 1945.

McCarthy, John. "Morality of Cremation—Catholic Teaching." *Irish Ecclesiastical Record* 65:188-92, March 1945.

Markham, Raphael J. "Apostolate To Assist the Dying." *Ecclesiastical Review* 87:130-36, August 1932.

Murray, Gerald C., C.SS.R. "Greater Esteem of Extreme Unction." *Catholic Mind* 43:174-78, March 1945.

O'Connor, William R. "Is the Limbo of Infants an Hypothesis?" *Homiletic and Pastoral Review* 47:373-79, February 1947.

—— "Lot of Infants Who Die without Baptism." *Ecclesiastical Review* 95:37-49, 152-64, July, August 1936.

Schaefers, William. "Catholic Physicians and the Sacrament of Extreme Unction." *Ecclesiastical Review* 91:469-74, November 1934.

"Telling a Patient He Is Going To Die." *Ecclesiastical Review* 86:637-39, June 1932.

Toner, P. J. "Extreme Unction." *Catholic Encyclopedia,* vol. V, pp. 716-30.

Van Roo, William A., S.J. "Infants Dying without Baptism: Survey of Recent Literature and Determination of the State of the Question." *Gregorianum* 35:406-73, 1954.

Walsh, James J., M.D., "Life and Death and the Sacraments." *Ecclesiastical Review* 93:36-44, July 1935.

CODES OF ETHICS

For the benefit of physicians who may wish to have them available for consultation, we here reproduce the declarations of ethical principles that have been published by three influential groups. These groups are the Catholic Hospital Association of the United States and Canada, the American Medical Association, and the American College of Surgeons.

ETHICAL AND RELIGIOUS DIRECTIVES FOR CATHOLIC HOSPITALS[1]

INTRODUCTION

RESPONSIBILITY OF HOSPITAL AUTHORITIES

1. Catholic hospitals exist to render medical and spiritual care to the sick. The patient adequately considered, and inclusive of his spiritual status and his claim to the helps of the Catholic religion, is the primary concern of those entrusted with the management of Catholic hospitals. Trustees and administrators of Catholic hospitals understand that this responsibility extends to every patient and that it is seriously binding in conscience. A partial statement of this basic obligation is contained in these Ethical and Religious Directives. All who associate themselves with a Catholic hospital, and particularly the members of the medical and nursing staffs, must understand the moral and religious obligations binding on those responsible for the management and operation of the hospital

[1] With permission of the Catholic Hospital Association of the United States and Canada.

393

and must realize that they are allowed to perform only such acts and to carry out only such procedures as will enable the owners and administrators to fulfill their obligations.

VITALITY OF DIRECTIVES

2. The principles underlying or expressed in these Directives are not subject to change. But in the application of principles the Directives can and should grow and change as theological investigation and the progress of medical science open up new problems or throw new light on old ones.

EXTENT OF PROHIBITIONS

3. As now formulated, the Directives prohibit only those procedures which, according to present knowledge of facts, seem certainly wrong. In questions legitimately debated by theologians, liberty is left to physicians to follow the opinions which seem to them more in conformity with the principles of sound medicine.

SOLUTIONS OF MORAL DOUBTS

4. Cases can arise in which the morality of some procedure is doubtful, either because the Directives do not seem to cover the case or because their application is not clear. In such cases, consultation is obligatory, if possible; and the hospital reserves the right to insist on this and to choose or to approve the consultants. In urgent cases that allow no time for consultation, the physician in charge should do what seems most proper to his own conscience. Having done what he honestly judges best in such an emergency, the physician has no just cause for anxiety of conscience; but he should refer the matter to the hospital authorities to obtain guidance for future emergencies of the same nature.

SECTION I: ETHICAL DIRECTIVES

GENERAL

5. These Ethical Directives concern all patients, regardless of religion, and they must be observed by all physicians, nurses, and others who work in the hospital.

6. Even the procedures listed in this section as permissible require the consent, at least reasonably presumed, of the patient or his guardians. This condition is to be understood in all cases.

7. Everyone has the right and the duty to prepare for the solemn moment of death. Unless it is clear, therefore, that a dying patient is

already well-prepared for death as regards both temporal and spiritual affairs, it is the physician's duty to inform him of his critical condition or to have some other responsible person impart this information.

8. Adequate consultation is required, not only when there is doubt concerning the morality of some procedure (as stated in n. 4), but also with regard to all procedures involving serious consequences, even though such procedures are listed here as permissible. The hospital reserves the right to insist on such consultation.

9. The physician is required to state definitely to the supervisor of the department concerned the nature of the operation he intends to perform or of the treatment he intends to give in the hospital.

10. All structures or parts of organs removed from patients must be sent at once and in their entirety to the pathologist for his examination and report. If the physician requests it, the specimens will be returned to him after examination.

(NOTE: In the event of an operation for the removal of a diseased organ containing a living fetus, the fetus should be extracted and baptized before the excised organ is sent to the pathologist.)

11. The obligation of professional secrecy must be carefully fulfilled not only as regards the information on the patients' charts and records but also as regards confidential matters learned in the exercise of professional duties. Moreover, the charts and records must be duly safeguarded against inspection by those who have no right to see them.

DIRECTIVES CONCERNING SPECIFIC PROCEDURES

I. Procedures Involving Serious Risk to, or Destruction of, Life

12. The direct killing of any innocent person, even at his own request, is always morally wrong. Any procedure whose sole immediate effect is the death of a human being is a direct killing.

13. Risk to life and even the indirect taking of life are morally justifiable for proportionate reasons. Life is taken indirectly when death is the unavoidable accompaniment or result of a procedure which is immediately directed to the attainment of some other purpose, e.g., to the removal of a diseased organ.

14. Every unborn child must be regarded as a human person, with all the rights of a human person, from the moment of conception.

15. Direct abortion is never permitted, even when the ultimate purpose is to save the life of the mother. No condition of pregnancy constitutes an exception to this prohibition. Every procedure whose sole immediate effect is the termination of pregnancy before viability is a direct abortion.

16. Operations, treatments, and medications during pregnancy which have for their immediate purpose the cure of a proportionately serious pathological condition of the mother are permitted when they cannot be safely postponed until the fetus is viable, even though they indirectly cause an abortion.

17. Regarding the treatment of hemorrhage during pregnancy and before the fetus is viable: Procedures that are primarily designed to empty the uterus of a living fetus still attached to the mother are not permitted; procedures primarily designed to stop hemorrhage (as distinguished from those designed precisely to expel the living and attached fetus) are permitted insofar as necessary, even to the extent of risking an abortion. In this case the abortion would be indirect.

18. Cesarean section for the removal of a viable fetus is permitted, even with some risk to the life of the mother, when necessary for successful delivery. It is likewise permitted, even with some risk for the child, when necessary for the safety of the mother.

19. Cranial and other operations for the destruction of fetal life are forbidden. Procedures designed to preserve fetal life (e.g., aspiration for hydrocephalus) are permitted even before delivery when such procedures are medically indicated.

20. In extrauterine pregnancy the affected part of the mother (e.g., an ovary or Fallopian tube) may be removed, even though the life of the fetus is thus indirectly terminated, provided the operation cannot be postponed without notably increasing the danger to the mother.

21. Euthanasia ("mercy killing") in all its forms is forbidden.

22. The failure to supply the ordinary means of preserving life is equivalent to euthanasia.

23. It is not euthanasia to give a dying person sedatives merely for the alleviation of pain, even to the extent of depriving the patient of the use of sense and reason, when this extreme measure is judged necessary. Such sedatives should not be given before the patient is properly prepared for death (in the case of a Catholic, this means the reception of the Last Sacraments); nor should they be given to patients who are able and willing to endure their sufferings for spiritual motives.

24. Hysterectomy, in the presence of pregnancy and even before viability, is permitted when directed to the removal of maternal pathology which is distinct from the pregnancy and which is of such a serious nature that the operation cannot be safely postponed until the fetus is viable.

25. Post-mortem examinations must not be begun until real death is morally certain.

(NOTE: The main point here is that the physician should be reasonably certain that the subject is not merely apparently dead before he starts the post-mortem. More precise information concerning the moment of real death is desirable. Lacking such information theologians usually allow the following intervals for the conditional administration of the sacraments: one-half hour to one hour, in the case of death after a lingering illness; and two or even more hours, in the case of sudden death.)

26. For a very serious reason labor may be induced immediately after the fetus is viable. In a properly equipped hospital the fetus may sometimes be considered viable after 26 weeks (6 calendar months); otherwise, 28 weeks are required.

27. In all cases in which the presence of pregnancy would render some procedure illicit (e.g., curettage), the physician must make use of such pregnancy tests and consultation as may be needed in order to be reasonably certain that the patient is not pregnant.

28. Radiation therapy of the mother's reproductive organs is permitted during pregnancy only when necessary to suppress a dangerous pathological condition.

II. Procedures Involving Reproductive Organs and Functions

(NOTE: The subsequent Ethical Directives suppose that there is no special risk to life, either for the patient or—in the case of a pregnant woman—for a fetus; otherwise the principles previously given must be applied.)

29. The unnatural use of the sex faculty (e.g., masturbation) is never permitted, even for a laudable purpose.

30. Continence, either periodic or continuous, is the only form of birth control not in itself morally objectionable.

31. Procedures that induce sterility, whether permanent or temporary, are permitted when:

a) they are immediately directed to the cure, diminution, or prevention of a serious pathological condition;

b) a simpler treatment is not reasonably available; and

c) the sterility itself is an unintended and, in the circumstances, an unavoidable effect.

32. Castration, surgical or otherwise, is permitted when required for the removal or diminution of a serious pathological condition, even in other organs. Hence: oophorectomy or irradiation of the ovaries may be allowed in treating carcinoma of the breast and metastasis therefrom; and orchidectomy is permitted in the treatment of carcinoma of the prostate. In all cases the procedure least harmful to the reproductive organs should be used, if equally effective with other procedures.

33. All operations, treatments, and devices designed to render conception impossible are morally objectionable. Advising or otherwise encouraging contraceptive practices is not permitted.

(NOTE: Continence is not contraception. A physician is entitled to advise and explain the practice of periodic continence to those who have need of such knowledge.)

34. Hysterectomy is permitted when it is sincerely judged to be the only effective remedy for prolapse of the uterus, or when it is a necessary means of removing some other serious pathology.

35. Hysterectomy is not permitted as a routine procedure after any definite number of cesarean sections. In these cases the pathology of each patient must be considered individually; and care must be had that hysterectomy is not performed as a merely contraceptive measure.

36. Even after the childbearing function has ceased, hysterectomy is still a mutilation, and it must not be performed unless sound medical reasons call for it.

37. If procedures designed to correct uterine malpositions induce sterility, the conditions given in n. 31 must be fulfilled; if they do not induce sterility the principle of proportionate good, as stated in n. 40, is to be applied.

38. Sterility tests involving the procurement of the male specimen by masturbation or unnatural intercourse are morally objectionable.

39. The use of artificial means to enable the natural marital act to be fertile (e.g. the cervical spoon) is permitted. No other form of artificial insemination is in accord with the divine plan for human procreation. Especially objectionable are donor insemination and unnatural methods of obtaining semen.

III. Other Procedures

40. Any procedure harmful to the patient is morally justified only insofar as it is designed to produce a proportionate good.

Ordinarily the "proportionate good" that justifies a directly mutilating procedure must be the welfare of the patient himself. However, such things as blood transfusions and skin grafts are permitted for the good of others. Whether this principle of "helping the neighbor" can justify organic transplantation is now a matter of discussion. Physicians are asked to present practical cases for solution, if such cases exist.

41. The removal of an apparently healthy appendix while the abdomen is open for some other reason may be allowed at the discretion of the physician.

42. Experimentation on patients without due consent and not for the benefit of the patients themselves is morally objectionable. Even when experimentation is for the genuine good of the patient, the physician must have the consent, at least reasonably presumed, of the patient or his legitimate guardian.

43. Ghost surgery, which implies the calculated deception of the patient as to the identity of the operating surgeon, is morally objectionable.

44. Lobotomy and similar operations are morally justifiable when medically indicated as the proper treatment of serious mental illness or of intractable pain. In each case the welfare of the patient himself, considered as a person, must be the determining factor. These operations are not justifiable when less extreme remedies are reasonably available or in cases in which the probability of harm to the patient outweighs the hope of benefit for him.

45. The use of narcosis or hypnosis for the cure of mental illness is permissible with the consent at least reasonably presumed of the patient, provided due precautions are taken to protect the patient and the hospital from harmful effects, and provided the patient's right to secrecy is duly safeguarded.

46. There is no objection on principle and in general to psychoanalysis or any other form of psychotherapy. The psychiatrists and psychotherapists, however, must observe the cautions dictated by sound morality, such as: avoiding the error of pan-sexualism; never counseling even material sin; respecting secrets that the patient is not permitted to reveal; avoiding the disproportionate risk of moral dangers.

47. Shock-therapy is permitted when medically indicated.

48. Unnecessary procedures, whether diagnostic or therapeutic, are morally objectionable. A procedure is unnecessary when no proportionate reason requires it for the welfare of the patient; *a fortiori* unnecessary is any procedure that is contraindicated by sound medical standards. This directive applies especially, but not exclusively, to unnecessary surgery.

SECTION II: THE RELIGIOUS CARE OF PATIENTS

I. Baptism

49. Except in cases of emergency (i.e., danger of death), all requests for baptism made by adults or for infants should be referred to the chaplain of the hospital, who will see that the prescriptions of canon law are observed.

50. Even cases of emergency should be referred to the chaplain or to some other priest if one is available. If a priest is not available, anyone having the use of reason can and should baptize.

51. The ordinary method of conferring emergency baptism is as follows: Water is poured on the head in such a way that it will flow on the skin, and not merely on the hair; and while the water is being poured these words are pronounced: *I baptize you in the Name of the Father, and of the Son, and of the Holy Ghost.* The water will more easily flow on the skin if it is poured on the forehead. The same person who pours the water should pronounce the words.

52. When emergency baptism is conferred, the fact should be noted on the patient's chart, and the chaplain should be notified as soon as possible so that he can properly record it.

II. *Other Sacraments*

53. It is the mind of the Church that the sick should have the widest possible liberty to receive the sacraments frequently. The generous co-operation of the entire hospital staff and personnel is requested for this purpose.

54. While providing the sick abundant opportunity to receive Holy Communion, there should be no interference with the perfect freedom of the faithful according to the mind of the Church to communicate or not to communicate; and moreover there should be no pressure exerted that might lead to sacrilegious Communions.

55. Those in danger of death are not obliged to keep the Eucharistic fast. Regarding other privileges available to the sick and hospital personnel, the chaplain or some other priest should be consulted.

56. Sufficient privacy should be provided for confession in wards and semi-private rooms, or the patient moved elsewhere for confession, if this is possible.

57. When possible, one who is critically ill should receive Holy Viaticum and extreme unction while in full possession of his rational faculties. The chaplain must, therefore, be notified as soon as an illness is diagnosed as critical.

III. *Spiritual Care of Non-Catholics*

58. While avoiding odious proselytism, we must not be indifferent to the spiritual needs and desires of non-Catholics; and everything consonant with our principles must be done for them. In particular, when a non-Catholic patient asks to have his minister or rabbi called this request should be honored.

IV. *Disposal of Amputated Members*

59. Major parts of the body should be buried in a cemetery when it is reasonably possible to do so. Moreover, the members of Catholics should, if possible, be buried in blessed ground. When burial is not reasonably possible, the burning of such members is permissible.

V. *Disposal of Dead Fetus*

60. The normal manner of disposing of a dead fetus, regardless of the degree of maturity, is suitable burial. A fetus may be burned only if sanitation or some similarly serious reason requires it. In exceptional cases, there is no objection to retaining a fetus for laboratory study and observation; but it should not be preserved in its membranes unless it is so obviously dead that baptism would certainly be of no avail.

(NOTE: It is imperative that all who are concerned with the disposal of a fetus should know and observe pertinent prescriptions of civil law. If there seems to be a conflict between the provisions of civil law and the instructions given here the matter should be referred to the hospital authorities for clarification.)

PRINCIPLES OF MEDICAL ETHICS
OF THE AMERICAN MEDICAL ASSOCIATION[1]

PREAMBLE

These principles are intended to serve the physician as a guide to ethical conduct as he strives to accomplish his prime purpose of serving the common good and improving the health of mankind. They provide a sound basis for solution of many of the problems which arise in his relationship with patients, with other physicians, and with the public. They are not immutable laws to govern the physician, for the ethical practitioner needs no such laws; rather they are standards by which he may determine the propriety of his own conduct. Undoubtedly, interpretation of these principles by an appropriate authority will be required at times. As a rule, however, the physician who is capable, honest, decent, courteous, vigilant, and an observer of the Golden Rule, and who conducts his affairs in the light of his own conscientious interpretation of these principles, will find no difficulty in the discharge of his professional obligations.

[1] With permission of the American Medical Association.

CHAPTER I

GENERAL PRINCIPLES

Character of the Physician

SECTION 1.—The prime object of the medical profession is to render service to humanity; reward or financial gain is a subordinate consideration. Whoever chooses this profession assumes the obligation to conduct himself in accord with its ideals. A physician should be "an upright man, instructed in the art of healing." He must keep himself pure in character and be diligent and conscientious in caring for the sick. As was said by Hippocrates, "He should also be modest, sober, patient, prompt to do his whole duty without anxiety; pious without going so far as superstition, conducting himself with propriety in his profession and in all the actions of his life."

The Physician's Responsibility

SEC. 2.—The avowed objective of the profession of medicine is the common good of mankind. Physicians faithful to the ancient tenets of this profession are ever cognizant of the fact that they are trustees of medical knowledge and skill and that they must dispense the benefits of their special attainments in medicine to all who need them. Physicians dedicate their lives to the alleviation of suffering, to the enhancement and prolongation of life, and to the destinies of humanity. They share whatever they have learned and whatever they may discover with their colleagues in every part of the globe. They recognize instinctively that the need for improvement of medical knowledge and skills is never at an end, and while they strive toward satisfaction of this need they are zealous in making available to physicians of good character who possess the desire and the ability to learn the aggregate of progress in medical education, research, and discoveries as they may exist at the time. They do not remain content to limit their activities to the care of the infirm, since they recognize also their useful rank among the vast concourse of citizens on whose shoulders the destiny of our nation rests. At the same time they will resist attempts to debase their services by diverting them to ignoble purposes. In their relationships with patients, with colleagues, and with the public, they maintain under God, as they have down the ages, the most inflexible standards of personal honor.

Groups and Clinics

SEC. 3.—The ethical principles actuating and governing a group or clinic are exactly the same as those applicable to the individual. As a group or clinic is composed of individual physicians, each of whom, whether employer, employee or partner, is subject to the principles of ethics herein elaborated, the uniting into a business or professional organization does not relieve them either individually or as a group from the obligation they assume when entering the profession.

Advertising

SEC. 4.—Solicitation of patients, directly or indirectly, by a physician, by groups of physicians or by institutions or organizations is unethical. This principle protects the public from the advertiser and salesman of medical care by establishing an easily discernible and generally recognized distinction between him and the ethical physician. Among unethical practices are included the not always obvious devices of furnishing or inspiring newspaper or magazine comments concerning cases in which the physician or group or institution has been, or is, concerned. Self laudations defy the traditions and lower the moral standard of the medical profession; they are an infraction of good taste and are disapproved.

The most worthy and effective advertisement possible, even for a young physician, especially among his brother physicians, is the establishment of a well merited reputation for professional ability and fidelity. This cannot be forced, but must be the outcome of character and conduct. The publication or circulation of simple professional cards is approved in some localities but is disapproved in others. Disregard of local customs and offenses against recognized ideals are unethical.

The Relationship of the Physician to Media of Public Information

SEC. 5.—Many people, literate and well educated, do not possess a special knowledge of medicine. Medical books and journals are not always easily accessible or readily understandable.

The medical profession considers it ethical for a physician to meet the request of a component or constituent medical society to write, act or speak for general readers or audiences. On the other hand, it may often happen that the representatives of popular news media are the first to perceive the adaptability of medical material for presentation to the public. In such a situation the physician may be asked to release to the public some information, exhibit, drawing or photograph. Refusal to release this material may be considered a refusal to perform a public service, yet compliance may bring the charge of self-seeking or solicitation.

An ethical physician may provide appropriate information regarding important medical and public health matters which have been discussed during open medical meetings or in technical papers which have been published, and he may reveal information regarding a patient's physical condition if the patient gives his permission, but he should seek the guidance of appropriate officials and designated spokesmen of component or constituent medical societies. Spokesmen should be empowered to give prompt and authoritative replies and a list should be issued which identifies them and discloses the manner in which they may be reached. These provisions are made with full knowledge that the primary responsibility of the physician is the welfare of his patient but proper observation of these ethical provisions by the physician concerned should protect him from any charge of self-aggrandizement.

Scientific articles written concerning hospitals, clinics or laboratories which portray clinical facts and technics and which display appropriate illustrations may well have the commendable effect of inspiring public confidence in the procedure described. Articles should be prepared authoritatively and should utilize information supplied by the physician or physicians in charge with the sanction of appropriate associates.

When any sort of medical information is released to the public, the promise of radical cures or boasting of cures or of extraordinary skill or success is unethical.

An institution may use means, approved by the medical profession in its own locality, to inform the public of its address and the special class, if any, of patients accommodated.

Payment for Professional Services

SEC. 6.—The ethical physician, engaged in the practice of medicine, limits the sources of his income received from professional activities to services rendered the patient. Remuneration received for such services should be in the form and amount specifically announced to the patient at the time the service is rendered or in the form of a subsequent statement.

Unethical methods of inducement to refer patients are devices employed in a system of patronage and reward. They are practiced only by unethical physicians and often utilize deception and coercion. They may consist of the division of a fee collected by one physician ostensibly for services rendered by him and divided with the referring physician or physicians or of receiving the entire fee in alternate cases.

When patients are referred by one physician to another, it is unethical for either physician to offer or to receive any inducement other than

404

the quality of professional services. Included among unethical inducements are split fees, rebates, "kickbacks," discounts, loans, favors, gifts, and emoluments with or without the knowledge of the patient. Fee splitting violates the patient's trust that his physician will not exploit his dependence upon him and invites physicians to place the desire for profit above the opportunity to render appropriate medical service.

Billing procedures which tend to induce physicians to split fees are unethical. Combined billing by physicians may jeopardize the doctor-patient relationship by limiting the opportunity for understanding of the financial arrangement between the patient and each physician. It may provide opportunity for excessive fees and may interfere with free choice of consultants, which is contrary to the highest standards of medical care.

Patents and Copyrights

SEC. 7.—A physician may patent surgical instruments, appliances, and medicines or copyright publications, methods, and procedures. The use of such patents or copyrights or the receipt of remuneration from them which retards or inhibits research or restricts the benefits derivable therefrom is unethical.

Dispensing of Drugs and Appliances by Physicians

SEC. 8.—It is not unethical for a physician to prescribe or supply drugs, remedies, or appliances as long as there is no exploitation of the patient.

Rebates and Commissions

SEC. 9.—The acceptance of rebates on prescriptions and appliances or of commissions from those who aid in the care of patients is unethical.

Secret Remedies

SEC. 10.—The prescription or dispensing by a physician of secret medicines or other secret remedial agents, of which he does not know the composition, or the manufacture or promotion of their use is unethical.

Evasion of Legal Restrictions

SEC. 11.—An ethical physician will observe the laws regulating the practice of medicine and will not assist others to evade such laws.

CHAPTER II

Duties of Physicians to Their Patients

Standards, Usefulness, Nonsectarianism

Section 1.—In order that a physician may best serve his patients, he is expected to exalt the standards of his profession and to extend its sphere of usefulness. To the same end, he should not base his practice on an exclusive dogma or a sectarian system, for "sects are implacable despots; to accept their thralldom is to take away all liberty from one's action and thought."* A sectarian or cultist as applied to medicine is one who alleges to follow or in his practice follows a dogma, tenet or principle based on the authority of its promulgator to the exclusion of demonstration and scientific experience. All voluntarily associated activities with cultists are unethical. A consultation with a cultist is a futile gesture if the cultist is assumed to have the same high grade of knowledge, training, and experience as is possessed by the doctor of medicine. Such consultation lowers the honor and dignity of the profession in the same degree in which it elevates the honor and dignity of those who are irregular in training and practice.

Patience, Delicacy, and Secrecy

Sec. 2.—Patience and delicacy should characterize the physician. Confidences concerning individual or domestic life entrusted by patients to a physician and defects in the disposition or character of patients observed during medical attendance should never be revealed unless their revelation is required by the laws of the state. Sometimes, however, a physician must determine whether his duty to society requires him to employ knowledge, obtained through confidences entrusted to him as a physician, to protect a healthy person against a communicable disease to which he is about to be exposed. In such instance, the physician should act as he would desire another to act toward one of his own family in like circumstances. Before he determines his course, the physician should know the civil law of his commonwealth concerning privileged communications.

Prognosis

Sec. 3.—The physician should neither exaggerate nor minimize the gravity of a patient's condition. He should assure himself that the patient, his relatives or his responsible friends have such knowledge of the pa-

* Nicon, father of Galen.

tient's condition as will serve the best interests of the patient and the family.

The Patient Must Not Be Neglected

Sec. 4.—A physician is free to choose whom he will serve. He should, however, respond to any request for his assistance in an emergency or whenever temperate public opinion expects the service. Once having undertaken a case, the physician should not neglect the patient, nor should he withdraw from the case without giving notice to the patient, his relatives or his responsible friends sufficiently long in advance of his withdrawal to allow them to secure another medical attendant.

CHAPTER III

DUTIES OF PHYSICIANS TO THE PROFESSION AT LARGE

Upholding the Honor of the Profession

SECTION 1.—A physician is expected to uphold the dignity and honor of his vocation.

Membership in Medical Societies

Sec. 2.—For the advancement of his profession, a physician should affiliate with medical societies and contribute of his time, energy and means so that these societies may represent the ideals of the profession.

Safeguarding the Profession

Sec. 3.—Every physician should aid in safeguarding the profession against admission to it of those who are deficient in moral character or education.

Exposure of Unethical Conduct

Sec. 4.—A physician should expose, without fear or favor, incompetent or corrupt, dishonest or unethical conduct on the part of members of the profession. Questions of such conduct should be considered, first, before proper medical tribunals in executive sessions or by special or duly appointed committees on ethical relations, provided such a course is possible and provided, also, that the law is not hampered thereby. If doubt should arise as to the legality of the physician's conduct, the situation under investigation may be placed before officers of the law, and the physician-investigators may take the necessary steps to enlist the interest of the proper authority.

CHAPTER IV

PROFESSIONAL SERVICES OF PHYSICIANS TO EACH OTHER

Dependence of Physicians on Each Other

SECTION 1.—As a general rule, a physician should not attempt to treat members of his family or himself. Consequently, a physician should cheerfully and without recompense give his professional services to physicians or their dependents if they are in his vicinity.

Compensation for Expenses

SEC. 2.—When a physician from a distance is called to advise another physician about his own illness or about that of one of his family dependents, and the physician to whom the service is rendered is in easy financial circumstances, a compensation that will at least meet the traveling expenses of the visiting physician should be proffered him. When such a service requires an absence from the accustomed field of professional work of the visitor that might reasonably be expected to entail a pecuniary loss, such loss may, in part at least, be provided for in the compensation offered.

One Physician in Charge

SEC. 3.—When a physician or a member of his dependent family is seriously ill, he or his family should select one physician to take charge of the case. The family may ask the physician in charge to call in other physicians to act as consultants.

CHAPTER V

DUTIES OF PHYSICIANS IN CONSULTATIONS

Consultations Should Be Encouraged

SECTION 1.—In a case of serious illness, especially in doubtful or difficult conditions, the physician should request consultations.

Consultation for Patient's Benefit

SEC. 2.—In every consultation, the benefit to the patient is of first importance. All physicians interested in the case should be candid with the patient, a member of his family or a responsible friend.

408

Punctuality

Sec. 3.—All physicians concerned in consultations should be punctual. When, however, one or more of the consultants are unavoidably delayed, the one who arrives first should wait for the others for a reasonable time, after which the consultation should be considered postponed. When the consultant has come from a distance, or when for any other reason it will be difficult to meet the physician in charge at another time, or if the case is urgent, or it be the desire of the patient, his family or his responsible friends, the consultant may examine the patient and mail his written opinion, or see that it is delivered under seal to the physician in charge. Under these conditions, the consultant's conduct must be especially tactful; he must remember that he is framing an opinion without the aid of the physician who has observed the course of the disease.

Patient Referred to Consultant

Sec. 4.—When a patient is sent to a consultant and the physician in charge of the case cannot accompany the patient, the physician in charge should provide the consultant with a history of the case, together with the physician's opinion and outline of the treatment, or so much of this as may be of service to the consultant. As soon as possible after the consultant has seen the patient he should address the physician in charge and advise him of the results of the consultant's investigation. The opinions of both the physician in charge and the consultant are confidential and must be so regarded by each.

Discussions in Consultation

Sec. 5.—After the physicians called in consultation have completed their investigations, they and the physician in charge should meet by themselves to discuss the course to be followed. Statements should not be made nor should discussion take place in the presence of the patient, his family or his friends, unless all physicians concerned are present or unless all of them have consented to another arrangement.

Responsibility of Attending Physician

Sec. 6.—The physician in charge of the case is responsible for treatment of the patient. Consequently, he may prescribe for the patient at any time and is privileged to vary the treatment outlined and agreed on at a consultation whenever, in his opinion, such a change is warranted. However, after such a change, it is best to call another consultation; then the physician in charge should state his reasons for departing from the course decided at the previous conference. When an emergency occurs during the absence of the physician in charge, a consultant may assume authority until the arrival of the physician in charge, but his authority should not extend further without the consent of the physician in charge.

Conflict of Opinion

SEC. 7.—Should the physician in charge and a consultant be unable to agree in their view of a case, another consultant should be called or the differing consultant should withdraw. However, since the patient employed the consultant to obtain his opinion, he should be permitted to state it to the patient, his relative or his responsible friend, in the presence of the physician in charge.

Consultant and Attendant

SEC. 8.—When a physician has acted as consultant in an illness, he should not become the physician in charge in the course of that illness, except with the consent of the physician who was in charge at the time of the consultation.

CHAPTER VI

DUTIES OF PHYSICIANS IN CASES OF INTERFERENCE

Misunderstandings To Be Avoided

SECTION 1.—A physician, in his relationship with a patient who is under the care of another physician, should not give hints relative to the nature and treatment of the patient's disorder; nor should a physician do anything to diminish the trust reposed by the patient in his own physician. In embarrassing situations, or whenever there seems to be a possibility of misunderstanding with a colleague, a physician should seek a personal interview with his fellow.

Social Calls on Patient of Another Physician

SEC. 2.—When a physician makes social calls on another physician's patient he should avoid conversation about the patient's illness.

Services to Patient of Another Physician

SEC. 3.—A physician should not take charge of, or prescribe for another physician's patient during any given illness (except in an emergency) until the other physician has relinquished the case or has been formally dismissed.

410

Criticism To Be Avoided

Sec. 4.—When a physician does succeed another physician in charge of a case, he should not disparage, by comment or insinuation, the one who preceded him. Such comment or insinuation tends to lower the confidence of the patient in the medical profession and so reacts against the patient, the profession and the critic.

Emergency Cases

Sec. 5.—When a physician is called in an emergency because the personal or family physician is not at hand, he should provide only for the patient's immediate need and should withdraw from the case on the arrival of the personal or family physician. However, he should first report to the personal or family physician the condition found and the treatment administered.

Precedence When Several Physicians Are Summoned

Sec. 6.—When several physicians have been summoned in a case of sudden illness or of accident, the first to arrive should be considered the physician in charge. However, as soon as is practicable, or on the arrival of the acknowledged personal or family physician, the first physician should withdraw. Should the patient, his family or his responsible friend wish some one other than he who has been in charge of the case, the patient or his representative should advise the personal or family physician of his desire. When, because of sudden illness or accident, a patient is taken to a hospital without the knowledge of the physician who is known to be the personal or family physician, the patient should be returned to the care of the personal or family physician as soon as is feasible.

A Colleague's Patient

Sec. 7.—When a physician is requested by a colleague to care for a patient during the colleague's temporary absence, or when, because of an emergency, a physician is asked to see a patient of a colleague, the physician should treat the patient in the same manner and with the same delicacy that he would wish used in similar circumstances if the patient were his responsibility. The patient should be returned to the care of the attending physician as soon as possible.

Substitution in Obstetric Work

Sec. 8.—When a physician attends a woman who is in labor because the one who was engaged to attend her is absent, the physician summoned in the emergency should relinquish the patient to the first engaged, on his arrival. The one in attendance is entitled to compensation for the professional services he may have rendered.

Disputes between Physicians

SEC. 9.—Whenever there arises between physicians a grave difference of opinion, or of interest, which cannot be promptly adjusted, the dispute should be referred for arbitration, preferably to an official body of a component society.

CHAPTER VII

COMPENSATION

Limits of Gratuitous Service

SECTION 1.—Poverty of a patient, and the obligation of physicians to attend one another and the dependent members of the families of one another, should command the gratuitous services of a physician. Institutions and organizations for mutual benefit, or for accident, sickness and life insurance, or for analogous purposes, should meet such costs as are covered by the contract under which the service is rendered.

Conditions of Medical Practice

SEC. 2.—A physician should not dispose of his services under conditions that make it impossible to render adequate service to his patients, except under circumstances in which the patients concerned might be deprived of immediately necessary care.

Contract Practice

SEC. 3.—Contract practice as applied to medicine means the practice of medicine under an agreement between a physician or a group of physicians, as principals or agents, and a corporation, organization, political subdivision or individual, whereby partial or full medical services are provided for a group or class of individuals on the basis of a fee schedule, or for a salary or for a fixed rate per capita.

Contract practice *per se* is not unethical. Contract practice is unethical if it permits of features or conditions that are declared unethical in these Principles of Medical Ethics or if the contract or any of its provisions causes deterioration of the quality of the medical services rendered.

412

Free Choice of Physician

Sec. 4.—Free choice of physician is defined as that degree of freedom in choosing a physician which can be exercised under usual conditions of employment between patients and physicians. The interjection of a third party who has a valid interest, or who intervenes between the physician and the patient does not *per se* cause a contract to be unethical. A third party has a valid interest when, by law or volition, the third party assumes legal responsibility and provides for the cost of medical care and indemnity for occupational disability.

Purveyal of Medical Service

Sec. 5.—A physician should not dispose of his professional attainments or services to any hospital, lay body, organization, group or individual, by whatever name called, or however organized, under terms or conditions which permit exploitation of the services of the physician for the financial profit of the agency concerned. Such a procedure is beneath the dignity of professional practice and is harmful alike to the profession of medicine and the welfare of the people.

CHAPTER VIII

DUTIES OF PHYSICIANS TO THE PUBLIC

Physicians as Citizens

SECTION 1.—Physicians, as good citizens, possessed of special training, should advise concerning the health of the community wherein they dwell. They should bear their part in enforcing the laws of the community and in sustaining the institutions that advance the interests of humanity. They should cooperate especially with the proper authorities in the administration of sanitary laws and regulations.

Public Health

Sec. 2.—Physicians, especially those engaged in public health work, should enlighten the public concerning quarantine regulations and measures for the prevention of epidemic and communicable diseases. At all times the physician should notify the constituted public health authorities of every case of communicable disease under his care, in accordance with the laws, rules, and regulations of the health authorities. When an epidemic prevails, a physician must continue his labors without regard to the risk to his own health.

Pharmacists

SEC. 3.—Physicians should recognize and promote the practice of pharmacy as a profession and should recognize the cooperation of the pharmacist in education of the public concerning the practice of ethical and scientific medicine.

A STATEMENT OF THE AMERICAN COLLEGE OF SURGEONS ON CERTAIN UNETHICAL PRACTICES IN SURGERY[1]

WHEREAS the essential of ethical financial relations in the medical profession is simple honesty, which requires the patient to be informed of the amount which is due to each physician for services rendered; and

WHEREAS the secret division of a fee between two physicians (commonly called "fee-splitting") is dishonest, against the public interest, and has long been considered unethical by responsible doctors of medicine; and

WHEREAS the payment of a referring physician by a surgeon for assistance during the operation without the knowledge of the patient, or the payment to the referring physician even with the knowledge of the patient, of an assistant's fee in excess of the amount customarily allowed for the service itself (commonly known as "inducement"), is likewise dishonest and unethical; and

WHEREAS deception of the patient as to the identity of the physician who performs an operation (a practice known as "ghost surgery") is likewise dishonest and unethical; and

WHEREAS the overcharging of a patient by a surgeon is unjust and encourages fee-splitting; and

WHEREAS the presentation of a combined unitemized bill by two physicians not formally associated each with the other is equivalent to fee-splitting; and

WHEREAS an itemized combined statement designating the amount due each physician, but out of proportion in any item to individual services rendered, is equally unethical; and

WHEREAS the payment or acceptance by physicians of rebates of fees for technical services or appliances has long been held to be unethical;

[1] With permission of the American College of Surgeons. The College has no code of ethics separate from that of the American Medical Association.

Therefore, be it resolved that the American College of Surgeons make it a matter of record that it is unalterably opposed to all of the unethical practices enumerated above; and

Be it further resolved that the American College of Surgeons shall foster, promote, and practice the following measures to combat unethical practices in medicine:

1. Education of the public upon the value of the services of all physicians (including surgeons), emphasizing that each should be paid adequately and directly.

2. Education of the medical student, intern, resident, and young practitioner upon the evils of unethical relations through definite instruction in medical schools, hospitals, and medical societies.

3. Education of the surgeon as to the opposition of the American College of Surgeons to exorbitant fees, the presentation of unitemized combined statements, the presentation of itemized combined statements out of proportion to individual services rendered, the payment of referring physicians used as surgical assistants or anesthetists without such payments being known to the patient, and the employment of a referring physician on a salary which is related in any way to the number of referred patients.

4. Encouragement of governing boards of hospitals, which are in any way uncertain as to the possibility of fee-splitting by a staff member, or applicant, in the adoption of the requirement for staff membership of a statement by a qualified public accountant that no evidence of unethical financial relations appears on the books of the staff member or applicant.

5. Encouragement of hospitals, which are having difficulty in identifying the responsible surgeons, in the enforcement of a regulation that the patient or his legal representative shall sign, before operation, a properly executed and witnessed permit, in which the responsible surgeon is indicated.

6. Notification to clinics and their representative organizations that the College considers placement of referring physicians on the part-time pay roll of a clinic as a dangerous practice subject to strong suspicion as to ethics.

7. Punishment of any Fellow of the College who is known to be violating the principles stated above, under Article VIII, Section 3, of Bylaws as amended to April 15, 1952.

Abdominal pregnancy. *See* Pregnancy, ectopic
Abnormal infants. *See* Infants, malformed
Abortion, attempted
  curettage after (Case 103), 212-13
  procedure after (Case 100), 209
Abortion, criminal. *See* Abortion, direct
Abortion, direct
  argument of unborn child as aggressor, 90, 93-94, 227
  as murder, 191-94
  avoiding apparent approval of (Case 43), 114
  avoiding cooperation in (Case 33), 107
  carcinoma of breast as cause for (Case 99), 208
  Catholic position on, 191-97
  change in medical attitude toward, 197-203, 208
  criminal, defined, 189
  defined, 188
  eclampsia as cause for (Case 96), 206-07
  emotional attitude toward, 15
  giving harmless drug as supposed abortifacient (Case 43), 114
  hemorrhage as cause for (Case 97), 207; (Case 104), 213
  hydatidiform mole as cause for (Case 102), 211-12
  hyperemesis gravidarum as cause for (Case 98), 207-08
  in an ectopic pregnancy (Case 116), 227-28
  indirect. *See* Abortion, indirect

kidney infection as cause for (Case 95), 206
mother-or-child dilemma, 195-97
oligohydramnios as cause for (Case 93), 205
physician's answer to request for, 203-04
rape as cause for (Case 94), 205-06
reasons given for, 190
referral of patient to abortionist (Case 42), 114
signing for therapeutic (Case 36), 108-09
spontaneous. *See* Miscarriage
therapeutic, 189, 195-203
Abortion, indirect
  baptism of fetus as cause of, 364-65
  carcinoma of uterus as cause for (Case 105), 215-16; (Case 107), 216-17; (Case 110), 217-18
  danger of from ergot (Case 91), 187
  gangrenous fibroid tumor as cause for (Case 111), 218
  hemorrhage as cause for (Case 113), 219
  in ectopic pregnancies, 220-30
  myoma of uterus as cause for (Case 112), 218-19
  principle of twofold effect in, 214
  rupture of uterus as cause for (Case 113), 219
  scarred uterus as cause for (Case 114), 219-20
Abortion, spontaneous. *See* Miscarriage

Chauffard, A., on continence and
health, 119
Child, unborn not aggressor, 90, 93-
94, 227
Childbirth. *See* Delivery; Labor;
Pregnancy
Children
adopted, 348-50
effect of on marriage, 317-21
illegitimate as result of artificial
insemination, 152-53
masturbation in, 346-48
obligation of to care for aged
parents, 351-52
parents' respect for rights of, 80-82
respecting secrets of, 52-53
sex training of, 329-40
spacing births of, 321-22
surgery in (Cases 24, 25, 26), 86-
88
when old enough to choose treatment, 81-82
See also Infants
Children's Bureau, United States, 350
Cholecystectomy. *See* Gall bladder
Chorea gravidarum, typhoid-
paratyphoid vaccine in, 235-36
Christ
example of suffering, 268
presence of in Eucharist, 373-74
Christianity, Freud's attitude toward,
285
See also Catholic Church
Church. *See* Catholic Church
Circumcision of newborn males
(Case 55), 128-29
Cleidotomy, licitness of (Case 140),
251-52
Clergyman, summoning for dying
patient (Case 40), 111-12
See also Priest
Clifford, John J.
on preventive castration, 126 *note*
on sterility tests, 149 *note*
Climate, change of, as means to preserve life, 77-78; (Case 23), 86
Cobb, Stanley, on continence and
health, 119
Code of ethics
of American College of Surgeons,
29, 414-15
of American Medical Association,
13, 401-14
of Catholic Hospital Association,
393-401

Codex juris canonici
on baptism of fetus delivered from
dead mother, 249 *note*
on doubtful impediment, 137 *note*
Coitus. *See* Sexual intercourse
Colostomy, removal of at risk of life
(Case 15), 76
Coma
caesarean section on patient in
(Case 136), 248
means of prolonging life in (Case
16), 80
Commissions accepted from phar-
macies (Case 6), 33
See also Fee splitting
Communion. *See* Eucharist
Concealing information. *See* Information, concealing; Secrets
Conditional baptism, 360; (Case
163), 370-71; (Case 169), 373
Condom, perforated, use of in obtaining sample of semen, 149
Confidential information. *See* Secrets
Consanguinity in marriage, 316-17
Consent
in marriage, 311
to brain surgery, 288
to narcotherapy, 291
to surgery, 123
to use of experimental drug, 21
to use of hypnotism, 265
to wire recording, 55
Consultants, obligation of to respect
secrets, 52
Consultations, obligation of physician
concerning, 29
Contagious disease. *See* Infectious
disease
Continence
and health, 116-19
in marriage, 324
periodic. *See* Rhythm
Contraceptives
cooperation in sale of, 105-06
inserting diaphragm in patient
(Case 37), 109-10
instructing patient in use of (Case
38), 110
selling of by physician, 96-97
use of in obtaining semen samples,
147
See also Birth control
Convicts, experimental use of new
drug by (Case 150), 261-62
See also Crime

421

423

431

433

Psychoanalysis
Catholic Church and, 283-84
dangers of, 286-87
Freud's teaching on, 280-82
morality of, 282-87
Psychoneurosis
lobotomy in (Case 157), 288-89
unnecessary surgery in, 56-57
Psychosis, lobotomy in with probable
loss of reason (Case 160), 289-
90
Psychosurgery, 287-90
Psychotherapy. *See* Hypnotism; Narcotherapy; Psychiatry; Psychoanalysis
Puberty, explaining to children, 339-
40
Pubiotomy, licitness of, 249
Public institutions, remedies for patients in (Case 1), 21-22
Puiula, Jacobus, on therapeutic abortion, 197 *note*
Puncture of fetal membranes
and hydramnios, 236-38
in baptizing, 364
Purity. *See* Chastity; Sex training of
children
Pyromania, hypnotism as cure for,
264

Quinine, use of during pregnancy,
185; (Cases 89, 90), 186-87

Rabinowitch, I. M., on euthanasia,
269
Rape
abortion because of (Case 94),
205-06
curettage after, 275
douche after, 275-78
Ratcliffe, J. D., on danger of drugs
in childbirth, 243 *note*
Ravdin, I. S., on ghost surgery, 26
note
Reading matter, irreligious and immoral in reception room (Case
41), 113
Reason
as guide to ethical goodness, 9-10,
15
probable loss of in transorbital
lobotomy (Case 160), 289-90
Reception room, irreligious and immoral magazines in (Case 41),
113

Redlich, Frederick C., on recording
of psychotherapeutic interviews,
55 *note*
Referral
for contraceptive instruction (Case
38), 110
to abortionist (Case 42), 114
unnecessary (Case 4), 32
See also Fee splitting
Religion
Freud's attitude toward, 283
physician's attitude toward, 354-55
See also Catholic Church; Sacraments
Remedies
for patients in public institutions
(Case 1), 21-22
selection of, 20-24
See also Drugs
Renal disease and surgery. *See* Kidneys
Respiration, artificial, as means of
preserving life, 70-71; (Case 27),
88-89
Respirator as means of preserving
life, 70-71; (Case 27), 88-89
Reward and punishment, belief in
as postulate, 3
Rh factor and marriage, 314-16
Rhesus factor, 314-16
Rhythm, 162-67, 325
as aid in fertility, 167
instruction on, 325
licitness of use of, 164-65
morality of, 163-67
reasons for using, 166-67
theory of ovulation and, 162-63
validity of marriage and, 163-64
Rice, Frederick W., on birth control,
157 *note*
Richmond, Winifred V., on continence and health, 116 *note*
Rights of man, 10-12
Rituale Romanum on diabolical possession, 292 *note*
Rock, John, on *in vitro* fertilization,
273 *note*
Roman Catholic Church. *See* Catholic Church
Roman Ritual on diabolical possession, 292
Rosen, James R., on artificial insemination, 152 *note*
Rosin, Jacob, on world food resources, 161 *note*

Surgery
  alleviative, 124-25
  as ordinary and as extraordinary
    means of saving life, 72-76
  avoidance of unnecessary, 56-57
  brain, 287-90
  corrective, 129-38
  doubtful, cooperating in (Case
    34), 107-08
  ethics of, 123-24
  ghost, 25-26
  illicit operation, assisting at (Case
    32), 106-07; (Case 162), 307
  illicit revelation during (Case 11),
    54
  in children (Cases 24, 25, 26),
    86-88
  in mental disorders, 287-90
  in pregnancy, 230-33
  in transvestism (Case 62), 135
  mistake in, calling attention to
    (Case 35), 108
  needless (Case 49), 124
  obligation of physician not to prac-
    tice unless qualified, 14-15
  plastic, 138
  preventive, 125-28
  problems connected with, 121-45
  to correct hermaphroditism, 133-
    35; (Case 61), 133
  to improve personal appearance,
    138-39
  when obligatory to save life, 63-67
  See also under names of organs
Sydenham's chorea. See Chorea
  gravidarum
Symphysiectomy or symphysiotomy,
  licitness of, 249
Syphilis
  licitness of marriage to syphilitic,
    312-13
  revealing to protect another, 49

Tamponing
  and indirect abortion, 239
  and placenta praevia, 238-39
Tampons, 278-79
Taussig, Frederick, on abortion, 202,
  203 note
Te Linde, Richard W., on thera-
  peutic abortion, 190
Temperature, basal body, 167-68
Terminal illnesses. See Dying persons
Tesson, Eugène, on brain surgery,
  288 note

Testes
  biopsy of for fertility test, 149
  excision of in transvestism (Case
    62), 135
  orchiectomy in carcinoma of pros-
    tate (Case 52), 126
  transplantation of, 142
Tests
  blood pressure, concealing results
    of from patient (Case 9), 44
  for pregnancy, 170-71
  for sterility, 146-50
  See also Experimentation
Therapeutic abortion
  attitude toward, 189-91
  definition of, 189
  needlessness of, 195-203
  signing for (Case 36), 108-09
  See also Abortion, direct
Thomas, John L., on marriage failure
  and size of family, 318 note
Thornton, Madeline J., on vaginal
  tampons, 279 note
Throat surgery in minor (Case 26),
  88
Thurston, Herbert, on miracles, 384
  note
Titus, Paul, on caesarean section, 246
  note
Tompkins, Pendleton, on body temperature and ovulation, 168 note
Tonsillectomy as ordinary means to
  preserve life, 75
Toxemia of pregnancy, hastening
  delivery because of (Case 131),
  245
Transfusions, blood, as means of
  preserving life (Case 22), 85-86
Transorbital lobotomy (Case 160),
  289-90
Transplantation of organs, 139-42
  from dead body, 141-42
  from living body, 139-41
  human to animal, 271-72; Case
    156), 274-75
Transverse presentation, embryotomy
  in (Case 138), 251
Transvestism, surgery in (Case 62),
  135
Travel as means to preserve life, 77-
  78; (Case 23), 86
Treatment. See Drugs; Remedies;
  Surgery; and so forth
Tredgold, A. F., on inheritance of
  mental defects, 302-03